OXFORD ENGLISH MONOGRAPHS

General Editors

ROS BALLASTER
PAULINA KEWES
LAURA MARCUS
HEATHER O'DONOGHUE
MATTHEW REYNOLDS
FIONA STAFFORD

Middle English Medical Recipes and Literary Play, 1375–1500

HANNAH BOWER

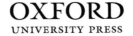

Great Clarendon Street, Oxford, OX2 6DP,
United Kingdom

Oxford University Press is a department of the University of Oxford.
It furthers the University's objective of excellence in research, scholarship,
and education by publishing worldwide. Oxford is a registered trade mark of
Oxford University Press in the UK and in certain other countries

© Hannah Bower 2022

The moral rights of the author have been asserted

First Edition published in 2022

Impression: 1

Some rights reserved. No part of this publication may be reproduced, stored in
a retrieval system, or transmitted, in any form or by any means, for commercial purposes,
without the prior permission in writing of Oxford University Press, or as expressly
permitted by law, by licence or under terms agreed with the appropriate
reprographics rights organization.

This is an open access publication, available online and distributed under the terms of a
Creative Commons Attribution – Non Commercial – No Derivatives 4.0
International licence (CC BY-NC-ND 4.0), a copy of which is available at
http://creativecommons.org/licenses/by-nc-nd/4.0/.

Enquiries concerning reproduction outside the scope of this licence
should be sent to the Rights Department, Oxford University Press, at the address above

Published in the United States of America by Oxford University Press
198 Madison Avenue, New York, NY 10016, United States of America

British Library Cataloguing in Publication Data
Data available

Library of Congress Control Number: 2021953107

ISBN 978-0-19-284949-6

DOI: 10.1093/oso/9780192849496.001.0001

Printed and bound by
CPI Group (UK) Ltd, Croydon, CR0 4YY

Links to third party websites are provided by Oxford in good faith and
for information only. Oxford disclaims any responsibility for the materials
contained in any third party website referenced in this work.

Acknowledgements

This book is based upon my DPhil, completed at the University of Oxford. I would like to thank my supervisors, Marion Turner and Daniel Wakelin, for their support, guidance, and unfailing enthusiasm. I left each supervision with an even greater curiosity about my subject and a continual eagerness to pursue new avenues of research. I miss our supervisions greatly. Secondly, I would like to thank my examiners, Vincent Gillespie and Lisa Cooper, for the useful and thoroughly enjoyable discussion we had during my viva. Helen Barr and Daniel McCann also provided invaluable feedback during my transfer and confirmation-of-status interviews. I am very grateful too to the English Faculty at Oxford for providing such a welcoming intellectual environment. I had numerous conversations at the weekly research seminars, which exerted a formative influence upon my work, helping me to see connections that I otherwise would have missed. These conversations have continued during my Junior Research Fellowship at Churchill College at the University of Cambridge. I feel very lucky to have had the time, resources, and support to produce this book.

My thesis was funded by the generous support of the Wellcome Trust and I benefited greatly from the many opportunities they provided for professional and academic development, including funding for attending conferences. At these conferences, I met mentors who have offered many helpful suggestions; I am particularly grateful to Julie Orlemanski. I also met friends and kindred recipe-lovers, such as Chelsea Silva, whose enthusiasm for all things medical has given me much food for thought. Indeed, the humour of friends often injected the DPhil with some light-heartedness and a sense of perspective; special thanks there to Raphaela Rohrhofer. I must also thank the many libraries I have visited, especially the Bodleian Library and the Huntington Library for the opportunity to carry out archival research with funding provided by the Erika and Kenneth Riley Fellowship. In addition, the funding I received from the Jeremy Griffiths Memorial Studentship during my Master's degree at St Hilda's College, Oxford enabled me to explore manuscript remedy books for the first time, sowing the seeds of my doctoral project.

Finally, I would like to thank my friends and family. Ciaran has been a perpetual sounding board for ideas; always enthusiastic about my interests, he has often helped me to think through a problem and to see the world—past and present—from a different perspective. Lastly, I would like to thank my parents and my sister for their patience, support, and endless generosity with their time: as proofreaders, computer fixers, and all-round supporters, they are always willing to enter into my world whilst reminding me that an important world exists outside of medieval recipes.

Contents

List of Illustrations   ix
Conventions and Abbreviations   xi
   Introduction   1

I. LITERARY FRAGMENTS

1. The Poetics of Prose Cures   31
2. Making Verse Remedies   71

II. COLLECTING FRAGMENTS

3. The Idea of the Remedy Collection   107

III. FRAGMENTS IN PLAY

4. Recipe Time: (Re)Imagining Bodies   141
5. Experiencing Boundaries   180
   Conclusion   207

Appendix 1: Vernacular Medical Collections Used in Sample   215
Bibliography   217
Index of Manuscripts   253
General Index   255

List of Illustrations

I.1. Remedy collection associated with 'Nicholas Neesbett'. The Bodleian Libraries, University of Oxford, MS Ashmole 1438, Part I, p. 57 — 14

1.1. Rubricated remedy for a healing salve. The Bodleian Libraries, University of Oxford, MS Douce 84, f. 38v — 43

3.1. A numbered recipe collection. The Bodleian Libraries, University of Oxford, MS Rawlinson C.506, ff. 96v–97r — 120

3.2. Accumulated recipes for removing hair. York Minster, MS XVI.E.32, f. 17v — 125

4.1. Recipes surviving alongside a devotional poem. The Bodleian Libraries, University of Oxford, MS Douce 78, f. 17v — 175

4.2. A devotional poem copied next to recipes. The Bodleian Libraries, University of Oxford, MS Douce 78, f. 18r — 176

C.1. Recipe collection with titles in a more elaborate display script. The British Library Board, BL MS Additional 19674, f. 5r — 210

C.2. Recipe collection using red and blue rubrication. Cambridge University Library, MS Kk.6.33, f. 30r — 211

Conventions and Abbreviations

Transcriptions

In my own transcriptions of medieval recipes, I have chosen to retain the original punctuation of the scribe; this is because many of my close readings allude to the rhythm and syntactic structures of recipes, as well as their manuscript representation. To ease the reading process, however, I have expanded abbreviations silently and decapitalized majuscule initials which are not serving a clear semantic or syntactic purpose; ambiguous cases are acknowledged with a footnote. I have also modernized word division for ease of reading.

When it is relevant to the discussion, rubricated text or display script is marked in bold. Text added by me to complete the sense of a quotation is enclosed in square brackets [] and text added to clarify the meaning of a quotation is enclosed in round brackets (). Text crossed out by a scribe or reader is enclosed in angle brackets <>. When text that has been crossed out can no longer be read, I signal this with a question mark enclosed in angle brackets <?>. When the text is illegible because of script, trimming, or the binding of the manuscript, I signal this with a question mark enclosed in square brackets [?]. Text written above the main body is enclosed by upper caret marks ^^. I use strokes to signal virgules executed by scribes (/) and a vertical line to signal the end of a line of verse (|).

When quoting modern printed editions, I have removed all italics and silently expanded any unexpanded abbreviations and ampersands.

List of Abbreviations

BL   British Library, London
BodL Bodleian Library, Oxford
BRB   Beinecke Rare Book and Manuscript Library, New Haven, CT
CMC   Magdalene College Pepys Library, Cambridge
CUL   University Library, Cambridge

xii CONVENTIONS AND ABBREVIATIONS

DIMEV An Open-Access Digital Edition of the *Index of Middle English Verse*, ed. by Linne R. Mooney and others, accessed online at www.dimev.net

DMLBS *Dictionary of Medieval Latin from British Sources*, ed. by Richard Ashdowne, David Howlett, and R.E. Latham (Oxford, 2018), accessed online at http://clt.brepolis.net/dmlbs/Default.aspx

DOST *The Dictionary of the Older Scottish Tongue*, accessed online at www.dsl.ac.uk

EETS Early English Text Society

eVK2 Patricia Kurtz and Linda Ehrsam Voigts, *Scientific and Medical Writings in Old and Middle English: An Electronic Reference*, accessed online at https://indexcat.nlm.nih.gov/vivisimo/cgi-bin/query-meta?v%3aproject=indexcat&v%3asources=etkevk2& and https://cctr1.umkc.edu/search

HEHL Huntington Library, San Marino

IMEP *The Index of Middle English Prose* (Woodbridge, 1984–present) (see Bibliography for details of individual volumes)

Manual George R. Keiser, *A Manual of the Writings in Middle English 1050–1500: Volume 10—Works of Science and Information*, ed. by J.B. Severs and A.E. Hartung (New Haven, CT, 1998)

MED *The Middle English Dictionary*, ed. by Robert E. Lewis and others (Ann Arbor, MI, 1952–2001); online edition consulted in the *Middle English Compendium*, ed. by Frances McSparran and others (Ann Arbor, MI, 2000–18), accessed online at http://quod.lib.umich.edu/m/middle-english-dictionary

NIMEV *A New Index of Middle English Verse*, ed. by Julia Boffey and A.S.G. Edwards (London, 2005)

NLW National Library of Wales, Aberystwyth

OED *The Oxford English Dictionary*, accessed online at www.oed.com

PML Pierpont Morgan Library, New York

SKB Kungliga Biblioteket, Stockholm

TCC Trinity College, Cambridge

WT Wellcome Trust, London

YM York Minster, York

Introduction

> It must not be poetry that I read that night, but a devotional or even a cookery book. Perhaps the last was best for my mood, and I chose an old one of recipes and miscellaneous household hints. I read about the care of aspidistras and how to wash lace and black woollen stockings, and I learned that a package or an envelope sealed with white of egg cannot be steamed open. *Though what use that knowledge would ever be to me I could not imagine.*
>
> Barbara Pym, *Excellent Women* (1952)[1]

Useful texts can be useless to particular readers at particular moments or new uses can be discovered for them: in the above passage, the narrator of Pym's novel imagines that a book of recipes would calm and distract her better than a book of poetry or devotional writings.[2] In a disorientating way, Pym's narrator blurs the certain ('I chose...I read...') with the speculative ('It must not be...Perhaps...') as she writes (or rewrites) an account of how she spent one evening; recipes are the means through which she fills time literally, narratively, and imaginatively.

Today, practical writings are often read for pleasure or distraction and possessed for reasons other than the practical: we own recipe books because we feel we should own them, because they signal a well-organized household, or because we think that, one day, they *could* be useful. They allow us to manage our fears and insecurities, to enjoy the feeling of acquiring and possessing knowledge, and to imagine transformations in our lives: if I read this cookery book, I can imagine making this expensive dish or becoming like the book's healthy, glamorous, or down-to-earth author.

---

[1] Barbara Pym, *Excellent Women* (London, 1952), p. 171, italics mine.
[2] The research for this monograph was supported by a Wellcome Trust Medical History and Humanities Scholarship [grant no. 108641/Z/15/Z], a Junior Research Fellowship at Churchill College, Cambridge, and a short-term Erika and Kenneth Riley Fellowship at the Huntington Library, California.

Middle English Medical Recipes and Literary Play, 1375–1500. Hannah Bower, Oxford University Press.
© Hannah Bower 2022. DOI: 10.1093/oso/9780192849496.003.0001

This study contends that a similarly diverse range of motivations, uses, and interpretations informed the writing, reading, possessing, and imagining of a particular kind of late medieval recipe: medical remedies. These recipes taught readers to prepare healing treatments but they could, this study argues, also act as nexus points for the intersection (and playful redefinition) of different written and spoken styles, spaces, and identities. Although medical recipes are often overlooked by modern readers, they were one of the most frequently copied text-types in late medieval England, as the following comparison highlights: more than eighty fifteenth-century manuscripts survive of all or part of Chaucer's vernacular story collection, *The Canterbury Tales*, and that is the highest number for any of his works.[3] In contrast, one substantial database records over 1,800 extant medical recipes or recipe collections copied in English in the fifteenth century.[4] A vast number of other uncounted recipes were copied by medieval scribes on spare manuscript pages or in the margins of other medieval texts. Although the comparison with *The Canterbury Tales* is skewed by the fact that not all of these manuscripts contain the same or similar remedies, the figures do suggest that recipes were an integral part of many people's social and textual lives and that they deserve to be more prominent in discussions of medieval textual culture.

It might seem unlikely that such recipes could be used for anything other than bodily healing. Indeed, authors and scribes of medieval medical texts are usually quite clear about medicine's practical function: echoing Isidore of Seville's definition of medicine, a fifteenth-century prologue to a medical treatise defines medicine's use as: 'Lechecraft is man to hele . of all maner sekenesse | And to kepe hym hool þat is hol . as fer as craft may'.[5] Prologues to remedy collections often align recipes' function with the first, restorative part of this definition:

---

[3] Derek Pearsall, *The Canterbury Tales* (London, 1985), p. 8.

[4] See https://indexcat.nlm.nih.gov/vivisimo/cgi-bin/query-meta?v%3aproject=indexcat&v%3asources=etkevk2& (an electronic version of *eVK2*) [accessed 19/11/2021]. I reached this number through an advanced search on the terms 'medical recipe' and '+15c' (1,861 results). The database also gives sixty-eight results for the search terms 'medical recipe' and '+14c', but I have omitted these from the count so as not to skew the comparison with fifteenth-century manuscripts of Chaucer. It should also be noted that in *eVK2*, Kurtz and Voigts have only recorded groups of three recipes or more and individual recipes of interest.

[5] BL, MS Sloane 340, f. 65v. The prologue—though prose—is lineated like verse (as discussed in Chapter 2). For Isidore of Seville's definition, see *Isidori Hispalensis Episcopi: Etymologiarvm sive originvm, Vol. 1—Libros I–X*, ed. by W.M. Lindsay (Oxford, 1911), Bk IV, p. 165, lines 1–3: 'Medicina est quae corporis vel tuetur vel restaurat salutem' ('Medicine is that which protects or restores the health of the body').

Here beginnes gode medicines for diuers euille þat men has for god lechis has drawin þem out of many gode bokys galien and asclopus for þei were þe best lechis in þe werld and who so will do as þe bok techis he may be sekir to be hole of his euille[6]

[*diuers euille* = diverse sicknesses; *galien* = Galen; *asclopus* = Asclepius or Asclepiades; *sekir* = certain; *hole* = recovered]

The prologue promises that, if the recipes are followed properly, they will return the patient to health. This statement makes it hard to imagine any other function for the texts. It is also hard because of the subject matter: one can understand why luxury foodstuffs might be pleasing to contemplate, but would a reader really leaf through a book about scabs, boils, and broken bones for pleasure, distraction, reassurance, or imaginative inspiration?

This study suggests that medieval readers did just that. It also contends that, though many medieval remedies might be considered inefficacious by modern standards and by their own self-proclaimed healing standards, they might have been considered effective by some contemporary readers: a remedy might not make a patient 'hole', but reading, owning, or applying it might distract, empower, and soothe. Scholars have recognized the placebo effect's capacity to redeem medieval medical practice, but they have not studied in depth how the words and structures of *texts* could contribute to it.[7] This study redresses that oversight. However, it also challenges the assumption that healing was always recipes' sole intention or effect, contending that the imaginative and aesthetic elements of recipes might sometimes exceed, or even *impede*, their self-proclaimed practical purpose.

Offering the first book-length study of medieval English remedies and building on recent reappraisals of other kinds of practical, technical, or specialist knowledge, I thus present a challenge to recipes' traditional reputation as mundane, unartful texts written and read *solely* for the sake of directing practical action. Crucially, I seek to relocate some of these understudied texts and overlooked manuscripts within the complex and fragmentary networks of medieval textual culture, demonstrating that medical recipes could be linguistically, formally, and imaginatively interconnected with other late medieval discourses: writers of remedies and writers of more

---

[6] BL, MS Sloane 213, f. 138r.
[7] See, for example, Anne van Arsdall, 'Challenging the "Eye of Newt" Image of Medieval Medicine', in *The Medieval Hospital and Medical Practice*, ed. by Barbara S. Bowers (Aldershot, 2007), pp. 195–205.

consistently literary or imaginative texts influenced one another in more precise ways than have hitherto been acknowledged, and both groups partook in shared cultural modes of creative expression. Tracing possible connections and overlaps will allow us to arrive at a more nuanced, holistic understanding of what 'practical', 'careful', 'imaginative', and 'playful' might have meant for late medieval writers and readers. It will showcase the literary, linguistic, and historical gains to be made by reinserting medical recipes into the tangled webs of medieval textual culture.

Recipes in Their Medical Context

Before reassessing these discursive boundaries, we must establish how recipe collections fit into the social and textual cultures constituting 'medicine' in late medieval England. Individuals seeking medical treatment, and endowed with the finances required to facilitate choice, were confronted with a wealth of different therapeutic models and practitioners in late medieval England, including university-educated physicians, guild-trained surgeons, barbers, apothecaries, itinerant practitioners, amateur lay healers, and family members.[8] As Julie Orlemanski remarks, 'England's growing culture of medical literacy and care was...a bricolaged, miscellaneous, and constantly renegotiated set of practices.'[9] This shifting patchwork of expertise was matched by the impressive variety of medical writings circulating in Latin and English: remedies, regimen, uroscopies, surgical handbooks, medical treatises, physiognomy guides, charms, and astrological writings provide a few examples.[10] A preliminary—but often blurred—distinction can be drawn between theoretical and practical writings: theoretical texts described the body's physiological and anatomical workings, while practical texts described treatments.

The humoral theory frequently deployed in these activities of understanding and curing diseases is well known, but a brief overview will help to

---

[8] For an overview, see Faye Getz, *Medicine in the English Middle Ages* (Princeton, NJ, 1998), pp. 3–19.
[9] Julie Orlemanski, *Symptomatic Subjects: Bodies, Medicine and Causation in the Literature of Late Medieval England* (Philadelphia, PA, 2019), p. 21.
[10] On these genres, see Linda E. Voigts, 'Medical Prose', in *Middle English Prose: A Critical Guide to Major Authors and Genres*, ed. by A.S.G. Edwards (New Brunswick, NJ, 1984), pp. 315–35.

contextualize remedies.[11] Medieval conceptions of the body revolved around four primary qualities (hot, cold, wet, and dry), two of which were predominant in each of the four elements: air was hot and wet; fire was hot and dry; water was wet and cold; and earth was cold and dry. A combination of these elements, with one always predominant, formed all terrestrial matter, including the human body and the substances within it. Consequently, four types of fluid substance, known as humours, were identified with the four elements and their qualities: black bile (cold and dry), yellow bile (hot and dry), phlegm (wet and cold), and blood (hot and wet). In each body, these humours existed in different proportions and each individual had their own equilibrium, a state in which the qualities existed in ideal proportion with one another, though not necessarily in equal amounts. That proportion was equivalent to a state of health. Illness occurred when the ideal proportion of humours and qualities was disrupted by an external force or factor, such as injury, astrological influence, or excess food. The proportion had to be restored through substances that possessed the opposite quality to that in excess or deficiency: thus, a learned practical medical compendium begins, 'If þe hed-ache be of hete, lete him vse coolde þingis, as watir of endyue or of roses'.[12]

Between the Norman Conquest in 1066 and the late fourteenth century, all kinds of medical texts—practical and theoretical—were predominantly written, copied, and read in Latin by academic and religious communities; some medical texts also circulated in Old English, but these declined greatly after the Norman Conquest hailed the ascendence of French and Latin.[13] Behind all of these writings in England, there was a long history of Roman, ancient Greek, Byzantine, Persian, and Arabic medical thought.[14] For instance, the Roman writer Pliny the Elder influenced Latin, Old English, and later Middle English texts.[15] Greek thinkers, who were more focused on theoretical explanations of the body's workings than the therapeutically minded Romans, were slower to influence Western medicine but, once they

[11] On this theory, see Joel Kaye, *A History of Balance, 1250–1375: The Emergence of a New Model of Equilibrium and Its Impact on Thought* (Cambridge, 2014), pp. 128–240.
[12] *Healing and Society in Medieval England: A Middle English Translation of the Pharmaceutical Writings of Gilbertus Anglicus*, ed. by Faye Getz (Madison, WI, 1991), p. 1. 'Endyue' may be sowthistle or wild lettuce: see *MED*, *endive*, n., entry 1.
[13] On Old English medical writings, see Emily Kesling, *Medical Texts in Anglo-Saxon Literary Culture* (Cambridge, 2020).
[14] On the overlooked innovations and influences of Byzantine medical thought, see Petros Bouras-Vallianatos, *Innovation in Byzantine Medicine: The Writings of John Zacharias Aktouarios (c. 1275–c. 1330)* (Oxford, 2020).
[15] Faye Getz, *Medicine in the English Middle Ages* (Princeton, NJ, 1998), pp. 45–8.

did, the effects were long-lasting.[16] Two Greek medical theorists are of particular importance. The first is Hippocrates (born c. 460 BC), whose name became associated with a group of Greek medical writings, now referred to as the Hippocratic Corpus. Hippocratic medicine, which considered every natural phenomenon to have a rational cause, is credited with the earliest written description of all four humours.[17] The second influential thinker is the second-century Greek philosopher, Galen. He developed the theory of the primary qualities by emphasizing the intricate relativity of the body: bodies were not only healthy when the primary qualities were well proportioned in each corporeal substance, individual organ, and body part; the complexions of these parts also had to exist in healthy proportion to one another.[18]

Aspects of this Greek pharmacy were incorporated into Roman medical encyclopaedias in the Latin West before the decline of the Western Roman Empire altered connections between East and West.[19] However, much of the theory was removed by the Romans. This, along with declining Western knowledge of Greek after the fall of the Western Roman Empire, meant that many Greek medical texts and theoretical writings became relatively unknown in the Latin and vernacular cultures of early medieval Western Europe (or known through heavily mediated Latin forms). That changed from the eleventh century: with the reconquest of parts of Muslim Spain, Latin scholars discovered translations of Greek writings by Arabic-speaking thinkers, including Al-Farabi and Avicenna. Scholars such as Constantine the African, Gerard of Cremona, and Adelard of Bath set about reproducing the Arabic texts in Latin and centres of translation developed in Toledo, Montpellier, Salerno, and Bologna. In the Italian city-states, medical learning had a long tradition which pre-existed the universities.[20] In Oxford and Cambridge, however, the first recorded medical graduates only date from the early fourteenth century and provision for medical learning remained small throughout the Middle Ages.[21] The only major medical writer

---

[16] Getz, *Medicine in the English Middle Ages*, p. 45 notes that Pliny often defined his writings in opposition to those of his Greek predecessors, who he considered excessively interested in the body.

[17] Kaye, *History of Balance*, p. 168.

[18] On other aspects of Galen's relativity, see Kaye, *History of Balance*, pp. 128–82.

[19] On the transfer of scientific knowledge and texts between Greek and Latin-speaking cultures, see William Eamon, *Science and the Secrets of Nature: Books of Secrets in Medieval and Early Modern Culture* (Princeton, NJ, 1994), pp. 15–37.

[20] Getz, *Medicine in the English Middle Ages*, p. 65.

[21] Faye Getz, 'The Faculty of Medicine before 1500', in *The History of the University of Oxford: Volume II—Late Medieval Oxford*, ed. by J.I. Catto and T.A.R. Evans (Oxford, 1993),

explicitly associated with an English university in surviving documentation is John of Gaddesden.[22] Nevertheless, medicine started to develop into a mobile and transferable discipline: in medieval Oxford, students enrolled in other degrees were able to take some medical courses as well.[23]

Between 1375 and 1500, the period with which this study is concerned, medicine's mobility took on a new and explosive impetus *outside* of the university: many of these Latin medical works were translated into English for the first time and new medical writings (or new compilations of old ones) were written in the vernacular for the first time since the Norman Conquest.[24] Several factors contributed to this: from the late fourteenth century, literacy levels among lay craftsmen and merchants increased, leading to a greater commercial market for vernacular books, as well as more amateur book production for personal use.[25] Furthermore, the cost of paper declined, leading to the production of cheaper, more accessible books for lay urban classes.[26] These things were both a cause and a consequence of increased vernacular text production in many areas of culture: poetry was composed in English by more writers and the Wycliffite Middle English translation of the Bible was produced. Astronomy, astrology, alchemy, physiognomy, and other areas of science also began to flourish in the vernacular. But the increase in vernacular *medical* texts was especially noticeable: six

---

pp. 373–405 (p. 381); Carole Rawcliffe, *Medicine and Society in Later Medieval England* (Stroud, 1995), pp. 108–9.

[22] Peter Murray Jones, 'Language and Register in English Medieval Surgery', in *Language in Medieval Britain: Networks and Exchanges—Proceedings of the 2013 Harlaxton Symposium*, ed. by Mary J. Carruthers (Donnington, 2015), pp. 74–89 (p. 78).

[23] Vern Bullough, 'Medical Study at Mediaeval Oxford', *Speculum*, 36 (1961), 600–12 (p. 603).

[24] On English as a scientific language see *Medical and Scientific Writing in Late Medieval English*, ed. by Irma Taavitsainen and Päivi Pahta (Cambridge, 2004); Tony Hunt, 'The Languages of Medical Writing in Medieval England', in *Medieval and Early Modern Literature, Science and Medicine*, ed. by Rachel Falconer and Denis Renevey (Tübingen, 2013), pp. 79–101; Linda E. Voigts, 'Multitudes of Middle English Medical Manuscripts, or the Englishing of Science and Medicine', in *Manuscript Sources of Medieval Medicine*, ed. by Margaret R. Schleissner (New York, 1995), pp. 183–95; H.S. Bennett, 'Science and Information in English Writings of the Fifteenth Century', *The Modern Language Review*, 39 (1944), 1–8; Peter Murray Jones, 'Information and Science', in *Fifteenth-Century Attitudes: Perceptions of Society in Late Medieval England*, ed. by Rosemary Horrox (Cambridge, 1994), pp. 97–111 (pp. 103–4).

[25] Malcolm Parkes, 'The Literacy of the Laity', in *Literature and Western Civilisation: The Medieval World*, ed. by David Daiches and Anthony Thorlby (London, 1973), pp. 555–77; Malcolm Richardson, *Middle Class Writing in Late Medieval London* (London, 2011); Carol Meale, 'Amateur Book Production and the Miscellany in Late Medieval East Anglia', in *Insular Books: Vernacular Manuscript Miscellanies in Late Medieval Britain*, ed. by Margaret Connolly and Raluca Radulescu (Oxford, 2015), pp. 157–73.

[26] Eric Kwakkel, 'A New Type of Book for a New Type of Reader: The Emergence of Paper in Vernacular Book Production', *The Library*, 4 (2003), 219–48.

times as many English medical writings survive from the fifteenth century than from the fourteenth century.[27]

Learned Latin texts were not merely translated into English during this period: they were often adapted, abridged, rearranged, and combined by anonymous readers to produce new texts. In particular, recipes embedded in longer theoretical writings were extracted and copied alongside remedies from other sources in patchwork processes of compilation. Faye Getz has illuminated this process in relation to Gilbert the Englishman's *Compendium medicinae*, a learned thirteenth-century handbook combining practical advice with condensed theoretical explanations. By taking one recipe from the Latin *Compendium* and tracing its reappearance in multiple compilations and anonymous vernacular remedy books, Getz has shown just how influential and wide-reaching Gilbert's text was.[28] Conversely, Margaret Ogden has found parallels for recipes in a late medieval vernacular remedy collection, often known as the *Liber de diversis medicinis*, in a wide range of learned Greek, Arabic, Latin, Anglo-Norman, and English sources.[29]

This piecemeal process of extraction produced remedy books that were, stylistically, quite different from the extended, theoretical treatises from which they frequently derived. Compare this discussion of red eyes in a fifteenth-century English translation of Gilbert the Englishman's extensive *Compendium* to an extract from part of a remedy book concerned with eye ailments. Although the former is not the source of the latter, the juxtaposition aptly illustrates the stylistic differences between the two modes of writing:

> A mannes iȝen ben oþirwhiles rede or infecte. Redenes comeþ of blode; infeccion comeþ of oþer humours and of oþer sikenes, as of þe ȝelewe yvele, or of stopping of þe splene, or of heting of þe lyver. To hele suche infeccions, firste þou muste hele þe sekenes þat ben cause of hem... Of blode comeþ redenes, and not al oneli, but oþerwhiles a gobet of fleisshe growing on þe iȝe. And oþerwhiles, for grete plente of blode and feblenes

---

[27] This estimate, which originated with Dorothy Waley Singer, has been reproduced in many studies including Faye Getz, 'Gilbertus Anglicus Anglicized', *Medical History*, 26 (1982), 436–42 (p. 436) and Murray Jones, 'Information and Science', p. 101. Rossell Hope Robbins, 'A Note on the Singer Survey of Medical Manuscripts in the British Isles', *Chaucer Review*, 4 (1969), 66–70, questions the accuracy of Singer's figures but agrees that, proportionally, the increase was dramatic.

[28] Getz, 'Gilbertus Anglicus Anglicized', pp. 441–2.

[29] *The 'Liber de diversis medicinis' in the Thornton Manuscript*, ed. by Margaret Ogden, EETS os 207 (London, 1938), pp. xx–xxviii.

of þe iȝe, þe blode lieþ y-congelid on þe iȝe and makeþ þe iȝen rede. Oþerwhiles þei ben rede for grete plente of blode þat is in þe veynes… And if þe yȝe be kitte in þe whijt of þe yȝe, or if þe whijt be y-broke, heel it herwith: Take sarcacol, mastike, encense, sandragon, emachite. And tempere hem with sangrinary þat is clepid sheppardis purse, or planteyn.[30]

For him þat may not wel see and hath rede eyn. Tak whiȝte gynger and rubbe it on a weston in a fayre basyn of metal and tak as meche salt as þow hast of powder and grynde hem wel togydder in þe basyn and tempere hem togydder wit whit wyn and let it stande a day and a nyȝt and þanne tak þe thynne þat stondyt aboue and do it a ful glas and when þe syke goth to bedde tak a fether and wet þerinne and onoynte wel þe sore eyn þerwyth and he schal be hool sekerly.[31]

The second extract exemplifies the kind of remedy that forms the main subject of this study. It is far less detailed and contains no information about the humoral causes of red eyes.[32] While the interest of Gilbert's translator in the various causes of red eyes is conveyed through the way he strings clauses together with the conjunctions 'or' and 'oþerwhiles', the remedy book is characterized by strings of imperatives linked paratactically by 'and'. The emphasis in the latter is not on the possibilities of theory but on the certainties of action.

Some of these simple, practically orientated remedy collections appear alongside culinary and domestic recipes, devotional writings, and poetry, suggesting that they were considered part of a 'household book', a term used literally and broadly by Julia Boffey to describe 'a book that was in use in a specific household'.[33] Recently, compilations which fit this criteria and which mix languages, genres, and epistemologies have received renewed critical attention as sites of experimentation, intertextual play, and aesthetic effect.[34] Another kind of compilation often containing simple medical

---

[30] Getz, ed., *Healing and Society*, pp. 54–5.
[31] WT, MS Wellcome 542, f. 1v. Rubrication is marked in bold.
[32] For an analogous comparison of the stylistic differences between scholastic and remedy-book registers in Latin surgical writing, see Murray Jones, 'Language and Register', pp. 74–89.
[33] Julia Boffey, 'Bodleian Library, MS Arch Selden B.24 and Definitions of the Household Book', in *The English Medieval Book: Studies in Memory of Jeremy Griffiths*, ed. by A.S.G. Edwards and others (London, 2000), pp. 125–34 (p. 129).
[34] E.g., *Robert Thornton and His Books: Essays on the Lincoln and London Thornton Manuscripts*, ed. by Susanna Fein and Michael Johnston (York, 2014); *Household Knowledges in Late Medieval England and France*, ed. by Glenn Burger and Rory Critten (Manchester, 2019); *Interpreting MS Digby 86: A Trilingual Book from Thirteenth Century Worcestershire*, ed. by

recipes has been labelled by Linda E. Voigts as a 'scientific book'.[35] Such books contain more homogenous subject matter, situating remedy collections alongside other medical, astronomical, astrological, and alchemical writings of a simple or sophisticated variety. The majority of remedy collections examined in this study belong to one or both of these broad categories; it can be futile to distinguish between the two, as compilations largely or solely made up of scientific writings could still have been used domestically or copied and compiled by interested members of the literate laity. Manuscripts could also metamorphosize between categories as new texts and genres were added or discrete quires were bound together.[36]

This begs the question: *who* was copying, owning, and reading vernacular remedy books? Counterintuitively, scholars have shown that many learned practitioners owned simple vernacular medical texts, perhaps as reminders or teaching aids.[37] At the same time, though, the vernacularization of medicine allowed all kinds of medical writings to reach audiences outside of academic institutions. For example, Cambridge, Gonville and Caius College, MS 176/97 is a manuscript containing Middle English medical treatises translated from canonical Latin texts. As Peter Murray Jones has pointed out, the manuscript begins with a prologue claiming that the texts were translated by a clerk for Thomas Plawdon, citizen and barber of London.[38] Barbers were not university-educated; instead, like surgeons, they were trained through guild-organized apprenticeships. However, they were usually trained to carry out more basic operations than surgeons, such as bloodletting.[39] The manuscript therefore suggests that there was a demand for medical texts—including those of a learned, theoretical kind—among vernacular readers with humbler medical training.

Susanna Fein (York, 2019). See especially Jennifer Jahner, 'Literary Therapeutics: Experimental Knowledge in MS Digby 86', in *Interpreting MS Digby 86*, ed. by Fein, pp. 73–86. On the aesthetics of compilation, see also Arthur Bahr, *Fragments and Assemblages: Forming Compilations of Medieval London* (Chicago, IL, 2015).

[35] Linda E. Voigts, 'Scientific and Medical Books', in *Book Production and Publishing in Britain, 1375–1475*, ed. by Jeremy Griffiths and Derek Pearsall (Cambridge, 1989), pp. 345–402.

[36] An excellent example of this is Robert Thornton's copy of the *Liber de Diversis Medicinis*, which seems to have been transformed from independent remedy book to scientific book to household miscellany: for this observation, see Julie Orlemanski, 'Thornton's Remedies and the Practices of Medical Reading', in *Robert Thornton and His Books*, ed. by Fein and Johnston, pp. 235–57 (pp. 241–6). See also the discussion of Oxford, BodL, MS Rawlinson C.506 in Chapter 3 of this study.

[37] See Rossell Hope Robbins, 'Medical Manuscripts in Middle English', *Speculum*, 45 (1970), 393–415 (pp. 408, 410) and Voigts, 'Scientific and Medical Books', pp. 383–4.

[38] Murray Jones, 'Medicine and Science', p. 435. [39] Ibid.

INTRODUCTION 11

Unfortunately, names as traceable as Plawdon's are rarely inscribed in the flyleaves of practically orientated remedy collections and these anonymous vernacular collections are not the kind of text usually recorded in wills and inventories. Susan Cavanaugh's *Study of Books Privately Owned in England 1300–1450* shows that, even in the increasingly literate later Middle Ages, the types of people who tended to record medical books in their wills were still male members of universities and religious houses and the books they recorded were often Latin texts by known canonical authorities such as Galen.[40] For example, although growing numbers of women were owning and reading books associated with religious instruction, Monica Green lists only ten late medieval women in England who are known to have owned medical writings.[41] She also translates a fifteenth-century note describing English books containing medical content that were owned by the Dutch noblewoman Jacqueline of Hainault (d. 1436) at her death.[42] After fleeing to the English court in 1421, Jacqueline married Humphrey, Duke of Gloucester. He was a great patron of literary and scientific writings and one of those in his favour was Gilbert Kymer, a university-qualified doctor of medicine who commissioned the copying of many medical works. This might explain why Jacqueline possessed medical books when so few other women appear to have done so.[43]

Vernacular manuscripts and amateur notebooks could, however, have circulated amongst women and lower-class laymen to a greater extent than we can establish from documentary evidence: the women in the Norfolk-based

---

[40] E.g., Susan Cavanaugh, *A Study of Books Privately Owned in England 1300–1450*, 2 vols (unpublished doctoral thesis, University of Pennsylvania, 1980), I, pp. 42, 121, 128. These are also the kind of medical books typically named in the library inventories of academic institutions, guilds, and hospitals; see, for example, the inventory of medical books in All Souls College, Oxford in 1443 in *The University and College Libraries of Oxford: Volume I*, ed. by Rodney M. Thomson, Corpus of British Medieval Library Catalogues, 16 (London, 2015), pp. 101–5, which includes texts by Rhazes, Avicenna, Constantine the African, Gilbert the Englishman, and John of Gaddesden and commentaries on Galen's works. For similar examples from guilds and hospitals, see *Hospitals, Towns and the Professions*, ed. by Nigel Ramsay and James M.W. Willoughby, Corpus of British Medieval Library Catalogues, 14 (London, 2009), pp. 107, 163, 168.

[41] Monica Green, 'The Possibilities of Literacy and the Limits of Reading: Women and the Gendering of Medical Literacy', in Green, *Women's Healthcare in the Medieval West* (Aldershot, 2000), pp. 1–76 (pp. 49–51).

[42] Transcribed in Cavanaugh, *A Study of Books Privately Owned*, I, p. 465 and translated in Green, 'The Possibilities of Literacy', p. 55, where it is also noted that one of Jacqueline of Hainault's medical books was sold eight years after her death to a travelling English merchant.

[43] Monica Green, *Making Women's Medicine Masculine: The Rise of Male Authority in Pre-Modern Gynaecology* (Oxford, 2008) shows that even medieval gynaecological texts rarely evoke a female audience in any uncomplicated way.

Paston family certainly possessed sufficient medical knowledge to send medical recipes to distant family members.[44] As Green notes, significantly more women and men could also have engaged with medical texts through oral conversations and readings: this is certainly the implication of a poem surviving in at least twenty-two manuscripts and normally appended to the beginning or end of remedy collections.[45] It begins:

> Þe man þat wyl of lechecraft lere
> Rede ouer þis boke and he may here
> Many a medcyn bothe goyd and trew
> Wylle hele sores bothe old and new[46]

The shift from 'rede' to 'here' in line 2 implies that the remedy collection could be read aloud to whoever wanted to 'lere'. The poem raises the possibility that this reader or listener will not only become a repository of knowledge about 'lechecraft', but also a practising healer themselves. In other recipe collections, the multiple subject positions available to readers are even more explicit: while academic writings normally address the reader consistently as an expert practitioner treating a sick patient, practical remedy compilations in both Latin and English—as Julie Orlemanski notes—frequently shift between addressing the reader as a practitioner who is consulting the text with intention to cure another, and somebody, possibly a more amateur individual, who wishes to heal him- or herself.[47] For instance, a fifteenth-century recipe to make a man sweat contains instructions that shift between second- and third-person pronouns: 'put it in a box and anoynte *þi* soles of *þi* fete and *þin* hondys aȝens a fere of charcole and let *hym* go to bedde and hele *hym* þat he take no cold'.[48] The recipe addresses the reader in quick succession as practitioner, self-healer, and patient.

---

[44] Elaine E. Whitaker, 'Reading the Pastons Medically', *English Language Notes*, 31 (1993), 19–27. On female book ownership, see also Carol Meale, '"alle the bokes that I haue of latyn, englisch, and frensch": Laywomen and Their Books in Late Medieval England', in *Women and Literature in Britain, 1150–1500*, ed. by Carol M. Meale (Cambridge, 1993), pp. 128–58.

[45] According to *eVK2* and Keiser's *Manual*, this poem survives in twenty-two known manuscripts, with two copies in BL, MS Sloane 468, ff. 7r, 80v and two copies in TCC MS O.1.13, ff. 45v, 166r–v. *eVK2* and *DIMEV* 5390 also record another possible manuscript which can no longer be traced.

[46] BodL, MS Ashmole 1444, Part III, p. 184.

[47] Julie Orlemanski, 'Jargon and the Matter of Medicine in Middle English', *Journal of Medieval and Early Modern Studies*, 42 (2012), 395–420 (p. 411).

[48] BodL, MS Ashmole 1438, Part II, p. 39, italics mine.

From the late fourteenth century onwards, amateur lay persons—be these merchants, literate craftsmen, or members of the gentry and nobility—were not only reading about, listening to, or practising medicine upon themselves, but sometimes copying those books as well. For instance, Robert Thornton, a member of the Yorkshire landed gentry, copied a herbal and the English recipe collection *Liber de diversis medicinis* alongside romances and devotional writings.[49] George Keiser has argued, however, that the mistakes Thornton made in his copying imply that he was not comfortable with the medical vocabulary he encountered.[50] We must remember, then, that vernacularization did not mean a smooth or uncomplicated dispersal of technical knowledge or a universal one. There were still many more challenges—financial, social, and intellectual—preventing female readers, lay artisans, and gentry families from accessing written medical texts than aristocratic, religious, or university-educated men.

Thornton's errors also testify to the importance of textual and codicological evidence when speculating about who wrote remedy collections and for whom. Engaging in this kind of close reading, however, often compels us to recomplicate the categories of 'lay' and 'learned' or 'amateur' and 'academic' only just clarified above. Consider an informal, scruffily copied fifteenth-century collection of remedies for wounds and fractures explored in more depth in Chapter 3 (see Figure I.1).[51] This is a practically orientated collection of straightforward prognostic tests and relatively simple recipes for ointments and plasters, seemingly accessible to readers with a basic knowledge of herb names. The text, which is punctuated by recipes copied in blank spaces by later hands, is in English with some Latin headings and it may have been copied by one 'Nicholas Neesbett' whose name is written at the top of the collection.[52] Notes interspersed amongst the recipes suggest the collection was going to be sent by the writer to another medical practitioner.[53] We cannot tell if this writer was an amateur or educated healer, but there is no evidence of an extensive medical education: all we can deduce is that he possessed a good knowledge of herb varieties, that he occasionally

---

[49] On Thornton's copying, see Orlemanski, 'Thornton's Remedies', pp. 235–57. For an edition of the manuscript, see Ogden, ed., *The 'Liber de diversis medicinis'*.

[50] George R. Keiser, 'Robert Thornton's *Liber de Diversis Medicinis*: Text, Vocabulary, and Scribal Confusion', in *Rethinking Middle English: Linguistic and Literary Approaches*, ed. by N. Ritt and H. Schnedel (Frankfurt, 2005), pp. 30–41.

[51] BodL, MS Ashmole 1438, Part I, pp. 57–71.

[52] Recipes seem to have been added in blank spaces by later hands on pp. 60, 62, 71, 72, and 73.

[53] For further discussion of this collection, see Chapter 3.

14 MIDDLE ENGLISH MEDICAL RECIPES AND LITERARY PLAY

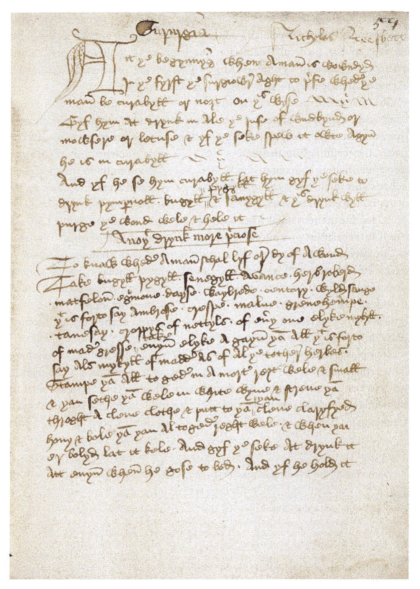

Figure I.1 Remedy collection associated with 'Nicholas Neesbett'. The Bodleian Libraries, University of Oxford, MS Ashmole 1438, Part I, p. 57. Reproduced with kind permission from the Bodleian Libraries, University of Oxford through the Creative Commons licence CC-BY-NC 4.0.

deployed slightly more technical words such as *sanatif* and *corrosif* (but nothing much more specialist), and that he seems to have had a particular interest in the medical treatment of the poor.[54] Finally, the lexical and orthographical features of his writing—if he was the composer as well as the scribe of the collection—can be linked to Lincolnshire.[55]

The text itself, however, provides us with some clues about Nicholas's intentions and his possible aspirations towards a more sophisticated form of medical discourse, despite the relative simplicity of his treatments: on two pages, the scribe begins the recipes with the words 'At þe begynnyng', using a large but amateurly decorated initial 'A'.[56] In addition to the obvious biblical echoes, this opening gives the recipe collection, in which recipes are roughly grouped into similar types, the semblance of having a logical order like that of longer, more theoretical writings. For example, a fifteenth-century Middle English translation of a surgical treatise by the university-educated practitioner Guy de Chauliac opens with summaries of each chapter, all of which start 'Here bygynneþ'.[57] Manuscripts such as the 'Nicholas Neesbett' collection remind us, then, that academic and lay learning or theoretical and practical discourses did not necessarily exist in strict opposition to one another, but, in terms of style and content, were part of the same continuum and could be mutually influencing.[58]

This play of influences works against any over-strict definition of a textual corpus; many of the features of recipes explored in this study place the texts in conversation with related modes of scientific and practical writing and with Latin and French remedy collections which, having been compiled for centuries, continued to circulate in the later Middle Ages.[59] Consequently,

---

[54] See BodL, MS Ashmole 1438, Part 1, p. 68 for 'sanatyf' and 'corvasyse'. On the oddness of this second spelling—which may suggest the scribe was not entirely comfortable with the word—see Chapter 3, note 75.

[55] M. Benskin and others, *An Electronic Version of a Linguistic Atlas of Late Medieval English*, accessed online at www.lel.ac.uk/ihd/elalme/elalme_frames.html [accessed 02/04/2018]. The collection comprises the *Atlas*'s linguistic profile 908. I have surmised that the scribe and/or addressee may have been particularly involved in treatment of the poor because the scribe writes that he could have written more 'costly' remedies but they are 'noȝt for a pure man'; he later declares a remedy to be 'a gude pure man salfe'. See BodL, MS Ashmole 1438, Part I, pp. 64–5, 65–6.

[56] BodL, MS Ashmole 1438, Part I, pp. 57, 59.

[57] *The Cyrurgie of Guy de Chauliac*, ed. by Margaret Sinclair Ogden, EETS os 265 (London, 1971), pp. 14–26.

[58] On the intersection of learned and household medical writing, see Michael Leahy, 'Domestic Ideals: Healing, Reading, and Perfection in the Late Medieval Household', in *Household Knowledges in Late Medieval England and France*, ed. by Burger and Critten, n.p., accessed online at www.perlego.com/home.

[59] Pearl Kibre and Lynn Thorndike, *A Catalogue of Incipits of Mediaeval Scientific Writings in Latin*, rev. edn (Cambridge, MA, 1963), accessed online at https://indexcat.nlm.nih.gov,

it might seem odd to focus this study predominantly on vernacular remedy books. However, the fifteenth-century explosion of English collections affirms that the vernacular was recognized as a suitable language in which to write the entirety or majority of a recipe collection, even if that medical language—as Sarah Star has demonstrated—was often developed through a creative repurposing and remaking of Latin words.[60] I believe, then, that vernacular collections merit attention as a corpus, but I nevertheless remain sensitive to the multilingual networks of inheritance and exchange surrounding them, noting significant traditions, revisions, and parallels.

I adopt the same approach in relation to culinary recipes, herbals, and other practical texts. Culinary recipes, containing diverse herbs, could be implicitly medical as food was one of the non-naturals affecting humoral balance and health.[61] Like miscellaneous recipes for making ink and parchment, dying clothes, or performing practical jokes, culinary recipes could be intermingled amongst medical recipes or culinary collections could, at some stage in the book's production and circulation, be bound together with medical ones. At the same time, a significant proportion of the recipe collections I have examined are largely or solely medical in content and they appear in manuscripts filled with astronomy, astrology, alchemy, and medicine, indicating that homogeneous 'scientific' subject matter could be as important to book compilers as miscellaneity or household utility. In the rest of this study, then, I try to juggle these two priorities, highlighting important discursive connections between different practical discourses, whilst drawing attention to instances of medicine's codicological, epistemological, and linguistic distinctiveness.

---

records Latin recipe collections from the ninth century. On the well-studied phenomenon of code-switching in medical texts, see Tony Hunt, 'Code-Switching in Medical Texts', in *Multilingualism in Later Medieval Britain*, ed. by D.A. Trotter (Cambridge, 2000), pp. 131–47; Päivi Pahta, 'On Structures of Code-Switching in Medical Texts from Medieval England', *Neuphilologische Mitteilungen*, 104 (2003), 197–210; and Päivi Pahta, 'Code Switching in Medieval Medical Writing', in *Medical and Scientific Writing*, ed. by Taavitsainen and Pahta, pp. 73–99.

[60] For Star's analysis of Henry Daniel's fourteenth-century medical vocabulary, see Sarah Star, 'Henry Daniel, Medieval English Medicine, and Linguistic Innovation: A Lexicographic Study of Huntington MS HM 505', *Huntington Library Quarterly*, 81 (2018), 63–105 (p. 69) and Sarah Star, 'The Textual Worlds of Henry Daniel', *Studies in the Age of Chaucer*, 40 (2018), 191–216.

[61] On the non-naturals, see Peregrine Horden, 'A Non-Natural Environment: Medicine Without Doctors and the Medieval European Hospital', in *The Medieval Hospital*, ed. by Bowers, pp. 133–45.

Re-evaluating Recipes

It should already be apparent that vernacular remedy collections are wonderfully plural and polyvocal, pieced together from a wealth of sources, copied next to a variety of other texts, and written in a language and idiom that are in continuous conversation with others. Herein lies their scholarly appeal: from the nineteenth century to the present, scholars have foregrounded the challenges and fascinations of an abundant, but obscure, Middle English medical vocabulary by producing editions with rich and detailed glossaries.[62] These resources have, in turn, encouraged linguists to plot the development of a vernacular medical vocabulary and create new dictionaries of Middle English medical terminology.[63] Admittedly, editors have not yet found a way of representing the complex relationships between similar recipes adapted between collections. Such variants have, however, become easier to trace in the last three decades through several finding aids: Linda E. Voigts and Patricia Kurtz's *Scientific and Medical Writings in Old and Middle English: An Electronic Reference*; *The Index of Middle English Prose*; and George Keiser's *Manual of the Writings in Middle English (1050–1500): Works of Science and Information*.[64] I have used these tools to locate remedy collections in over seventy manuscripts.

A substantial body of scholarship has also tried to piece together the social, intellectual, and corporeal contexts informing, and informed by, remedies. For instance, mid-twentieth-century German scholarship understood remedies as a type of *Fachliteratur* that, along with other kinds of agricultural and household texts, taught practical skills.[65] More recently, researchers have tested some cures and found them to be efficacious, whilst others have considered the possibility of a placebo effect.[66]

---

[62] E.g., *Ein Mittelenglisches Medizinbuch*, ed. by Fritz Heinrich (Halle, 1896); *A Leechbook or Collection of Medical Recipes of the Fifteenth Century: The Text of MS no. 136 of the Medical Society of London, Together with a Transcript into Modern Spelling*, ed. by Warren R. Dawson (London, 1934); Ogden, ed., *The 'Liber de diversis medicinis'*. See also Getz, ed., *Healing and Society* for an edition of Gilbert the Englishman's *Compendium*.

[63] On English as a scientific language, see note 24 of this chapter. For a recent and extensive dictionary, see Juhani Norri, *Dictionary of Medical Vocabulary in English, 1375–1550: Body Parts, Sicknesses, Instruments and Medicinal Preparations* (London, 2016).

[64] Full details of these aids are provided in the List of Abbreviations and Bibliography.

[65] E.g., Gerhard Eis, *Mittelalterliche Fachliteratur* (Stuttgart, 1962); *Fachliteratur des Mittelalters: Festschrift für Gerhard Eis*, ed. by Gundolf Keil and others (Stuttgart, 1968).

[66] www.nottingham.ac.uk/news/pressreleases/2015/march/ancientbiotics---a-medieval-remedy-for-modern-day-superbugs.aspx [accessed 21/10/2021]. On the placebo effect, see Van Arsdall, 'Challenging the "Eye of Newt" Image'; Toni Mount, *Dragon's Blood and Willow Bark: The Mysteries of Medieval Medicine* (Stroud, 2015), pp. 104–16. Michael Solomon, *Fictions of*

Recipes' contexts of production and circulation have also attracted interest: Claire Jones, Linda E. Voigts, and Irma Taavitsainen have connected the copying and use of specific medical manuscripts to certain practitioners, discourse communities, geographical regions, and copying houses, whilst Carrie Griffin has explored how the material form of instructional texts (both in manuscript and print) shapes readers' perceived sense of their purpose and significance.[67] Linne Mooney has paid similarly close attention to medical manuscripts, detecting physical signs of practical use, such as droplets of blood and fragments of herbs.[68] Undoubtedly, many such manuscripts *were* used to heal (or try to heal) real human bodies. And yet, traditionally, an assumption that this is the only function recipes served has led scholars to overlook clues to other imaginative and cultural roles they may have performed: in an essay on the problems inherent in cataloguing recipes, Henry Hargreaves made explicit this implied opposition between the practical and the poetic, the utilitarian and the imaginative, by proclaiming that remedies 'have, of course, not the slightest scintilla of literary interest'.[69]

The present study challenges Hargreaves' assured dismissal of recipe collections. In pursuing this focus, it is partially indebted to the recent endeavours of early modernists: Wendy Wall, Jayne Elisabeth Archer, Robert Appelbaum, and Mary Fissell have all traced the ways that recipes—of various kinds—intersect culturally, linguistically, and codicologically with early modern literary modes and rhetorical styles.[70] In their analysis of the various

Well-Being: Sickly Readers and Vernacular Medical Writing in Late Medieval and Early Modern Spain (Philadelphia, PA, 2010), has explored in vernacular Spanish writings how 'tropes of usefulness, professional competence and efficacy' might have encouraged readers of medical texts to construct a 'fiction of his or her imminent well-being' (pp. 7, 9).

[67] Claire Jones, 'Discourse Communities and Medical Texts', in *Medical and Scientific Writing*, ed. by Taavitsainen and Pahta, pp. 23–36; Irma Taavitsainen, 'Scriptorial "House-Styles" and Discourse Communities', in *Medical and Scientific Writing*, ed. by Taavitsainen and Pahta, pp. 209–40; Linda E. Voigts, 'The "Sloane Group": Related Scientific and Medical Manuscripts from the Fifteenth Century in the Sloane Collection', *The British Library Journal*, 16 (1990), 26–57; Carrie Griffin, *Instructional Writing in English, 1350–1650: Materiality and Meaning* (London, 2019).

[68] Linne Mooney, 'Manuscript Evidence for the Use of Medieval Scientific and Utilitarian Texts', in *Interstices: Studies in Middle English and Anglo-Latin Texts in Honour of A.G. Rigg*, ed. by Richard Firth Green and Linne Mooney (Toronto, 2004), pp. 184–202.

[69] Henry Hargreaves, 'Some Problems in Indexing Middle English Recipes', in *Middle English Prose: Essays on Bibliographic Problems*, ed. by A.S.G. Edwards and Derek Pearsall (New York, 1981), pp. 91–113 (p. 92).

[70] Wendy Wall, *Recipes for Thought: Knowledge and Taste in the Early Modern English Kitchen* (Philadelphia, PA, 2016); Jayne Elisabeth Archer, '"The Quintessence of Wit": Poems and Recipes in Early Modern Women's Writing', in *Reading and Writing Recipe Books 1550–1800*, ed. by Michelle DiMeo and Sara Pennell (Manchester, 2013), pp. 114–34; Robert

ways that poetic language can serve and supplement recipes' practical purposes, they have built upon the historical studies of Michelle DiMeo, Sara Pennell, and Elaine Leong, who have explored the social and communicative networks created through print and manuscript recipes, recipes' connection to early modern experimental culture, and their relationship to gender roles.[71] These scholars have raised invaluable questions for me about the interconnection of disciplines. However, they have done so through concepts of wit, poetry, book production, gender, and experimentation that are often distinctly early modern. Frequently, the studies contain no sustained consideration of the medieval manuscripts preceding their early modern examples. This study supplies that missing story by considering how earlier recipes shaped, and were shaped by, late medieval imaginations.

The essays of four medieval scholars have been particularly influential in approaching this task and therefore merit extended mention. Lisa Cooper's essay, 'The Poetics of Practicality', has been a vital launchpad for scholars interested in rethinking distinctions between genres and modes of reading.[72] Cooper carries out close readings on parts of medieval practical writings from different genres, suggesting that those writings contain rhetorical, narrative, and dialogic structures, and that they appeal to readers' imaginations by asking them to envisage themselves performing an activity or craft that they are not currently engaged in. In a second essay, Cooper has focused more explicitly on the recipe form, contending that the 'rhetoric of recipe' can be used in literary texts as an epistemological tool, a means of signalling that a text 'is not simply didactic but also *productive*'—that it does not just teach a reader 'about something' but also '*how* that something *is, can be* (or...*was*) made'.[73]

Appelbaum, 'Rhetoric and Epistemology in Early Printed Recipe Collections', *Journal for Early Modern Cultural Studies*, 3 (2003), 1–35; Mary E. Fissell, 'Readers, Texts, and Contexts: Vernacular Medical Works in Early Modern England', in *The Popularization of Medicine 1650–1850*, ed. by Roy Porter (London, 1992), pp. 72–96.

[71] See, for example, DiMeo and Pennell, eds., *Reading and Writing Recipe Books*; Elaine Leong, 'Collecting Knowledge for the Family: Recipes, Gender and Practical Knowledge in the Early Modern English Household', *Centaurus*, 55 (2013), 81–103; Elaine Leong, *Recipes and Everyday Knowledge: Medicine, Science and the Household in Early Modern England* (Chicago, IL, 2018); Sara Pennell and Elaine Leong, 'Recipe Collections and the Currency of Medical Knowledge in the Early Modern "Medical Marketplace"', in *Medicine and the Market in England and Its Colonies c.1450–c.1850*, ed. by Mark S.R. Jenner and Patrick Wallis (Basingstoke, 2007), pp. 133–52.

[72] Lisa H. Cooper, 'The Poetics of Practicality', in *Twenty-First Century Approaches to Literature: Middle English*, ed. by Paul Strohm (Oxford, 2007), pp. 491–505.

[73] Lisa H. Cooper, 'Recipes for the Realm: John Lydgate's "Soteltes" and *The Debate of the Horse, Goose, and Sheep*', in *Essays on Aesthetics in Medieval Literature in Honour of Howell Chickering*, ed. by John M. Hill, Bonnie Wheeler, and R.F. Yeager (Toronto, 2014), pp. 194–215 (p. 196).

In a later article, focused on the narrative qualities of a selection of medieval medical and culinary recipes, Carrie Griffin has also drawn attention to recipes' future-orientated temporality: their capacity to function aspirationally as 'wish-lists' for costly dishes or remedies.[74] One of the most helpful aspects of this essay is Griffin's critique of cataloguing systems that present recipe collections as coherent, organized, and integral units; she foregrounds instead the collections' unpredictable and shifting 'thematic focus', which can 'confound the distinctions we might want to make between short, individual instructive pieces and larger collections'.[75] Because many vernacular remedy collections came into being though a patchwork compilation process, the collections are rarely coherent in style and contents, even if they appear visually coherent on the manuscript page.[76] This study's focus on large collections containing over one hundred remedies is partly because that focus enabled me to access large numbers of recipes at one time, but also because it allowed me to explore further the impulses behind, and changing dynamics produced by, the form of the recipe *collection*.

When moving from questions of form to questions of language, the work of Sarah Star and Julie Orlemanski is especially illuminating. Star has meticulously reconstructed the textual landscape inhabited and reinvented by Henry Daniel, the fourteenth-century author of one of the earliest surviving uroscopy treatises in English.[77] Star highlights Daniel's linguistic ingenuity and polyvocal, compilational approach to medical learning and textual construction.[78] Orlemanski's recent book, focused on aetiology in medical narratives, is equally interested in the polyvocal, bricolaged nature of texts and practice.[79] Furthermore, her essay on Middle English medical jargon highlights how medieval parodies of recipes foreground the 'poetical energies' of 'a medical language turned aside from its healing purpose' and verging on incomprehensibility.[80] Her close reading of the sonic and semantic properties of such parodies is another model for the way that I analyse

---

[74] Carrie Griffin, 'Reconsidering the Recipe: Materiality, Narrative and Text in Later Medieval Instructional Manuscripts and Collections', in *Manuscripts and Printed Books in Europe, 1350–1550: Packaging, Presentation and Consumption*, ed. by Emma Cayley and Susan Powell (Liverpool, 2013), pp. 135–49 (p. 148). See also Carrie Griffin, 'Instruction and Inspiration: Fifteenth-Century Codicological Recipes', *Exemplaria*, 30 (2018), 20–34 for discussion of how codicological recipes similarly stimulate the imagination.

[75] Griffin, 'Reconsidering the Recipe', p. 147.

[76] The recipes are often written in prose with a rubricated title beginning 'For…'.

[77] Star, 'Henry Daniel', pp. 63–105 and Star, 'Textual Worlds', pp. 191–216.

[78] Star, 'Textual Worlds', pp. 191–216.   [79] Orlemanski, *Symptomatic Subjects*.

[80] Orlemanski, 'Jargon', p. 395.

sonic and semantic patterning in medical recipes that did, or could, serve a healing purpose.

Though indebted to these studies, this work builds on their insights in three important ways: firstly, instead of analysing particular case studies or individual examples of different practical genres, I have focused on *one* genre, in order to achieve a deeper understanding of how features like similes, couplets, and additive structures function there. Secondly, while this study follows Cooper's and Griffin's lead in exploring how practical purposes might be fulfilled (or exceeded) through poetic devices, it also explores how those devices might *fail* to fulfil, or might impede, the remedies' ostensible purpose of communicating and clarifying therapeutic knowledge. Here, I extend Orlemanski's focus on jargon to consider how other forms work against the communication of healing knowledge, speculating about how this ostensible 'failure' might lead us to consider alternative purposes and motivations for recipes. Finally, the study extends the scope of these articles by exploring a broader range of interconnections between recipes and poetic texts, comparing how they frame, theorize, and use figures of thought and speech. Rather than collapsing the boundary between the poetic and the practical, I argue that we should think about many of the texts as participating in larger, shared traditions of imaginative and aesthetic expression. These traditions were used in overlapping ways in all kinds of writing, but there are often important differences in the way that they were understood and deployed and the effects they might have had upon readers.

In making this argument, I contribute to a developing body of scholarship focused on linguistic and imaginative exchanges between medicine, religion, and literature.[81] My study, however, uniquely foregrounds the migration and

---

[81] E.g., Jeremy J. Citrome, *The Surgeon in Medieval English Literature* (New York, 2006); Marion Turner, 'Illness Narratives in the Later Middle Ages: Arderne, Chaucer and Hoccleve', in *Medical Discourse in Premodern Europe*, ed. by Marion Turner as a special issue of *The Journal of Medieval and Early Modern Studies*, 46 (2016), 61–87; Daniel McCann, 'Medicine of Words: Purgative Reading in Richard Rolle's Meditations on the Passion', *The Medieval Journal*, 5 (2015), 53–83; Daniel McCann, *Soul Health: Therapeutic Reading in Later Medieval England* (Cardiff, 2018); Joseph Ziegler, *Medicine and Religion c. 1300: The Case of Arnau de Vilanova* (Oxford, 1998), pp. 46–113; Virginia Langum, '"The Wounded Surgeon": Devotion, Compassion and Metaphor in Medieval England', in *Wounds and Wound Repair in Medieval Culture*, ed. by Larissa Tracy and Kelley Devries (Leiden, 2015), pp. 269–90; Virginia Langum, *Medicine and the Seven Deadly Sins in Late Medieval Literature and Culture* (New York, 2016); Sarah Star, 'Anima Carnis in Sanguine Est: Blood, Life and *The King of Tars*', *Journal of English and Germanic Philosophy*, 115 (2016), 442–62; Michael Leahy, '"To Speke of Phisik": Medical Discourse in Late Medieval English Culture' (unpublished doctoral thesis, Birkbeck College, University of London, 2015); Marie-Christine Pouchelle, *The Body and Surgery in the Middle Ages*, trans. by Rosemary Morris (Cambridge, 1990), pp. 91–205; Louise Bishop, *Words, Stones and Herbs: The Healing Word in Medieval and Early Modern England* (Syracuse, NY, 2007).

adulteration of *recipe* forms, words, and stylistic tics. Because so many remedy collections remain unedited and unread, important and surprising connections have been overlooked. Tracing these overlaps and exchanges between discourses will not only illuminate the contemporary reception of medical remedies: it will also help us to resituate more consistently poetic writings within the rich, transgeneric network of connotation and association through which they may have been interpreted by their first readers. So, although this study is about remedy writing, it also offers new ways of reading our most canonical poetic texts.

The Practical, the Poetic, and the Playful

The preceding discussion of discursive boundaries raises one final question to be addressed in this Introduction: how were the terms 'poetic', 'playful', and 'practical' understood in the Middle Ages and what was their relationship? Although they developed from older, equivalent terms in Latin and French, the noun or adjective *practik* and the adjective *practicale* were new additions to the English language in the late fourteenth and fifteenth centuries.[82] Often functioning as an antithesis to 'theorie' and signalling a method, active usage, or form of applied knowledge, they reaffirm that know-how was an increasingly prominent preoccupation of vernacular language and culture. My definition of *practical* in subsequent chapters draws on these medieval definitions but shifts the word more explicitly towards the cognitive, describing those aspects of a recipe that help a reader *translate* the text's instructions into real-world action: how did those features communicate, organize, clarify, and impress information upon readers' minds? Medieval writers and readers were clearly preoccupied with these cognitive processes, as testified to by the development of increasingly refined methods of textual *ordinatio* (organisation and arrangement) from

---

These studies are in conversation with a related body of work which has explored how other discourses traditionally considered non-literary, such as bureaucratic documents and grammar textbooks, have shaped and been shaped by literary practices and traditions: see, for example, Paul Strohm, *Theory and the Premodern Text* (Minneapolis, MN, 2000), pp. 3–19; Ethan Knapp, *The Bureaucratic Muse: Thomas Hoccleve and the Literature of Late Medieval England* (University Park, PA, 2001); Christopher Cannon, *From Literacy to Literature: England, 1300–1400* (Oxford, 2016); Emily Steiner, *Documentary Culture and the Making of Medieval English Literature* (Cambridge, 2003).

[82] *MED, praktik*, n., entries 1(a) and 1(b); *praktik*, adj., entry 1; *practical*, adj., entry 1.

the thirteenth century onwards.[83] What is more, such developments were accompanied by specific, formally motivated kinds of reflection and analysis: thirteenth-century Aristotelian-influenced commentaries contained careful delineation of a work's *forma tractatus*, analysing the shape and argumentative significance of its organization.[84] My close reading of finding aids, chapters, and organizing frameworks is a modern reinterpretation of this tradition.

The *practicality* of a text differs from its *efficacy*; we cannot know whether remedies actually healed people. Even though modern experiments demonstrate that some ingredients—such as garlic, snail slime, and spider webs—possess healing properties, medieval practitioners may not have used the same plant varieties or prepared them in the same conditions.[85] They may have supplemented the recipe with their own tacit knowledge. As Pierre Bourdieu notes in his theory of human practice, 'even the most strictly ritualized exchanges, in which all the moments of the action, and their unfolding, are rigorously foreseen, have room for strategies'.[86] Humans are agents who can adapt whatever script they find before them and it is for this reason that, when thinking about the use or usefulness of recipes, I heed the warning of David Pye in his theory of design: it is a mistake to '[talk] about function as though it were something objective: something of which it could be said that it belonged to a thing'.[87] Accordingly, I remain sensitive to the plural, shifting purposes recipes could serve.

The term *poetic*, often set by modern scholars in opposition to the practical, is more difficult to define because, in both modern and Middle English, it is associated with a wealth of subjects, modes, forms, and reader experiences. As Glending Olson and Jenni Nuttall have demonstrated, one strand of medieval thought distinguished between *poets* and *makers*: the first term, along with the nouns *poetrie* or *poesie*, did not designate writers of verse (as it does now) but was often reserved for classical or humanistic writers who wrote about classical subject matter in a metaphorical and allegorical style and for a philosophical, moral, or historical truth-telling purpose. On the

---

[83] Malcolm Parkes, *Scribes, Scripts and Readers: Studies in the Communication, Presentation and Dissemination of Medieval Texts* (London, 1991), pp. 35–70.
[84] See D. Vance Smith, 'Medieval Forma: The Logic of the Work', in *Reading for Form*, ed. by Susan J. Wolfson and Marshall Brown (Seattle, WA, 2015), pp. 66–79.
[85] Mount, *Dragon's Blood*, pp. 104–16.
[86] Pierre Bourdieu, *Outline of a Theory of Practice*, trans. by Richard Nice (Cambridge, 1977), p. 15. On tacit knowledge, see also Gilbert Ryle, 'Knowing How and Knowing That: The Presidential Address', *Proceedings of the Aristotelian Society*, 46 (1945-6), 1–16.
[87] David Pye, *The Nature and Aesthetics of Design: A Design Handbook* (London, 1978), p. 11.

other hand, *makers*, who were often vernacular writers, were associated less with specific content and considered more as a kind of craftsmen, who produced artefacts of formal complexity.[88] These artefacts could serve moral or philosophical purposes, but it was not a prerequisite. Concerned with the shaping of language rather than abstract intellectual pursuits, the term *maker* was often perceived as the less lofty of the two, but it created a connection—which could be positive as well as pejorative—between literary writers, urban artisans, and other manual craftsmen including surgeons, barbers, and physicians.[89]

This distinction between poets and makers inevitably blurred. For instance, Latin handbooks known as *artes poetriae* were used in grammar schools to teach boys how to compose ornate verse and prose; they presented poetry as a craft that could be learnt. A grammar-school reader would have been taught by such a manual how to structure his thoughts into text, how to memorize and perform that text, and, in between, how to achieve different effects and affects by embellishing his verse or prose with figures of thought and speech. As James Jerome Murphy notes, most of the precepts and figures listed in Geoffrey of Vinsauf's *Poetria nova*, the most influential poetic handbook in the late Middle Ages, are repeated in Geoffrey's later treatise on prose composition, suggesting that he thought both modes could be similarly ornate.[90] The emphasis in the *artes poetriae* was not, then, just upon treating classical matter in a metaphorical way; instead, they advise readers how to use a wide range of figurative language to produce eloquent prose or verse compositions on any subject matter.[91]

Similar handbooks taught adult readers how to compose sermons (*artes praedicandi*) and letters (*artes dictaminis*). Each type of writing was thus associated with a specific kind of craft or technique (*ars*). There are clear parallels here with modern formalist theories of literary language: defining literary language as a special, enhanced, or deviant kind of language, these

---

[88] Glending Olson, 'Making and Poetry in the Age of Chaucer', *Comparative Literature*, 31 (1979), 272–90; Jenni Nuttall, 'Poesie and Poetrie', paper presented at Middle English Literary Theory Workshop: Keywords and Methodologies, Centre for Early Modern and Medieval Studies at the University of Sussex, 16 June 2016, pp. 1–5, accessed online at http://stylisticienne.com/middle-english-literary-theory [accessed 28/02/2018].

[89] For a detailed study of this connection, see Lisa Cooper, *Artisans and Narrative Craft* (Cambridge, 2011).

[90] James Jerome Murphy, *Rhetoric in the Middle Ages: A History of Rhetorical Theory from Saint Augustine to the Renaissance* (Berkeley, CA, 1974), p. 172.

[91] On the lack of restriction in subject matter, see James Jerome Murphy, 'The Arts of Poetry and Prose', in *The Cambridge History of Literary Criticism: Volume I—The Middle Ages*, ed. by Alastair Minnis and Ian Johnson (Cambridge, 2005), pp. 42–67 (pp. 44, 50–1, 52, 53, 60, 62–3).

theories have often faced problems when trying to establish what ordinary language is: the approach has 'led not to a satisfactory account of literature but to an often extremely productive identification of literariness in other cultural phenomena—from historical narratives and Freudian case histories to advertising slogans'.[92] Was there an analogous situation in the late Middle Ages where different kinds of writing—letters, sermons, legal documents, poetic compositions, and recipes—were each associated with a distinctive kind of literary crafting?

Recipes certainly possess distinctive characteristics which were replicated by successions of scribes: as the remedy for red eyes quoted earlier illustrated, imperatives, ingredient lists, ordered stages of action, and efficacy guarantees are characteristic of English and Latin recipes.[93] Did medieval writers really recognize these features as part of a particular style? For much of the later Middle Ages, the words *stilus* (Latin) and *stile* (English) were frequently used in discussions, probably originating in the pseudo-Ciceronian text *Rhetorica ad Herennium*, about three different modes of rhetoric: the grand, middle, and plain styles.[94] The word is therefore intertwined with ideas about decorum and the rhetorical imperative to adapt one's language use to one's audience. The conventional format of many remedies seems to offer little room for such stylistic adaptation. Remedies might therefore be more productively compared to formularies of letters and legal documents: those contained fully fleshed-out exemplars into which readers inserted their names and details when copying. In the same way, writers could insert different ailments and ingredients into a conventional recipe format.[95]

Some recipes, though, do display evidence of heightened stylistic crafting, of having been shaped and phrased with a particular purpose or audience in mind: they might diverge from the formula on account of their excessive use of superlative language, unusual syntactic patterning, or notable sound play. Often, this just occurs in one recipe in a collection and the shift

---

[92] Jonathan Culler, *The Literary in Theory* (Stanford, CA, 2007), p. 25.
[93] On the defining features of medieval recipes, see Ruth Carroll, 'Middle English Recipes: Vernacularisation of a Text-Type', in *Medical and Scientific Writing in Late Medieval English*, ed. by Taavitsainen and Pahta, pp. 174–91.
[94] *MED*, stile, n. 2, entry (c). Maura Nolan, 'The Biennial Chaucer Lecture: The Invention of Style', *Studies in the Age of Chaucer*, 41 (2019), 33–71 shows that (though the concept has a long Latin history) this rhetorical meaning attaches to the English word in the later fourteenth century. Nolan also shows through the writings of Chaucer and Lydgate that, in the late fourteenth and fifteenth centuries, *stile* was also starting to be used to describe the style of a particular writer.
[95] Malcolm Richardson, 'The *Ars dictaminis*, the Formulary, and Medieval Epistolary Practice', in *Letter Writing Manuals and Instruction from Antiquity to the Present*, ed. by Carol Poster and Linda C. Mitchell (Columbia, SC, 2007), pp. 52–66.

might be the result of it deriving from a different source. Consequently, I suggest that we think in terms of stylistic fragments, with *pieces* of recipes and *parts* of collections sharing features with poetic writings. This captures well the sporadic, unpredictable, and inconsistent feel of remedy books, which coexists with their more formulaic elements. That coexistence of the sporadic and formulaic also points towards the usefulness of the multifaceted term 'play' when approaching recipes: like recipes, play—as formulated by John Huizinga—has its own rules and boundaries, but it is simultaneously disruptive, flexible, and adaptable.[96] Moreover, it gestures towards recipes' indeterminate and shifting relationships to aesthetics, practicality, and imagination: recipes can be activated or translated into action like instruments are *played*; they can be connected, ordered, and rearranged by imaginations *in play*; and they can be mischievous, comic, or play*ful* in content.[97]

The aim of this study, then, is to rotate the discursive features of remedies through many competing and coexisting medieval (and modern) conceptions of the rhetorical, poetic, playful, and imaginative. For example, in Chapter 1, I examine similes used in medical recipes through the lens of the imaginative syllogism, a concept integral to Arabic definitions of the poetic. As Vincent Gillespie has shown, this idea—which was highly influential upon late medieval Western thinkers—freed poetry from needing to serve an ethical purpose; although it could be co-opted for moral ends, the experience of figurative language was not *intrinsically* moral or rhetorical, producing, instead, instinctive somatic, emotional, and imaginative responses.[98] Aesthetic concepts like this in turn raise questions about the place of bodies, affects, and emotions in remedy collections. In the following chapters, I am particularly interested in the effects of *words* on minds and bodies and vice versa: how did the language of healing texts make readers think and feel and how did particular feelings, affects, and associations shape interpretations of medical language in complex and layered ways?[99] Of course, we can never

---

[96] For further discussion and citation of John Huizinga's theories, see Chapter 5.
[97] I am grateful to an anonymous peer-reviewer at Oxford University Press for drawing my attention in an earlier draft to this parallel with the playing of musical instruments.
[98] Vincent Gillespie, 'Ethice Subponitur: The Imaginative Syllogism and the Idea of the Poetic', in *Medieval Thought Experiments: Poetry, Hypothesis and Experience in the European Middle Ages*, ed. by Phillip Knox, Jonathan Morton, and Daniel Reeve (Turnhout, 2018), pp. 297–327.
[99] A model for my mode of analysis is McCann, *Soul Health*, p. 11: he explores the 'multi-layered manner' in which emotions are encoded into and evoked by devotional texts; through the framework of the non-naturals, these can constitute a composite 'medicine of words'. For a similar argument on a smaller scale and about a specific type of medical writing, see

reconstruct these bodies, but we can use medieval models of the body and contemporary understandings of affective habits to speculate about the interplay between word, body, and thing.

Because of this study's emphasis on close reading words, textual forms, and codicological structures *through* multiple, coexisting (and competing) historically informed contextual lenses, it intersects closely with scholarship grouped under the capacious critical umbrella New Formalism.[100] It also dovetails with the contributions to Robert Meyer-Lee and Catherine Sanok's recent volume, *The Medieval Literary: Beyond Form*.[101] This collection shows 'that form, liberated from fixed taxonomies that axiomatically index the literary, can serve instead as a lens for recognizing fluid points of contact and influence across aesthetic, linguistic, textual and conceptual registers'.[102] However, the title of the volume also points to the importance of thinking 'beyond form'. This is of crucial importance for recipes: although they have been shaped and crafted, they can simultaneously appear under-shaped, sparse, and elliptical, bringing the central terms of formalism into confusion.[103] Recipes are, like exempla, also highly mobile, contextually dependent texts: their meaning can change radically from context to context, even if their form stays the same. I argue, therefore, that the collections invite the kind of dynamic, reader-orientated formalism that Arthur Bahr terms 'read[ing] compilationally': this describes a subjective mode through which readers interpret textual fragments in a manuscript as belonging to 'an interpretably

---

Mary C. Flannery, 'Emotion and the Ideal Reader in Middle English Gynaecological Texts', in *Medieval and Early Modern Literature, Science and Medicine*, ed. by Falconer and Renevey, pp. 103–15. Another model is Bishop, *Words, Stones and Herbs*, though Bishop does not always engage in sustained close readings of the medical texts she discusses: see, for instance, her discussion of charms on pp. 70–6.

[100] On the broad and problematic nature of the label New Formalism, see Marjorie Levinson, 'What Is New Formalism?', *PMLA*, 122 (2007), 558–69 (p. 561). Close models for my work include Christopher Cannon's insistence upon the designed*ness* of apparently unformed or perverse early Middle English texts in Christopher Cannon, 'Form', in *Twenty-First Century Approaches*, ed. by Strohm, pp. 177–90. I also share Paul Strohm's interest in breaking down traditional relations between 'text' and 'context' by finding ways of using different kinds of literary, historical, legal, and practical writings to illuminate each other in 'post-Copernican' analytical constellations: see Paul Strohm, *Hochon's Arrow: The Social Imagination of Fourteenth-Century Texts* (Princeton, NJ, 1992), p. 8.

[101] *The Medieval Literary Beyond Form*, ed. by Robert J. Meyer-Lee and Catherine Sanok (Cambridge, 2018). The essays in this volume by Jessica Brantley, Ingrid Nelson, and Claire Waters on the thoughtfulness of apparently mundane, ubiquitous forms are of particular interest and are discussed more fully in subsequent chapters.

[102] Robert J. Meyer-Lee and Catherine Sanok, 'Introduction', in *The Medieval Literary Beyond Form*, ed. by Meyer-Lee and Sanok, pp. 1–12 (p. 12).

[103] I am indebted to one of the anonymous peer-reviewers at Oxford University Press for helping me to draw together this insight.

meaningful arrangement' with its own aesthetics.[104] Bahr's work showcases the gains made by extending formalist close-reading techniques into the realm of the material.[105]

Given the centrality of fragments and compilations to my way of understanding recipes, it is no surprise that they are also integral to this study's structure: Part I, 'Literary Fragments', explores the sporadic and intermittent appearance of poetic elements in both prose and verse remedies, recontextualizing key features—including particular similes, rhymes, and puns—within larger linguistic and cultural networks. Part II, 'Collecting Fragments', shifts the emphasis from individual fragments to larger, piecemeal structures, considering the diverse impulses that motivated various kinds of remedy compilation. It also probes how the accumulative form of collections might parallel various literary models, becoming an opaque and polysemous form in its own right. This approach is extended in the final part, 'Fragments in Play'. Here, I use the thematic lenses of time, taboo, and metamorphosis to consider the particular ways that recipes— and their formal arrangement or sequencing—might have stimulated readers' imaginations, bringing the marvellous and the mundane into complicated interplay. In these chapters, I posit possible imaginative exchanges between remedies, romances, and fabliaux and contend that recipes can defy straightforward interpretation and 'elud[e] the certainties of conceptual thought' as resolutely as literary texts.[106]

---

[104] Bahr, *Fragments*, p. 3.
[105] On the intersection of formalism and book history, see Arthur Bahr and Alexandra Gillespie, 'Medieval English Manuscripts: Form, Aesthetics, and the Literary Text', *Chaucer Review*, 47 (2013), 346–60; Helen Marshall and Peter Buchanan, 'New Formalism and the Forms of Middle English Literary Texts', *Literature Compass*, 8 (2011), 164–72; Daniel Wakelin, *Scribal Correction and Literary Craft: English Manuscripts 1375–1510* (Cambridge, 2014).
[106] Peggy Knapp, *Chaucerian Aesthetics* (New York, 2008), p. 3. Knapp has argued that the appeal of Chaucer's writings lies in the way he brings ideas and concepts into unresolved play, never promoting fixed moral messages, but playfully 'elud[ing] the certainties of conceptual thought'. This aesthetics of balance, tension, and play will be integral to my analysis of the dynamics of recipe collections.

PART I
LITERARY FRAGMENTS

1
The Poetics of Prose Cures

The later Middle Ages witnessed a growing preference for prose over verse as the language of lay instruction: pastoral handbooks, household manuals, and accessible medical guides were increasingly likely to be written in the vernacular and in prose, perhaps suggesting that a growing literate proportion of society was less dependent on rhymed verse, memory, and oral transmission for the circulation of such knowledge.[1] In these apparently practical text-types, the preference was established more rapidly than in more explicitly fantastical, entertaining genres such as romance.[2] This emerging fifteenth-century association between prose and practicality may explain why prose recipes' unpredictable and quirky craftsmanship has been overlooked: scholars—also biased by formally weighted modern critical vocabulary—are inclined to see those remedies as 'prosaic', as 'plainly or simply worded', and as less carefully crafted than verse.[3]

This chapter contends, however, that prose recipes do have their own sporadic, intermittent, and fragmentary poetics and that prose itself could promote particular kinds of textual crafting in medical texts, such as elaborate syntactic structures.[4] Many of these structures show how repetition can be the foundation for creativity, variation, and embellishment. Other forms, such as similes and puns, have no obvious intrinsic connection to prose but,

---

[1] See George Keiser, 'Scientific, Medical and Utilitarian Prose', in *A Companion to Middle English Prose*, ed. by A.S.G. Edwards (Woodbridge, 2004), pp. 231–47; Laurel Braswell, 'Utilitarian and Scientific Prose', in *Middle English Prose: A Critical Guide*, ed. by Edwards, pp. 337–87; Vincent Gillespie, 'Anonymous Devotional Writings', in *A Companion to Middle English Prose*, ed. by Edwards, pp. 127–49; Voigts, 'Medical Prose', pp. 315–35.

[2] Helen Cooper, 'Prose Romances', in *A Companion to Middle English Prose*, ed. by Edwards, pp. 215–30 (pp. 215–16).

[3] *OED*, *prosaic*, adj., entries 2(a) and 2(b).

[4] Parts of this chapter, especially the section on similes, are revised and developed from Hannah Bower, 'Similes We Cure By: The Poetics of Late Medieval Medical Texts', *New Medieval Literatures*, 18 (2018), 183–210. Boydell and Brewer, the journal publishers, have kindly granted me permission to reuse parts of that article.

perhaps because of the greater number of surviving prose texts, those forms appear more frequently in prose remedies than verse ones.[5]

As we will see, these forms exist in a complex, textured, and multi-layered relationship with the recipes' proclaimed practical purpose of directing healing action. They simultaneously fulfil, exceed, and impede that purpose in ways that encourage scholars to diversify and enrich their sense of what these texts offered medieval readers, how they might have shaped healing action, and how they might have inflected the experience of acquiring medical know-how. These poetic fragments also function as points of contact with more consistently crafted texts, ranging from the poetry of Chaucer to the devotional writings of Julian of Norwich. By highlighting precise parallels between such diverse texts, this chapter suggests that remedy writers and poets drew upon a shared, commonplace tradition of figurative language, which was not the property of one particular type of writing but was used in various modes and texts for distinct but overlapping purposes. Each piece of this textual puzzle (however incompletable it may be) enables us to understand the other pieces—and their medieval reception—more fully.

Fragments

The sporadic manner in which these similes, syntactic structures, and puns appear across remedy collections was probably a result of the piecemeal process through which recipes were extracted from longer texts and arranged in compilations. That inconsistency seems to set the recipes at odds with medieval conceptions of the poetic which stress stylistic unity. For instance, in Horace's *Ars poetica*, a touchstone for the medieval *artes poetriae*, the importance of stylistic consistency is communicated through the image of a monstrous hybrid: for Horace, a text lacking stylistic unity is like a painting depicting a monster formed from parts—or fragments—of human, horse, bird, and fish.[6]

The fragmentary and piecemeal was, then, an integral part of medieval conceptions of the literary, even if it was often used to illustrate how it should *not* be done. Like most injunctions, such prohibitions contain within

---

[5] For more discussion of the numbers of surviving prose and verse texts, see Chapter 2. The only simile I have encountered in a verse remedy compares ringing in a person's ears to the sound of horns being blown. See TCC, MS R.14.51, f. 2r.

[6] Horace, *Satires, Epistles and Ars Poetica*, trans. by H.R. Fairclough (Cambridge, MA, 1952), pp. 450–1.

them an admission of the desirability of the very thing they prohibit: Horace's monstrous creation is as imaginatively tantalizing as it is troubling. Indeed, medieval thinkers regularly theorized the powers of the human imagination using just such hybrid creations; the imaginative faculty was not only defined by its capacity to reproduce images in the mind without sense stimuli, but also by its ability to combine mental images to produce never-before-seen combinations.[7] St Augustine wrote that, if the image of a crow is brought to mind, 'it may be brought, by the taking away of some features and the addition of others, to almost any image such as was never seen by the eye'.[8] Later, the Arabic thinker Avicenna (d. 1037) illustrated these compositional powers through the image of a golden mountain and a chimera formed from a lion's head, goat's body, and serpent's tail.

These conceptions of fragmentary imaginative inventions were framed by larger metaphysical prohibitions against *creation ex nihilo*: scholastic thinkers argued that the crucial difference between God and man was that God could create out of nothing, whilst humans had to create out of the materials available to them; consequently, all human creations were composite mishmashes of bits and pieces. As Patricia Ingham notes, 'submission to the ideal of divine creativity produced not only a rather astonishing array of "adulterated" new things, poems, tales, and images; but also a persistent return to problems of "adulteration"'.[9] Bold and varied adulterations such as gargoyles, manuscript marginalia, and deviant grammatical constructions all highlighted the potential of the human imagination for creation and perversion. It was partly for this reason, and because of Augustinian critiques of the imagination's susceptibility to diabolic manipulation, that in Western medieval psychology 'a full theory of imaginative aesthetics never did develop'.[10] Nevertheless, as Michelle Karnes notes, 'although... the medieval west offers no developed theory of the creative imagination or wonder as a literary value, this hardly means that either went untheorized'.[11]

---

[7] On the capacities of the imagination, see Aranye Fradenburg, 'Imagination', in *A Handbook to Middle English Studies*, ed. by Marion Turner (Chichester, 2013), pp. 15–32; Alastair Minnis, 'Medieval Imagination and Memory', in *The Cambridge History of Literary Criticism*, ed. by Minnis and Johnson, pp. 237–74; Michelle Karnes, *Imagination, Meditation and Cognition in the Middle Ages* (Chicago, IL, 2011); Michelle Karnes, 'Wonder, Marvels and Metaphor in the Squire's Tale', *ELH*, 82 (2015), 461–90.

[8] Augustine, *Letters: Volume I (1–82)*, trans. by Sister Wilfrid Parsons (New York, 1951), p. 18. Also cited in Minnis, 'Medieval Imagination', p. 241.

[9] Patricia Clare Ingham, *The Medieval New: Ambivalence in an Age of Innovation* (Philadelphia, PA, 2015), p. 44.

[10] Minnis, 'Medieval Imagination', p. 243.

[11] Karnes, 'Wonder, Marvels, and Metaphor', p. 484.

Intriguingly, medicine—both in language and practice—seems to have been a popular realm for exploring, testing, and tentatively theorizing ideas of stylistic unity and imaginative adulteration. Consider Book II of Chaucer's *Troilus and Criseyde*: Pandarus warns Troilus not to 'jompre' ('jumble') any 'discordant thyng' in his love letter to Criseyde, particularly 'termes of phisik' (II. 1037–8). He then repeats Horace's advice that 'if a peyntour wolde peynte a pyk/With asses feet, and hedde it as an ape,/It cordeth naught'.[12] Medicine is held up here as the prime example of disruptive discourse. As Orlemanski notes, Pandarus's warning implies that medicine's 'at least imaginary cordoning off from other conceptual vocabularies...was a comprehensible one' to medieval readers.[13] Love poetry and medicine apparently should not mix.

The same point is made in reverse in Francesco Petrarch's *Invective contra medicum* (*Invectives against the Physician*), four polemical letters which the fourteenth-century Italian poet addressed to an unnamed physician for his incompetent and crooked treatment of Pope Clement VI. Petrarch condemns the physician's use of seductive rhetoric, not merely because it deceives patients but also because it constitutes an improper mixing of the mechanical arts (physic) with the liberal arts (rhetoric). Medicine's status as a manual craft, art, or science was much debated in the Middle Ages, with many physicians keen to elevate it above the purely practical, hands-on procedures frequently associated with surgeons and barbers.[14] Petrarch, however, uses another string of hybrid, adulterate creations to reassert that such rhetorical elevation should not accompany the physician's manual work: 'Tam decet ornatus medicum, quam asellum falere...Quisquis te disertum dixerit, idem et nitidam suem, et volucrem testudinem at candidum corvum dicat' ('Ornate speech suits a doctor just as a caparison suits a donkey...If someone calls you eloquent, let him also call the hog elegant, the turtle winged and the crow snow-white').[15] Just as medicine should not infiltrate poetry, poetry should not infiltrate medicine.

Petrarch's bitter reassertion of the unnaturalness of mixing these two styles is, of course, an admission that such mixing has come to seem natural.

---

[12] Geoffrey Chaucer, *Troilus and Crisedye*, in *The Riverside Chaucer*, ed. by Larry D. Benson, 3rd edn (Oxford, 2008), II. 1041–3.
[13] Orlemanski, *Symptomatic Subjects*, p. 1.
[14] Murray Jones, 'Medicine and Science', p. 433; Michael McVaugh, 'The Nature and Limits of Medical Certitude at Early Fourteenth-Century Montpellier', *Osiris*, 6 (1990), 62–84.
[15] Francesco Petrarch, *Invectives*, ed. and trans. by David Marsh (Cambridge, MA, 2003), pp. 136–7.

THE POETICS OF PROSE CURES   35

Similarly, Pandarus's injunction cannot avoid sounding ironic to Chaucer's readers given that, throughout his poetry, Chaucer deploys medical concepts, terms, and metaphors to convey his protagonists' narratives. The creative and perverse potential of such discursive mixing is simultaneously apparent. Nowhere is this more obvious and more directly applicable to recipe-writing than in 'Sum Practysis of Medecyne', a set of parodic medical recipes composed by one of Chaucer's Scottish successors, the late fifteenth-century poet Robert Henryson. 'Sum Practysis' is composed of four parodic remedies addressed by an outraged narrator to a quack physician who has falsely declared the narrator 'dottit' or crazed.[16] The narrator uses the mock-remedies to imitate and ridicule the physician's lack of genuine healing knowledge, accusing him of being a peddler of meaningless medical jargon. For instance, the remedy for a befouled rectum reads:

> Dia Culcakit
>
> Cape cuk maid, and crop the colleraige,
> Ane medecyne for the maw and ʒe cowth mak it
> With sueit satlingis and sowrokis, þe sop of the sege,
> The crud of my culome, with ʒour teith crakit,
> Lawrean and linget seid, and the luffage,
> The hair of the hurcheoun nocht half deill hakkit,
> With þe snowt of ane selch, ane swelling to swage:
> This cure is callit in our craft *dia culcakkit*.
> Put all thir in ane pan with pepper and pik.
> Syne sett in to this,
> The count of ane sow kis;
> Is nocht bettir, I wis,
> For þe collik.
>
> (26–39)
>
> [*cukmaid* = fresh dung; *colleraige* = water pepper; *maw* = stomach; *sueit satlingis* = sweet dregs; *sowrokis* = sorrel; *sop of the sege* = sap of sage; *crud of my culome* = dirt of my anus; *lawrean* = laurel; *linget* = seed of flax; *luffage* = lovage; *hurcheon* = hedgehog; *selch* = seal; *pik* = pitch]

---

[16] Robert Henryson, 'Sum Practysis of Medecyne', in *The Poems of Robert Henryson*, ed. by Denton Fox (Oxford, 1981), line 3. Future references are included within the text; glosses are also based on this edition.

The other mock-recipes follow a similar pattern. Typically, they combine disgusting bodily substances like 'the crud of my culome' with absurdly precise ingredients (such as 'the hair of the hurcheoun nocht half deill hakkit') or bits of animals that are not usually used in medical preparations (such as 'þe snowt of ane selch'). Subsequent remedies in the series push and confound readers' imaginations even further, mixing the abstract and concrete in ingredients like 'the gant of an grey mair' ('the yawn of a grey horse', 41) and offending readers' sense of scale as they ask for 'ane vnce of ane oster poik at þe nether parte' ('an ounce of an oyster's stomach at the lower part', 71). Similar parodic medical texts survive in French and German and all confound categories and combine bodies, things, and scales in this nonsensical way.[17] Genuine remedies, of course, often do something similar, mingling together in extensive lists material fragments of very different kinds: a remedy for head pain instructs readers to 'take encence and coluere dunge and whete floure' ('take incense, dove excrement, and wheat flour').[18] Outside of medical practice, incense would not be associated with dove excrement or flour. Consequently, such lists have the power, in Michel Foucault's words, to '[break] up all the ordered surfaces and all the planes with which we are accustomed to tame the wild profusion of existing things'.[19]

Julie Orlemanski has aptly summarized this ambivalent attitude in 'Sum Practysis' to medicine's perverse poetics: on the one hand, Henryson's alliterating combinations of obscure, impossible, or revolting ingredients underline the semantic debasement afflicting medical discourse when it descends into incomprehensible jargon and empty sound; that language then becomes as material, physical, and base as the fleshly matter it is supposed to treat. On the other hand, and on a more positive note, Henryson's poem flaunts the 'peculiar musicality' and 'poetical energies' of 'a medical language turned aside from its healing purpose'; the sounds of the ingredients' names come into greater prominence when we are unable to imagine them as material referents.[20] I would add to this reading that 'Sum Practysis'

---

[17] See the speech of the quack apothecary or physician who intrudes upon the action of a fourteenth-century Innsbruck Easter play in *Das Innsbrucker Osterspiel; Das Osterspiel von Muri: Mittlhochdeutsch und Neuhochdeutsch*, ed. and trans. by Rudolf Meier (Stuttgart, 1962), lines 828–37. On French parodic texts containing similar constructions see Denton Fox, 'Henryson's "Sum Practysis"', *Studies in Philology*, 69 (1972), 453–60 (pp. 453–4).

[18] WT, MS Wellcome 136, f. 1v.

[19] Michel Foucault, *The Order of Things: An Archaeology of the Human Sciences* (New York, 1994), p. xvi. See also Eric Griffiths, 'Lists', in *If Not Critical*, ed. by Freya Johnston (Oxford, 2018), pp. 8–28.

[20] Orlemanski, 'Jargon', p. 395.

also showcases the wonderful and perverse powers of the imagination's composite abilities: there is a creative—if pointless—challenge in the act of pairing together the most inappropriate or revolting things one can think of which begin with the same letter. The satirical framing of Henryson's poem suggests that he, like Petrarch, considered such rhetorical and imaginative skill to be misapplied in the world of physic. But his very decision to amplify and exaggerate such language into a poetic effect shows that he recognized some creative worth within it.

So, whilst Latin rhetoricians and the authors of the *artes poetriae* considered consistency and unity to be vital aspects of poetic success, these late medieval poets saw the piecemeal, fragmentary, and inconsistent as *integral* to the peculiar poetics and imaginative dynamics of medical writing—to medicine's own confounding of categories *and* its capacity to adulterate and fragment other discourses. For Chaucer and Henryson, these qualities were improper and ridiculous and, at the same time, alluring and enjoyable. Of course, as poets, they were trained to notice patterns, figures, and other creative deviations in language, whether that language was deployed in 'ordinary' or 'extraordinary' contexts. However, that does not make their conception of medical poetics any less valid. What is more, that conception provides a useful framework for approaching many of the discursive features examined in this chapter: similes, puns, and embellished lists not only disrupt and diversify recipes' formulaic structures, but also encourage readers to use their imaginations to transgress and confound conceptual boundaries in ways that can be both troubling and pleasing. Readers of recipes did not need to be trained poets to experience that fragmentary poetics.

Shaping Syntax

As we have seen, lists can disorientate readers of remedies, blurring distinctions between human, animal, plant, and thing and bringing diverse areas of life together through material fragments such as dove excrement, incense, and flour. Lists are not exclusive to scientific prose but, for purposes of clarity and comprehension, they often seem better suited to it than verse; it also takes greater skill to transform long lists of specialist terms into rhymed verse. Consider Chaucer's *Canon's Yeoman's Tale*, a parody of alchemical recipes and treatises which is written (predominantly) in rhymed decasyllabic lines and is well known for its extensive, overwhelming lists of alchemical processes and ingredients, including herbs commonly used in medical recipes. A small extract suffices to illustrate the effect:

> Watres rubifiyng, and boles galle,
> Arsenyk, sal armonyak, and brymstoon;
> And herbes koude I telle eek many oon,
> As egremoyne, valerian, and lunarie[21]

Here, Chaucer highlights the impenetrable, jargon-heavy nature of alchemical discourse: the Yeoman, who proclaims that he cannot 'reherce' the items within his list 'by ordre' (786), knows the alchemical terms but not their semantic relationship to one another.[22] The verse form heightens this sense of confusion for readers: because the terms are jammed into—and used to disrupt—the rhythm of a ten-syllable line, readers have little opportunity to try to decode the jargon before the next term, or line, is upon them. Chaucer's poem therefore illustrates the formal tension between the confines of verse lines and extensive, overrunning lists of polysyllabic terms. Prose, being unbounded, can be a more appropriate form for rendering such lists clear and comprehensible; it offers readers time to reflect upon the words before them and, in the case of medical recipes, sometimes creates room for writers to give multiple names for a herb or ingredient, increasing the chances that at least one name will be familiar to readers.[23]

This tension between form and content probably explains why verse remedies often only contain short lists of three or four ingredients: 'For hedwerk...To takyn eysyl pulyole ryale | And camamylle and sethe with all' ('For headache...take vinegar, pennyroyal, and camomile and boil [it] all together').[24] In contrast, prose recipes often include longer lists such as 'tak sayn wormode aueroygne tansey yuy tereste betoyne egrymoyne...' ('Take

---

[21] Geoffrey Chaucer, *The Canon's Yeoman's Tale*, in *Riverside*, ed. by Benson, lines 797–800. Future references are included in the text.

[22] On alchemy's connection to craft discourse, see Christopher Cannon, 'Chaucer and the Language of London', in *Chaucer and the City*, ed. by Ardis Butterfield (Cambridge, 2006), pp. 79–95 (pp. 82–9).

[23] See, for example, the recipe for wounds and swellings discussed later on in this chapter.

[24] *Extracts in Prose and Verse from an Old English Medical Manuscript, Preserved in the Royal Library at Stockholm*, ed. by George Stephens (London, 1844), p. 350, lines 18–20. The verse remedy collection extends over pp. 349–63. Exceptional remedies containing longer lists of ingredients occur on pp. 356–7, lines 227–34; p. 358, lines 267–71; p. 359, lines 323–8, and p. 361, lines 390–5.

tut-saine,[25] wormwood, southernwood, tansy, ground ivy, betony, agrimony...').[26] Extravagantly long prose lists sometimes contain over one hundred herbs.[27] It is not, then, merely extra-textual factors, such as efficacious plant combinations, which determine the content of a remedy: the prose or verse form can also determine how many ingredients are used. It is already apparent that verse and prose are not merely passive moulds into which medical material is deposited, but active shapers of that material.

Lengthy lists were deployed by many medieval poets, rhetoricians, and preachers and could be used to prolong a particular lyric or narrative moment, display the extent of one's learning, or create an enchanting rhythm.[28] But lists do not guarantee pleasing sound patterns: sometimes the sounds of items in a list clash unpleasantly or create a breathless feeling of claustrophobia. The extract below from a remedy for wounds, swellings, and other external injuries exemplifies how lists in recipes can swerve towards, and then away from, explicit craftsmanship and poeticity. Consequently, this individual remedy encapsulates in microcosm the sporadic, fragmentary, and inconsistent style of recipe collections:

Take bugle, synagle, avance, violett, waybrede, lely and henbayne and morell, gume of the sour plumtre, wax, white pik þat thir spicers calles pik album and fresche grese of a swyn or a bare and fresche suete of an herte and fresch talghe of a moton, of ilkan elike mekill. Do all thies thynges in a pan and welle tham wele.[29]

[*bugle* = blue-flowered herb of the mint family; *synagyle* = European sanicle; *avance* = plant of the genus Geum, possibly wood avens; *waybrede* = plant of the plantain family; *lely* = lily; *morell* = a herb of the Solanum family; *white pik* = resin; *suete* = fat; *talghe* = fatty tissue, tallow; *welle* = to boil]

---

[25] I cannot find 'sayn' listed by itself in the MED, Tony Hunt, *Plant Names of Medieval England* (Cambridge, 1989), or Norri, *Dictionary of Medical Vocabulary*. The Middle English *tut-saine* can refer to tutsan (St. John's wort) or agnus castus: see *MED, tut-saine*, n., entry 1(a). The plant names given in medieval recipes often have lots of possible modern equivalents; I have tried to give a likely gloss, but other possibilities can be tracked through Hunt, *Plant Names*.
[26] YM, MS XVI. E. 32, f. 15v.
[27] See Chapter 4 for more detailed discussion of these hyper-long remedies.
[28] See Stephen A. Barney, 'Chaucer's Lists', in *The Wisdom of Poetry: Essays in English Literature in Honour of Morton W. Bloomfield*, ed. by Larry D. Benson and Siegfried Wenzel (Kalamazoo, MI, 1982), pp. 189–223.
[29] Ogden, ed., *The 'Liber de diversis medicinis'*, p. 54. Quoted in Orlemanski, 'Jargon', p. 402 where Orlemanski comments on the importation of Latin and French words, rather than the sound play. Her essay does explore, though, similar sound play in parodic recipes.

As Orlemanski notes, the writer responsible for the explanation of the Latin term 'pik album' clearly foresaw that the multitude of English, Latin, and French words available for individual medical substances might confuse a reader, turning that part of the text into empty, jargonistic noise.[30] But, in fact, even if a reader were comfortable decoding the recipe, explicit sound play might have drawn his or her attention away from its content: aside from the visual and sonic echo 'welle tham wele' (which shall be discussed later), there is also the half-rhyme 'bugle' and 'synagle', which initiates a string of less harmonious items. The tripartite rhyme 'bugle, pygle, sanygle' is a frequent occurrence in prose recipes, suggesting that it was a formulaic pattern.[31] Another reoccurring pattern is detectable in the tripartite repetition 'fresche grese...fresche suete...fresch talghe...'. This structure has a parallel in a remedy for poor hearing, which requires 'þe fressh grece of a fressh blak ele of the fresshe water'.[32] Such echoes and resemblances—often altered or distorted—might suggest more than a shared love of sound patterning amongst remedy writers and scribes: they might imply a complex web of borrowing, modification, and hybridization.[33] Copied and recopied between manuscripts and probably passed on by word of mouth too, such remedies seem to be woven through with subtle, and perhaps unconscious, echoes of each other.

The fragments of prose rhythm that the above sound play creates also recall the explicit sound patterns of charms, a kind of medical text which has been much more extensively discussed by scholars.[34] Such charms are frequently composed in rhyming couplets designed to be performed aloud or, in some cases, written on material substances: for instance, a rhyming charm for sore teeth begins 'Byfore the gate of Galile. Saynte Petur there sate hee. Vppon a colde marbull stone . And hilde his honde vnder his cheke bone'.[35] Such charms were believed to work upon the body through divine power; this power was apparently channelled through the charm's words,

---

[30] Orlemanski, 'Jargon', pp. 402–3.
[31] Similar patterns appear on BodL, MS Douce 84, ff. 37r, 40r; BodL, MS Ashmole 1444, pp. 179, 180; BodL, MS Hatton 29, ff. 82v, 84v, 86r; BL, MS Harley 2378, f. 143r; BL, MS Harley 1602, f. 20r; BL, MS Additional 33996, f. 143r; HEHL, MS HM 58, ff. 62v, 85r-v; HEHL, HM 19079, ff. 3v, 4v.
[32] BL, MS Additional 19674, f. 46r.
[33] On comparable echoes and distortions in charms, see Lea Olsan, 'Latin Charms of Medieval England: Verbal Healing in a Christian Oral Tradition', *Oral Tradition*, 7 (1992), 116–42 (pp. 124–8).
[34] E.g. Olsan, 'Latin Charms'; Don Skemer, *Binding Words: Textual Amulets in the Middle Ages* (Philadelphia, PA, 2006); Bishop, *Words, Stones and Herbs*, pp. 44–76, 97–100.
[35] HEHL, MS HM 64, ff. 145ra–145rb (letters refer to columns).

rhymes, and rhythms. The patterning of the above recipe may have convinced patients in a similar way that the remedy possessed an intrinsic and occult healing power; although the text does not evoke divine power, it may have been understood as a kind of natural magic.

From the thirteenth century onwards, natural magic was increasingly recognized as an acceptable alternative to demonic magic: it did not involve spirits, but exploited the hidden (and God-given) powers of plants, animals, stones, words, and other substances. The effects these substances had upon one another and upon human bodies could not be explained through humoral theory or physical form; they were only observable in practice.[36] The mystery of their workings may actually have increased some readers' conviction of their efficacy; modern research into the placebo effect has shown that thinking one will be healed can be a vital part of healing oneself. Charms and patterned remedies like the example above therefore sensitize readers to the ways in which patterned language might get things done in the world, already eroding any fixed opposition between poetry and practicality.[37] As Louise Bishop has argued in relation to charms specifically, such writings also testify to words' palpable materiality and perceived material efficacy on bodies in the Middle Ages.[38]

Given their potential potency, it is not surprising that authors and scribes were keen to maintain these crafted structures. Daniel Wakelin has shown that scribes of recipe collections sometimes revisit syntactic doublets that they have copied in order to insert prepositions into the doublet. Examples from his study include: 'Take the Ius of verneyne and ^of^ celidoyne' and 'kutt with swerd or ^with^ knyfe'.[39] As Wakelin points out, these additions can be necessary to clarify the meaning of an instruction: in the first example the preposition indicates that it is the *sap* (or 'ius') of both plants which is to be used.[40] In the second example, though, the added 'with' does not make the instruction any clearer; instead, the preposition seems to have been added in order to create a pleasingly balanced structure. I have found many other examples of lists in remedy collections where practical concerns seem to shade imperceptibly into a more gratuitous concern with stylistic crafting, and these sometimes also showcase how visual, material

---

[36] Sophie Page, *Magic in Medieval Manuscripts* (London, 2004), pp. 18–28.
[37] Claire M. Waters, 'What's the Use? Marian Miracles and the Workings of the Literary', in *The Medieval Literary Beyond Form*, ed. by Meyer-Lee and Sanok, pp. 15–34 (p. 26) makes a similar point about the functionality of repetition in Marian miracles.
[38] Bishop, *Words, Stones and Herbs*, pp. 44–76.
[39] Wakelin, *Scribal Correction*, p. 206.   [40] Ibid.

embellishment could work to highlight syntactic adornment. Consider this list in a remedy for a healing salve. Rubricated characters are reproduced in bold (see Figure 1.1 for a photo of the original):

> Take **b**rokkyis grece / **k**attys grece / **h**aris grece* swynys grece / **d**oggis grece / **c**apouns grece / **s**wet of a der / **s**chepis talwȝe of eche ylyche moche þen take þe ius of bismalue / of rewbarbe* of morel / of comferye / of daysyes / of Rewe / of plawnteyne / of matithen /of heyryffes / of matfelon* of dragaunce of eche ylyche moche[41]

> [*bismalue* = marshmallow; *comferye* = comfrey; *matithen*, possibly a variant spelling and duplication of *matfelon* or variant spelling of *maithe*;[42] *maithe* = stinking camomile; *matfelon* = knapweed; *heyryffes* = cleavers; *dragaunce* = dragonwort]

> *end of line in manuscript

As in Wakelin's example, the author or copier of this remedy has taken great care to clarify that the 'ius' of each plant is to be used by adding 'of' before each noun.[43] The repetition, then, is useful but, along with the repetition of 'grece', it also creates a pleasing rhythm. Furthermore, the scribe has gone to extra lengths to highlight this repetition: not only does he place virgules between each genitive construction but he also rubricates each virgule. It is only at line breaks that virgules are not added. This attention to the recipe's formal crafting exceeds the requirements of practicality; the scribe appears as a literary critic, drawing the reader's attention to the text's formal patterning by making that pattern visual as well as sonic.[44]

Lists are recipes' most common feature, but sometimes more intricate syntactic manipulations appear which not only bring the practical and poetic into conversation but also evoke other modes of medical and practical writing, thickening the patchwork texture of collections further. For instance, the following passage is from a remedy for a migraine. It deploys

---

[41] BodL, MS Douce 84. f. 38v.
[42] See *MED*, *mate-feloun*, n. (a variant spelling is listed as *matifoun*) and *MED*, *maithe*, n. (a variant spelling is listed as *maithen*).
[43] Similar repetitions occur in BodL, MS Douce 84, ff. 38r, 42r, 43r, 44r.
[44] See Julie Orlemanski, 'Physiognomy and Otiose Practicality', *Exemplaria*, 23 (2011), 194–218 for similar points about gratuitous, excessive, or unhelpful aspects of physiognomic manuals. However, Orlemanski does not usually focus on the manuscript presentation of the texts.

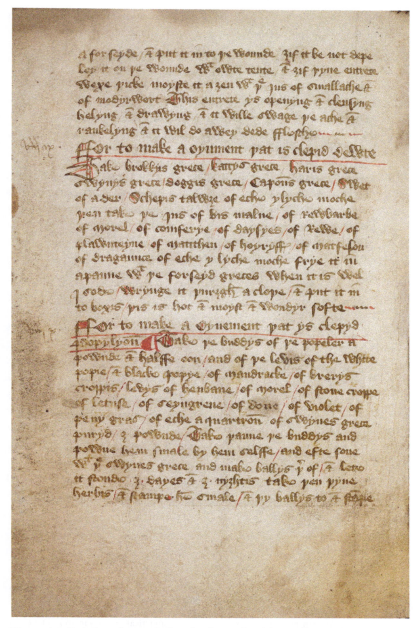

Figure 1.1 Rubricated remedy for a healing salve. The Bodleian Libraries, University of Oxford, MS Douce 84, f. 38v. Reproduced with kind permission from the Bodleian Libraries, University of Oxford through the Creative Commons licence CC-BY-NC 4.0.

homely culinary similes to explain instructions but, through its form, it evokes more academic medical writings:

> Then grynde alle þe forsayde materys on a marbulle stonne tille hit be as þik as a thynne pappe. and if hit be to þik be vertu of þe floure ⸵ þen put a litelle more of þe glayre þerto. and if be to thyn be vertu of þe glayre ⸵ þen þik hit with more of þe floure. til hit be as þik as a thyn pappe.[45]
>
> [*pappe* = porridge; *glayre* = egg white]

Antithesis, chiasmus, and parallelism are all at work here. Like the scribe who used virgules to draw attention to the syntactic patterning of a list, this scribe has used punctuation (in the form of the punctus and the punctus elevatus) to draw attention to the repetition of clausal structures and the juxtaposition of 'floure' and 'glayre' and 'þik' and 'thyn'.[46] These juxtapositions and repetitions may have been intended to make the recipe easier to comprehend or recite by heart.[47] But they may also be an echo of more consistently patterned academic and theoretical medical writings: in a fifteenth-century English translation of Gilbert the Englishman's *Compendium medicinae*, the different prognostic tokens associated with similar diseases are distinguished in this way: 'And in epilencie, tremblyng of þe bodi is an yuel signe, but in þe palesie it is a good signe. Fomyng here is a good signe, but in appoplexie it is an yvel signe.'[48] This chiastic structure, with its simultaneous emphasis upon similarity and difference, suits the text's learned and scholastic predilection for drawing precise distinctions between different ailments and symptoms. It is noteworthy, though, that in the remedy book the structure has been deployed to explain a practical, hands-on process, rather than a cognitive concern with interpretations and distinctions. Processes of recycling and adaptation clearly created texts that were allusive, fragmentary, and piecemeal and yet distinctive in their style and purposes.

---

[45] BodL, MS Douce 78, f. 11v.
[46] On scribal use of the punctus elevatus within balanced constructions, see Malcom Parkes, *Pause and Effect: An Introduction to the History of Punctuation in the West* (Aldershot, 1992), pp. 69, 73, and 153.
[47] On the breaking up of texts into smaller semantic and rhythmic units for the purposes of memorization, see Mary Carruthers, *The Book of Memory: A Study of Memory in Medieval Culture*, 2nd edn (Cambridge, 2008), p. 141.
[48] Getz, ed., *Healing and Society*, p. 21, lines 10–13.

In both texts, the chiastic structure produces a variety of effects: it not only communicates and impresses distinctions on readers' minds but also functions rhetorically to persuade them of the importance of making careful distinctions in practice or theory. Furthermore, the structures are peculiarly performative: merely reading or listening to their repetitions and juxtapositions makes a reader or listener feel as though he or she has already made the distinctions and cognitive judgements that the structures describe. A similarly performative effect is produced in other medical texts, when authors string words together in order to communicate to the reader onomatopoeically a particular kind of bodily substance, movement, or feeling: for instance, Henry Daniel, the author of one of the earliest uroscopies in English, claims that the surface of a specific type of bloody urine is 'as hit were gobatysch and cloddyssh and chiprysshe that in phisyke ys cald trumbous' ('as if it were lumpy, full of blood clots and fragments, which in medicine is described as *trumbous*').[49] Sarah Star has drawn attention to how elaborately and sonically patterned all of Daniel's medical writing is and the way in which he uses strings of synonyms to gloss one another, thereby rendering familiar an unfamiliar vernacular medical vocabulary.[50] In this particular example, sound and matter are closely allied as the tongue-twisting half-rhymes reproduce sonically the thick, clotted texture of the urine. The body is consequently involved in its own healing: with their ears and tongues, readers reproduce the claustrophobic fullness of the urine, which illuminates their visual imagining of it. In Middle English, 'to feel' encompassed a vast range of interconnected experiences, referring to sensual and emotional experiences as well as the experience of comprehending and knowing. This example of feeling new knowledge from Daniel's text aptly illustrates that 'integration of the somatic, affective and cognitive'.[51]

Sometimes, though, this mimetic aspect of syntactic patterning is absent and the structures are no longer affectively encoded *with* knowledge. Instead, they just convey the feeling *of* accumulating knowledge. In her study of physiognomic manuals, Orlemanski has recently developed the helpful concept of *otiose practicality*: she contends that the manuals contain information that cannot actually be translated into practice, but is nonetheless presented as if it can be.[52] Here, we can see the applicability of that idea

---

[49] HEHL, MS HM 505, f. 119v.   [50] Star, 'Textual Worlds', pp. 204–6.
[51] Sarah McNamer, 'Feeling', in *Twenty-First Century Approaches to Literature*, ed. by Strohm, pp. 241–57 (p. 247).
[52] Orlemanski, 'Physiognomy'.

at a more microscopic, textual level. For instance, in John Trevisa's fourteenth-century translation of Bartholomew the Englishman's Latin encyclopaedia *De proprietatibus rerum* (which describes, among many other things, the physiology of body parts and the causes and symptoms of diseases), pairs of verbs ending in '-ing' are used to communicate a wide variety of sensations and processes, including 'greet icchinge and fretinge', 'cracching and clawing', and 'norischinge and fedinge'.[53] The repetition of the '-ing' ending does not mimic all of the sensations described; instead, it just makes the reader *feel*, with each accumulated '-ing', that they have accrued a new insight into the pain. Consequently, the accumulation of knowledge is simulated, but not necessarily stimulated by the patterning.

Crafted syntactic structures may not, then, always have helped readers to interpret instructional texts, but only made those readers think they had helped. Sometimes, the structures may actually have hindered comprehension. For example, because the chiastic structures in the above migraine remedy are composed from clauses that are almost but not quite the same, they can obscure the very distinctions they are designed to clarify: when reading or reciting the lines from memory it is easy to lose one's place, think one has misread a particular clause, or confuse the elements within the structure, accidentally replacing one ailment, ingredient, or adjective with another. In other remedy books, we find instances where even seemingly straightforward structures can confuse scribes, the first readers of the recipe. Consider this cure for epilepsy:

> Do hym þat hase the ewylle clene be schryfen and do hym drynke tytemal with ale or with watyr and doyn hym saye a pater noster and an aue and late hym noght slepyn an howre efter þat / and if the ewylle comme aȝeyn do hym drynke anoder titemalle temperred with the iuce of rwe and do hym sayn thwo pater nosters and thwo aues and hyf hafe it the thyrde tyme do hym drynke annoder tytemalle with rewe iuce and centorye and doyn hym sayn thre pater noster and thre aues and if he hafe ^it^ the <thyrde tyme> fowrte tyme do hym drynke anoder tytemalle temperde with the ivce of rewe centurie and egrimonie and say iiij paternosters and foure aves and if he haf it the v tyme do hym drynke anodyr tytemal

---

[53] John Trevisa, *On the Properties of Things: John Trevisa's Translation of Bartholomæus Anglicus De Proprietatibus Rerum*, ed. by M.C. Seymour and others, 3 vols (Oxford, 1975–88), I, Bk 7, p. 345, lines 2, 3, and 26–7. On the lyrical, affective qualities of Trevisa's prose, see Emily Steiner, 'Compendious Genres: Higden, Trevisa and the Medieval Encyclopedia', *Exemplaria*, 27 (2015), 73–92 (pp. 83–9).

temperde with the iuce of rewe, ^e^grimone and suyele Et dicat v pater noster et v aue and þat he sleipe noght efter þat he hase taken the medycyn be the space of an owre[54]

[*tytemal* = a plant of the genus Euphorbia; *rwe* = rue; *aue* = Ave Maria; *centorye* = centaury; *egrimonie* = agrimony; *suyele* = variant spelling of *souel* or of *sorel?*; *souel* = a food eaten with bread, such as meat or pottage;[55] *sorel* = sour dock or sorrel]

Each time the illness returns, the number of prayers increases and a new ingredient is added to the herb *tytemal*. This repetitive structure recalls that of nursery rhymes and songs and may have assisted with oral transmission and memorization. It does not seem, however, to have assisted the scribe in copying the recipe: he still manages to miss out the herb centaury during the recipe's fifth and final repetition. In other recipes, similar structures actively cause the scribe to miscopy the text through eyeskip.[56] These examples show that the very forms that seem most explicitly crafted to promote comprehension, clarity, and retention are—on account of that crafting—sometimes the ones that hinder it. They are thus an important reminder that, in our analysis, we should use the features of instructional writing to open up rather than close down possibilities: close reading the intricate, counterintuitive, and varied ways in which those features work across recipes and manuscripts points to a reading experience that could be unpredictable, multi-layered, and affective.

Similes

Similes are another fragment in this bricolaged texture, which not only invite variegated responses from readers but also connect recipes to other kinds of late medieval literary experience, embedding them within broader textual networks. *Similitudo*—a broad term covering different kinds of similes and comparisons—is defined by Isidore of Seville as 'that by which the description of some less known thing is made clear by something better

---

[54] TCC, MS R.14.39, f. 56v. I have used the foliation in the top-right corner of the manuscript.
[55] See *MED*, *souel*, n. 2.
[56] E.g. CUL, MS Kk.6.33, f. 76r where, in an ointment for wounds, the scribe copies 'þer wil arise a watir' a second time when he should have written 'þer wil arise bame'.

known which is similar to it'.[57] Accordingly, similes are used in remedies to describe symptoms and explain the processes involved in preparing cures: head wounds are likened to a 'spynand webbe blewe or ellys rede' or 'a burbyl of water when þat it raynes'; a strangury patient's strained urine is compared to the way in which the gutters or 'eues of an house dropiþ [rainwater]'; cloths used to apply medicines are to be shaped like a 'litel scheld' and pinned like a 'dublet' ('doublet'), and the faeces of a patient suffering from dysentery are likened to 'þe shauyng of parchemyn'.[58] Just like the impossible sonic ingredients in Henryson's mock-remedies and the list containing dove dung, flour, and incense, comparisons such as these compel readers to destabilize categories, to blur boundaries between bodies and things.

The examples listed above come from a range of remedy collections and related medical texts. In academic, theoretically framed recipe collections such as Gilbert the Englishman's *Compendium medicinae*, similes are a consistent part of the text's style, frequently appearing as diagnostic aids. Such comparisons also appear in Latin and vernacular uroscopy texts and in encyclopaedic works such as Bartholomew the Englishman's *De proprietatibus rerum*.[59] Less theoretical vernacular remedy books absorbed influences from these genres. Consequently, similes appear within them but, once again, they occur in a more haphazard way.

Like the syntactic structures examined above, these descriptive similes seem designed to function as communicative tools. How successfully they fulfil that function depends in part on their ability to represent real-world phenomena with vividness. This requirement, not always clearly fulfilled, immediately brings the remedies into conversation with more consistently poetic writings, also concerned with the powers and limitations of figurative language. Medieval writers would have been familiar with the idea of figurative language as a shared ground between writings on different subjects: in the classes on grammar and rhetoric offered to most schoolboys,

---

[57] Isidore of Seville, *The Etymologies of Isidore of Seville*, ed. and trans. by Stephen A. Barney and others (Cambridge, 2006), pp. 63–4, Book I.xxxviii.31. On medieval conceptions of *imago*, *similitudo*, and *exemplum*, see John J. McGavin, *Chaucer and Dissimilarity: Literary Comparisons in Chaucer and Other Late Medieval Writing* (Madison, WI, 2000), pp. 31–57.

[58] Respectively BodL, MS Ashmole 1444, p. 179; TCC, MS O.1.13, f. 69v; Getz, ed., *Healing and Society*, p. 254, lines 13–14; TCC, MS O.1.65, f. 252v; TCC, MS O.1.65, f. 252v; Getz, ed., *Healing and Society*, p. 191, line 22.

[59] For a guide to uroscopy texts, see M. Teresa Tavormina, 'Uroscopy in Middle English: A Guide to the Texts and Manuscripts', *Studies in Medieval and Renaissance History*, 11 (2014), 1–154.

figurative language was portrayed as fundamental to any kind of eloquent and crafted composition, regardless of its topic.[60]

On the one hand, grammatical textbooks used to teach these pupils portrayed figurative constructions and patterned language as deviations from the grammatical norm, which only differed from barbarisms and solecisms because they had been deliberately (not erroneously) produced in order to cultivate a specific aesthetic or rhetorical effect. When learning about these structures, schoolboys studied examples from Latin poetry: these ranged from Virgil's *Aeneid* to more overtly instructional texts such as the *Distichs of Cato*, a collection of proverbs.[61] As a compilation of formulaic and pithy structures, this latter text has more obvious parallels with recipes' aesthetic.

On the other hand, in the teaching of rhetoric, tropes and syntactical manipulations were portrayed differently: instead of deviations from the grammatical norm, they were represented as embellishments that could be added to the surface of any text.[62] This model influenced the most widely copied of the *artes poetriae*, Geoffrey of Vinsauf's *Poetria nova*. Geoffrey's handbook divides the composition process into four stages: the gathering and selection of material; the ordering of it and the decision about how much weight to give each element by amplifying or abbreviating it; the addition of ornaments of style (types of figurative and patterned language), and advice on memorizing and performing the composition.[63] Within this model, and in many medieval reflections on rhetoric, tropes and figures are presented as added embellishments, as clothing, or as a kind of sweet exterior wrapped around the selected matter: Geoffrey claims that meaning should wear a 'precious garment' ('pretiosum…amictum').[64]

---

[60] On this tradition, see *Medieval Grammar and Rhetoric: Language Arts and Literary Theory AD 300-1475*, ed. by Rita Copeland and Ineke Sluiter (Oxford, 2015), pp. 1–60; Suzanne Reynolds, *Medieval Reading: Grammar, Rhetoric and the Classical Text* (Cambridge, 1996), pp. 17–41; Murphy, 'The Arts of Poetry and Prose', pp. 42–67; Martin Irvine and David Thomson, '*Grammatica* and Literary Theory', in *The Cambridge History of Literary Criticism*, ed. by Minnis and Johnson, pp. 15–41; Nicholas Orme, *Medieval Schools: From Roman Britain to Renaissance England* (New Haven, CT, 2006), pp. 86–127; Marjorie Curry Woods, 'A Medieval Rhetoric Goes to School—and to the University: The Commentaries on the *Poetria Nova*', *Rhetorica*, 9 (1991), 55–65.

[61] Cannon, *From Literacy to Literature*, pp. 159–98.

[62] Copeland and Sluiter, eds, *Medieval Grammar and Rhetoric*, p. 28.

[63] See *Les arts poétiques du XIIe et du Xiii^e siècle: Recherches et documents sur la technique littéraire du moyen âge*, ed. by Edmond Faral (Paris, 1924), pp. 197–262 for Geoffrey's Latin treatise; for an English translation, see Geoffrey of Vinsauf, *Poetria Nova*, trans. by Margaret F. Nims, rev. edn (Toronto, 2010), pp. 19–80.

[64] Faral, ed., *Les arts poétiques*, p. 220, line 756.

The uses and effects of figurative language were, however, more complex in practice than such analogies imply. In the *Poetria nova*, tropes such as personification and apostrophe are not actually included in the section on ornaments of style but in the section on *amplificatio* and *abbreviato*: they are part of the structural process through which different parts of the text are given different weight, shaping how much importance a reader attributes to a particular matter. Indeed, it is telling that Geoffrey's handbook begins with an analogy comparing the planning and invention of a poetic composition to the plan a builder makes before beginning to build his house: the fundamental first stage of composition—without which composition cannot begin—cannot be explained to the reader without an extended simile.[65] Consequently, figurative language appears less as superfluous ornament in this rhetorical tradition and more as the foundation for any successful communicative act.

Just how integral writers considered figurative language to be to successful exchanges of knowledge—and especially scientific knowledge—is demonstrated by the eagle in Chaucer's *House of Fame*. In an oft-cited passage, the eagle explains to the dreamer the properties of sound through a series of analogies with fire, water, and other things. He precedes these analogies with the introduction:

Now herkene wel, for-why I wille
Tellen the a propre skille
And a worthy demonstracion
In myn ymagynacion[66]

As the beginning of this chapter explained, *imaginacioun* was semantically wide-ranging in the Middle Ages, connoting creative resourcefulness and pejorative artfulness, as well as referring more technically to the area in the brain where mental images formed from sense data were created and combined.[67] The *imaginacioun* was therefore central to cognition: without it, information from the senses could not be turned into usable or retainable knowledge. So, by locating his analogies (which are combinations of mental

---

[65] Faral, ed., *Les arts poétiques*, p. 198, lines 43–8. On Chaucer's use of this analogy, see Cannon, 'Form', pp. 177–9.
[66] Geoffrey Chaucer, *The House of Fame*, in *Riverside*, ed. by Benson, lines 725–8.
[67] *MED*, *imaginacioun*, n., entry 1(a).

images) within the imagination, the eagle is emphasizing not just their artfulness but also how fundamental to teaching and learning they are.

The similes in recipes and other medical texts can also be considered pedagogical aids. Consider this prognostic text for a head wound which appears in a fifteenth-century remedy collection and contains two of the similes introduced earlier:

> if þou se þer on abouyn [the head] as it were a bolle of water þan it is a seyn of dethe and if þou se befor þe tey as it were a spynand webbe blewe or ellys rede þat is a seyn þat þe bon of his brayn is brokyn þat is a seyn of hasty dethe[68]
>
> [*boll* = bubble; *tey* = dura mater]

The first type of head wound is compared to the surface of water disrupted by a bubble and the second is compared to a spider's web (presumably referring to the exposed arachnoid layer of the brain underneath the dura mater).[69] In the same text in other recipe collections, the wound is compared more specifically to 'a burbyl of water when þat it raynes', which suggests that the head wound was supposed to resemble a pool of water disrupted by bubbles produced by incoming raindrops.[70] This added detail, along with the specification that the veiny, web-like structure be blue or red, conveys a sense of precision. The author of these comparisons vividly draws out the crucial characteristics of the bodily phenomena in order to make the reader feel able to identify the nature of the ailment with confidence and precision.

The comparisons often instil this confidence by likening aspects of medical treatments to things familiar from related practical crafts. For instance, a remedy for the skin affliction *saucefleume* instructs the reader to grind together boar's fat and quicksilver 'as thou woldest grynde vermelon',

---

[68] BodL, MS Ashmole 1444, p. 179. On this text, its different manuscript versions, and its anatomical accuracy, see M. Benskin, 'For a Wound in the Head: A Late Medieval View of the Brain', *Neuphilologische Mitteilungen*, 86 (1985), 199–215.

[69] On the arachnoid layer, see Benskin, 'For a Wound in the Head', p. 208; Irina Metzler, *Disability in Medieval Europe: Thinking about Physical Impairment during the High Middle Ages, c. 1100–1400* (London, 2006), p. 100.

[70] TCC, MS O.1.13, f. 69v. I have also consulted versions in BL, MS Harley 2378, f. 145r; HEHL, HM 58, f. 63r–v; HEHL, HM 19079, f. 5r; WT, MS London Medical Society 136, f. 8v; and HEHL, HM 64, f. 144ra, in which the scribe has misread *tey*, the dura mater, for *teeth*, making that part of the simile: 'And if thou see byfore hit as hit were tethe or as hit were a bloo spynynge webbe or redde'. On similar misreadings in other manuscripts, see Benskin, 'For a Wound in the Head', pp. 206–7.

meaning vermillion or cinnabar, which is used in medieval book-making recipes to create red pigment.[71] Analogies like these and analogies which refer to culinary processes and products (such as porridge or gingerbread) show how different kinds of medieval recipe could become intertwined with one another even if they were not in the same physical manuscript.[72] Phenomena familiar from nature (like spiders' webs or raindrops) or from domestic environments (such as clothing and heraldry) could also offer comparisons: in one late medieval recipe for improving digestion, the cloth used to apply the medicine is to be 'mad in þe manere of a litel scheld þat may keuere þyn stomak'.[73] The same cloth should be laid 'flat to þyn stomac... and broched croswyse in þe manere of a dublet'.[74] Doublets were clothing items worn in different varieties by most social classes. This imagery seems designed, then, to reflect the middle- and upper-class domestic spaces in which many remedy books were increasingly used.

Sometimes, these similes seem to have been specifically associated by late medieval writers and translators with vernacular voices. For example, Gilbert the Englishman's Latin *Compendium medicinae* often contains figurative language in order to help the reader identify afflictions correctly. However, as Faye Getz notes, many more figurative passages are added to the fifteenth-century English translation: one such passage—which makes explicit use of domestic imagery—is the following definition of vertigo: vertigo 'makeþ a man semen þat al-þinge þat he seeþ as it semeþ to dronken men: þat þe house goeþ aboute hem and þat þe weie riseþ vp aȝenst hem'.[75] The same image appears in Henry Daniel's vernacular *Liber Uricrisiarum*.[76] Indeed, uroscopies—which often follow on from, or appear embedded within, remedy collections—are frequently a site where figurative

---

[71] HEHL, MS HM 58, f. 47r.
[72] See CUL, MS Kk.6.33, f. 66r for a salve recipe instructing the reader to 'oyle þi handis as þou woldist do gyngerbrede'.
[73] TCC, MS O.1.65, f. 252v. Another version occurs in BL, MS Harley 2378, f. 28r. On the use of heraldry in foodstuffs and culinary recipes, see Claire Sponsler, *The Queen's Dumbshows: John Lydgate and the Making of Early Theater* (Philadelphia, PA, 2014), p. 155.
[74] TCC, MS O.1.65, f. 252v.
[75] Getz, ed., *Healing and Society*, p. xlvii. The passage in question occurs on WT, MS 537, f. 52v. For examples of continental medical writers adding homely figurative images to vernacular versions of Latin texts, see Chiara Crisciani, 'Histories, Stories, Exempla and Anecdotes: Michele Savonarola from Latin to Vernacular', in *Historia: Empiricism and Erudition in Early Modern Europe*, ed. by Gianna Pomata and Nancy G. Siraisi (Cambridge, MA, 2005), pp. 297–324.
[76] Henry Daniel, *Liber Uricrisiarum: A Reading Edition*, ed. by Ruth E. Harvey, M. Teresa Tavormina, and Sarah Star (Toronto, 2020), p. 123, lines 253–4.

vernacular voices interact with other languages.⁷⁷ In most uroscopies, the colour of the urine is identified through two means: a colour term and a simile, comparing the colour to everyday substances such as cabbage stalks, apple, milk, ink, and lead. These colour descriptions, which reoccur across the corpus of uroscopy texts, derive from classical Greek and early medieval Latin texts. In these earlier versions, though, the colour terms and the similes are in the same language; in the Middle English uroscopies, the colour term remains in Latin, while the simile is translated into the vernacular. For example, in a frequently copied uroscopy, the colour 'subrubycundus' ('reddish') is explained through the image 'vryne colowre as a blase of fyre'.⁷⁸ This means that, even though they are present in the Latin texts too, these Middle English figurative images look like glosses on the Latin terminology explicitly designed to help the vernacular reader decode an alien Latinate vocabulary.

As well as rendering the unfamiliar familiar, these similes offered medical practitioners a means of creating a common language of diagnosis and prognosis. When establishing what was afflicting a patient, the medieval practitioner normally depended upon his or her ability to read the visual and tactile clues presented by the exterior of that patient's body.⁷⁹ The senses, though, were considered fallible and subjective. These comparisons with common phenomena present readers with an attractive means of moving subjective, sensual experience towards the objective and verifiable. The comparative marker 'like' consequently carries a significant amount of rhetorical weight in the simile, persuading and reassuring the reader by making explicit the cognitive path from unfamiliar to familiar that they are being guided along.

This rhetorical weight was not, however, recognized in Geoffrey of Vinsauf's *Poetria nova*, which suggests that similes are less artful than metaphors because such comparative markers draw attention to the simile's formal construction:

> ...Respice quaedam
> Juncta satis lepide; sed quaedam signa revelant

---

⁷⁷ E.g. TCC, MS O.1.65, ff. 265v–269v.
⁷⁸ Ibid., f. 269v. Versions of this text survive in at least sixty-nine manuscripts: for a comprehensive list, see Tavormina, 'Uroscopy in Middle English', pp. 14–21.
⁷⁹ Faith Wallis, 'Medicine and the Senses: Feeling the Pulse, Smelling the Plague and Listening for the Cure', in *A Cultural History of the Senses*, ed. by Richard Newhauser (London, 2014), pp. 133–52.

> Nodum juncturae: collatio quae fit aperte
> Se gerit in specie simili, quam signa revelant
> Expresse. Tria sunt haec signa: magis, minus, aeque.
> Quae fit in occulto, nullo venit indice signo;
> Non venit in vulto proprio, sed dissimulato,
> Et quasi non sit ibi collatio, sed nova quaedam
> Insita mirifice transsumptio, res ubi caute
> Sic sedet in serie quasi sit de themate nata
>
> ...
>
> ...Plus habet artis
> Hic modus, est in eo longe sollemnior usus[80]

> Notice that some things are joined deftly enough, but certain signs reveal the point of juncture. A comparison which is made overtly presents a resemblance which signs explicitly point out. These signs are three: the words more, less, equally. A comparison that is made in a hidden way is introduced with no sign to point it out. It is introduced not under its own aspect but with dissembled mien, as if there were no comparison there at all, but the taking on, one might say, of a new form marvellously engrafted, where the new element fits as securely into the context as if it were born of the theme...This type of comparison is more artistic; its use is much more distinguished.[81]

The distinction Geoffrey makes is between forms such as metaphor, allegory, and synecdoche, which present one thing as another without highlighting the transferral that has taken place, and forms of comparison, such as similes, which draw explicit attention to the act of craftsmanship that has drawn the two things together. This distinction is also implicit in more general attitudes to artistic crafting: as Glending Olson and Jenni Nuttall have shown, it was often writers who were consistently metaphorical and allegorical who were described as *poets* by their contemporaries.[82] This alternative valuation of similes is an important reminder that, though recipes can have more in common with poetic discourse than has been acknowledged, the differences between medical and poetic discourse should not be elided

---

[80] Faral, ed., *Les arts poétiques*, pp. 204–5, lines 242–63.
[81] Geoffrey of Vinsauf, *Poetria nova*, pp. 26–7.
[82] Olson, 'Making and Poetry', pp. 272–90; Nuttall, 'Poesie and Poetrie', pp. 1–5.

and the former should not always be subordinated to the standards, judgements, and precepts of the latter. Although they overlap, the two discourses retain distinctive rationales for their stylistic choices and priorities.

Geoffrey's enthusiasm here for a 'new form marvellously engrafted' also points towards another way in which medical and poetic discourse could be considered to diverge. The phrase emphasizes the importance of novelty and surprise to poetic compositions: familiar words, tropes, and generic patterns might be recycled but they are adapted and turned towards new purposes. Ironically, making use of a medical analogy, Geoffrey commands readers: 'if a word is old, be its physician and give to the old a new vigour.'[83] In contrast to such rejuvenation, medical and scientific texts appear to repeat a stock set of images in a way that could circumscribe not only their literary qualities but also their practical capacity to communicate useful information. Take the example of the spider's web. Most famously, this simile is used in Chaucer's *Treatise on the Astrolabe*: as well as comparing the astrolabe to a hairnet, Chaucer makes explicit the etymology of the word *rete* (which means 'net' or 'web' in Latin) by declaring that the rete of the astrolabe is 'shapen in manere of a net or of a lopweb'.[84] That image has a long and varied history in medical and scientific terminology: for instance, it underpins the Latin medical term *rete mirabile* ('wonderful net' or 'web'), which was originally coined in Greek by Herophilus in 3 or 4 BC to refer to the web of blood vessels at the base of the animal brain he was dissecting; it was erroneously used by later writers to describe human anatomy.[85] Later, in his encyclopaedic *De proprietatibus rerum*, Bartholomew the Englishman glosses a Latin medical term describing the first of seven tunics encircling the eyeball; in John Trevisa's fourteenth-century translation, this is rendered as '[þe first tunic] hatte *tela aranea*, as it were "þe webbe of an attercoppe"'.[86]

The image was often associated with eyes: for instance, *web* was used metaphorically in remedy books as a name for cataracts or other filmy growths across the lens of the eye.[87] But it could also be used to represent

---

[83] Geoffrey of Vinsauf, *Poetria nova*, p. 41; for the Latin, see Faral, ed., *Les arts poétiques*, p. 220, lines 756–8: 'Ut res ergo sibi pretiosum sumat amictum,/Si vetus est verbum, sis physicus et veteranum/Redde novum'.
[84] Geoffrey Chaucer, *A Treatise on the Astrolabe*, in *Riverside*, ed. by Benson, Part I.21.2–3.
[85] *Herophilus: The Art of Medicine in Early Alexandria—Edition, Translation and Essays*, ed. and trans. by Heinrich von Staden (Cambridge, 1989), p. 179.
[86] Trevisa, *On the Properties of Things*, I, Bk 5, p. 178, lines 21–2. For the Latin version of the simile, see Bartholomaeus Anglicus, *Tractatus de proprietatibus rerum* (Nuremberg, 1483), Bk V, Section V.
[87] *MED*, *web*, n., entry 3(a).

very different bodily phenomena: we have already encountered a head wound resembling a spider's web and, in a prognostic text describing the urine of a leper, it is written, 'When ye looke thereto at the .3. ^de^ daye there wylle appeere abowe the vreyne as hit were a coppewebbe.'[88]

In examples such as the rete of the astrolabe or the web of blood vessels, it is easy to see why the spider's web image has been chosen: it bears a clear resemblance to the thing it is describing or is etymologically connected to the Latin term. And yet the repetitive and conventional nature of the image, which is applied to things as different as a head wound and the surface of urine, might make one question just how precise it really is: did the image represent the particularities and oddities of human bodies very accurately? Not everything, after all, can look like a spider's web.[89] Some writers and copyists of medical texts recognized this danger of conventional comparisons. For example, in his vernacular uroscopy, the *Liber Uricrisiarum*, Henry Daniel undoes a traditional simile which translates the Latin colour term *lacteus* as 'as it were of milk', by writing:

And his kallid lactea and mylke white // not for it is white as mylke . For so white is none vrin // but for hit gothe moste tawarde mylke[90]

Daniel points out the simile's figurative imprecision in order, ultimately, to make it more precise.

Other medical writers dealt with this imprecision by adding extra details to the similes: for instance, in one copy of a uroscopy text, the standard simile for *lacteus* is changed to the more specific comparison 'as mylke wanne hit is cold'.[91] Similarly, whilst one copy of a uroscopy translates the Latin colour *inops* (*oenopus*, 'wine coloured') as 'colour of lyuer' ('colour of

---

[88] HEHL, MS HM 64, f. 173ra.

[89] It is possible in some instances to conjecture about how a simile might have moved between different afflictions and text-types. For instance, Henry Daniel describes a type of urine characterized by bubbles that are 'riȝt as þou seest in water podelles when it reyneth'; in addition to signifying other ailments, the bubbles can 'seiþ disposicioun toward ake and sekenesse in þe hed' (see Daniel, *Liber Uricrisiarum*, p. 224, lines 23–4). This recalls the image of raindrops in puddles used in some remedy collections to describe a head wound. In one text-type, the simile is a sign of an internal headache and in the other it is a sign of external head trauma. Perhaps, just as certain motifs and biblical narratives become associated in charms with particular ailments, particular similes started to cluster around connected ailments.

[90] HEHL, HM 505, f. 54v.

[91] BodL, MS Ashmole 1393, f. 58r. Quoted from M. Teresa Tavormina, 'The Twenty Jordan Series: An Illustrated Middle English Uroscopy Text', *American Notes and Queries*, 18 (2005), 43–67 (p. 62).

liver'), another scribe or writer has chosen to translate this as the colour of 'a manis lyuer. or to olde rede wyne yturned into blackenes'.[92] This example shows that writers also tried to counter the imprecision of similes by offering multiple similes. Daniel adopts this tactic himself when using the spider's web simile to describe a type of urine. The urine is not that of a leper (as it is in the above remedy book), which reaffirms that the image was a conventional one, reused in different contexts:

> And apperyth mykylle vpon that [urine] as hit is seyde // Sometyme lyke as broþe of browes // And sumtyme ther gaddryth aboue þe vryne lyke powdere that were strawen þereon. or ellys lyke an arayns webbe in so mychille þat one may takyn hit of fro þe vryn with a yarde or a stykke right as þou seyst in a fesselle with hote potage[93]
>
> [*broþe of browes* = type of broth; *arayns webbe* = spider's web; *fessel* = vessel; *potage* = soup, stew, or porridge]

The surface of the urine is first compared to broth, then to the surface upon which a powdery substance has been strewn; next it is compared to a spider's web, and finally to the surface of stew or porridge. Perhaps Daniel felt that accumulating these similes would help him to create the most vivid image possible of the urine. The repetition of 'sometyme' suggests that the succession of images was also partly an attempt to capture subtle changes and variations occurring in the urine's appearance. However, each new simile simultaneously reads as an admission of the previous simile's limitations, of its inability to convey the urine's appearance with sufficient nuance or detail. It is also significant that the similes nearly come full-circle: the sequence begins with a comparison to broth and ends with an image of a broth- or stew-like substance. This suggests that Daniel found himself tracing and retracing a confined range of comparisons, all of which were highly appropriate and yet not quite appropriate enough. So, like the repetitive syntactic structures examined earlier, the simile does not function as a perfectly practical form in medieval medical texts and was not perceived to do so by medieval writers.

---

[92] BL, MS Sloane 7, f. 59v (quoted from Tavormina, 'Twenty Jordan Series', p. 60) and WT, MS 537, f. 18r (see Tavormina, 'Twenty Jordan Series', p. 61, n. 99 for other variants).
[93] HEHL, HM 505, f. 112r. See also Daniel, *Liber Uricrisiarum: A Reading Edition*, p. 227 for a more condensed description of the surface of the urine, using only three similes: the surface appears as if it has a spider's web, powder, or dust strewn across it.

Might it, however, have offered readers something other than an accurate representation of the ailing body before them? Here we return to the similes as rhetorical devices capable of convincing readers that unfamiliar, sick, and misbehaving bodies *could* be knowable and, therefore, treatable. Similes in medical texts do not just render that body familiar by likening it to everyday phenomena or by using similes that are widespread in scientific writings: some of the comparisons they use are actually commonplace comparisons which reappear in a wide variety of medieval genres. For example, in many late medieval uroscopies, the appearance and texture of particular kinds of urine are likened to specks of dust visible in the sunlight. One example reads:

> ȝif þere chewe þerinne as yt were smale motys as ben in þe sonne it betokeneth a rewme in þe heued / defnesse / posse / and heuynesse[94]

> [*chewe þerinne* = appears in the urine; *motys* = motes; *rewme* = watery fluid; *posse* = head cold]

Atthomi, meaning 'motes', are first discussed in early medieval Latin uroscopy texts emerging from the Salernitan school of medicine.[95] However, similes *explicitly* likening the particles to specks of dust in the sunlight seem to be a characteristic of Middle English uroscopies, appearing in texts such as Henry Daniel's *Liber Uricrisiarum* and, as the above example shows, *The Twenty Jordan Series*.[96] They do not appear (as far as I and others can ascertain) in earlier Latin, Greek, or Arabic texts.[97] One might speculate that the simile was inspired by the process of inspecting urine: medieval illustrations frequently depict physicians holding urine aloft and it is easy to assume that they are holding it up to the sunlight.[98] And yet, as M. Teresa Tavormina notes, references to light in uroscopy texts are ambiguous: Henry Daniel warns against examining the urine in over-bright light and cites the

---

[94] TCC, MS O.1.65, f. 266r.
[95] E.g. see BodL, MS Laud Lat. 106, ff. 209v–229r (f. 213rb) for a discussion of *atthomi* in a commentary on Gilles of Corbeil's *Carmen de urinis*. See also Daniel, *Liber Uricrisiarum: A Reading Edition*, p. 10 for more discussion of this development and earlier understandings of urine contents. As Bouras-Vallianatos, *Innovation in Byzantine Medicine*, p. 40 also notes, as early as the Hippocratic writings, 'the presence of suspended (enaiōrēma) particles and "clouds" (nephelē) is...noted, but no clear distinction is made between them'.
[96] E.g. HEHL, MS HM 505, f. 123r.
[97] For this knowledge of Greek, Arabic, and Latin uroscopy texts, I am indebted to M. Teresa Tavormina (private email exchange, 9 December 2017).
[98] Peter Murray Jones, *Medieval Medical Miniatures* (London, 1984), p. 56 and Elizabeth Lane Furdell, *Fatal Thirst: Diabetes in Britain until Insulin* (Leiden, 2009), p. 27.

recommendation of Isaac Israeli (d. 932 AD) for examining the urine in candlelight instead.[99]

A more obvious source for the simile is, then, a commonplace image that appears in multiple Middle English texts and usually connotes material abundance.[100] Chaucer's Wife of Bath opens her tale by declaring that, though it has not always been the case, 'lymytours and othere hooly freres' are now 'as thikke as motes in the sonne-beem'.[101] The same image is used in Margery Kempe's fifteenth-century *Book* to describe one of her visions: 'Sche sey ... many white thyngys flying al abowte hir on every syde, as thykke in a maner as motys in the sunne.'[102] Finally, the version of the Trojan myth now known as *The Laud Troy Book* claims that Hector felled the Greeks 'thikker, than the motes | In somer-tide fflyen In the sonne'.[103] In all of these examples, the comparison is used to represent real-world referents that are simultaneously insubstantial and substantial: the newly arrived friars, envisioned white things, and felled Greek warriors are (in their own ways) all fleeting, provisional, and weightless, but they are, simultaneously, weighty, sensually discernible, and material. The comparison may be commonplace but it is capable of conveying nuance, detail, and paradox in each situation. For this same reason, the comparison offers a fitting description of the urine: the *atthomi* within it may be delicate and in need of careful discernment but they are simultaneously as material and bodily as other *materia medica*.

The wide-ranging applicability of such comparisons may have affected a reader's response to medical similes as practical, rhetorical, and aesthetic devices: firstly, it probably meant that the things to which unfamiliar bodily phenomena were compared in the medical similes were doubly familiar—not only recognizable from everyday life but also from commonplace language. Secondly, as Christopher Cannon argues, the ubiquity of proverbs and commonplaces in medieval literary writings suggests that a widespread aesthetic attitude was built upon the premise that medieval readers derived pleasure from recognizing what they already knew.[104] Repetition of

---

[99] BL, MS Royal 17 D.i, f. 14ra. My attention was drawn to this ambiguity by M. Teresa Tavormina (private email exchange, 9 December 2017).
[100] Bartlett Jere Whiting, *Proverbs, Sentences and Proverbial Phrases: From English Writings Mainly Before 1500* (London, 1968), p. 413 (no. M709).
[101] Geoffrey Chaucer, *The Wife of Bath's Tale*, in *Riverside*, ed. by Benson, lines 866–8.
[102] *The Book of Margery Kempe*, ed. by Barry Windeatt (Cambridge, 2004), lines 2874–6.
[103] *Laud Troy Book*, ed. by Ernst Wülfing, EETS os 121 (London, 1902), lines 6848–9.
[104] Christopher Cannon, 'Proverbs and the Wisdom of Literature: *The Proverbs of Alfred* and Chaucer's *Tale of Melibee*', *Textual Practice*, 24 (2010), 407–34 (p. 408).

commonplace or formulaic imagery does not, then, necessarily diminish the fragmentary aesthetic of medical texts, but may well have constituted it for some medieval readers.

The fact that this commonplace image recurs in literary and devotional writings also provides a crucial reminder that medical writing participated in textual cultures alongside other genres: not only did those genres often occupy the same manuscript space, they also sometimes shared a common mode of creative expression. Stephanie Trigg has recognized the importance of commonplace similes for connecting and interpreting literary texts such as Chaucer's *Canterbury Tales* and Malory's *Morte d'Arthur*: she contends that the comparisons 'simultaneously [draw] attention to authorial exceptionality... while also testifying to normative and proverbial medieval ideas'.[105] The above examples suggest, however, that we need to go further, incorporating *medical* texts into our intertextual analysis.

Recognizing such connections might allow us to reread canonical poetic texts with a richer and more nuanced understanding of their potential meanings. Consider the following extract from Julian of Norwich's fourteenth-century devotional text, *A Revelation of Love*. In an oft-quoted passage, Julian describes Christ's crucified body through a series of unsettlingly familiar images. One of these likens Christ's gushing blood to the innumerable droplets of water falling from a gutter after a heavy rain shower:

> The plentuoushede [of Christ's blood] is like to the droppes of water that falle of the evesing of an house after a grete shower of raine, that falle so thicke that no man may number them with no bodely wit[106]

This same image is used in the fifteenth-century English translation of Gilbert the Englishman's *Compendium medicinae*, but it is there applied to the strained passing of urine by a patient suffering from strangury: the patient passes water as the 'eues of an house dropiþ'.[107] Both Julian and the translator of the *Compendium* seem to be deploying the commonplace

---

[105] Stephanie Trigg, 'Weeping Like a Beaten Child: Figurative Language and the Emotions in Chaucer and Malory', in *Medieval Affect, Feeling, and Emotion*, ed. by Glenn D. Burger and Holly A. Crocker (Cambridge, 2019), pp. 25–46 (p. 26).
[106] *The Writings of Julian of Norwich*, ed. by Nicholas Watson and Jacqueline Jenkins (Philadelphia, PA, 2006), ch. 7, lines 17–19.
[107] Getz, ed., *Healing and Society*, p. 254. This image seems to have been stimulated by a phrase in Gilbert's Latin: see Gilbertus Anglicus, *Compendium medicine* (Lyon, 1510), f. 274r: 'Unde sicut guttatim in vesicam cadit'.

Middle English simile, 'To run like gutters'.[108] One applies it to abundance and the other to scarcity, showing the image's pliability. Recognizing this parallel might help us to understand Julian's text better. The similes that Julian uses in this chapter of *A Revelation* often attract attention on account of their striking homeliness: Christ's body is represented through things as mundane as herring scales, rain gutters, and pellets of food or medicine. Knowing that the comparison to raindrops falling from a gutter was a commonplace that could be used by a medical writer to describe the passing of a patient's urine only makes this homeliness more pronounced, further emphasizing the stunning capaciousness and accessibility of Julian's imagery. Along with the description of the 'white thyngys' in *The Boke of Margery Kempe*, this parallel suggests that medieval writers were content to spring the highest thoughts off the most humble and widely circulating images.[109]

The image—if experienced as a commonplace—thereby enacts Julian's message that Christ and God are open to all. However, the shock one feels at the juxtaposition of the divine and mundane simultaneously works to reaffirm the otherness of the divine being; Julian underlines this when she emphasizes that 'no man' may count the number of blood droplets with 'bodely wit'.[110] A comparable dynamic is present in the recipes: the similes—tracing the movement from unfamiliar to familiar through the comparative marker 'like'—are also reminders that the sick bodies depicted by them risk becoming worryingly incomprehensible: a man unable to pass urine in a normal way is alien (albeit to a different degree) in the same way that Christ's crucified body is.

So, the comparisons in remedies function as markers of the alien *and* as means by which that otherness might be overcome. This dynamic is aptly illustrated by a modern source which has striking parallels with medieval remedy collections. In 1916, a schoolboy called Patrick Blundstone recounted the crash of an airship and the appearance of the victims' wounded bodies. He wrote:

---

[108] Whiting, *Proverbs*, p. 255 (no. G495). Whiting gives another example from the *Siege of Jerusalem*.

[109] This explains how in *The Boke of Margery Kempe*, God can sum up Margery's love for her fellow people with a commonplace cooking simile: 'thu wuldist ben hakkyd as small as flesche to the potte for her lofe' (Windeatt, ed., *The Book of Margery Kempe*, lines 6891–2).

[110] On the communication of this otherness, see Vincent Gillespie and Maggie Ross, 'The Apophatic Image: The Poetics of Effacement in Julian of Norwich', in *The Medieval Mystical Tradition in England: Exeter Symposium V*, ed. by Marion Glasscoe (Woodbridge, 1992), pp. 53–77 (p. 65).

I would rather not describe the condition of the crew, of course they were dead—burnt to death. They were roasted, there is absolutely no other word for it. They were brown, like the outside of Roast Beef. One had his legs off at the knees, and you could see the joint![111]

The letter gains expressive momentum as Patrick moves from reticence to talk, to culinary similes, to absolute clarity and literal transparency ('you could see the joint!'). The simile succeeds in making the unfamiliar and gruesome bodies familiar and utterable for the boy, even as the crossing of boundaries between bodies and cooked meat continues to unsettle readers.

Like modern scholars, medieval thinkers pondered the capacity of figurative language to transform perceptions and attitudes in this way.[112] For instance, Persian and Arabic-speaking philosophers Al-Farabi and Avicenna, who transmitted a lot of Greek medical thought to the West, explored the psychological effects of comparative devices such as metaphors and similes.[113] They claimed that the pleasure provoked by these devices triggered an act of compliance from the imagination, the mental faculty which mediated between the senses and higher intellectual powers. This compliance could be compared and contrasted to the conviction which logical syllogisms sought to extract from audiences' rational faculties because both responses were types of compliance that occurred in the mind.[114] However, while the goal of logical syllogisms was to produce conviction in the truth of the propositions, the goal of these poetic premises

---

[111] London, Imperial War Museum, Document No. 5508, accessed online at www.iwm.org.uk/collections/item/object/1030005513 [accessed 01/04/2020].

[112] For a summary and critique of the modern 'interaction theory' of metaphor, see Stephen C. Levinson, *Pragmatics* (Cambridge, 1983), pp. 148–51. The starting point for much of this research was George Lakoff and Mark Johnson, *Metaphors We Live By*, rev. edn (Chicago, IL, 2003), which demonstrated that metaphors embedded into cultures shape the way that inhabitants conceptualize things. See also George Lakoff, 'Mapping the Brain's Metaphor Circuitry: Metaphorical Thought in Everyday Reason', *Frontiers in Human Neuroscience*, 8 (2014), 1–14. An account of different approaches to metaphor can also be found in Bishop, *Words, Stones, and Herbs*, 77–83.

[113] Salim Kemal, *The Philosophical Poetics of Alfarabi, Avicenna and Averroës: The Aristotelian Reception* (London, 2003), pp. 82–127.

[114] *Avicenna's Commentary on the Poetics: A Critical Study with an Annotated Translation of the Text*, ed. and trans. by Ismail M. Dahiyat (Leiden, 1974), ch. 1.4, p. 63: 'Both imaginative assent and conviction are [kinds of] compliance. Imaginative assent, however, is a compliance due to the wonder and pleasure that are caused by the utterance itself, while conviction is a compliance due to the realization that the thing is what it is said to be.' See also Vincent Gillespie, 'Never Look a Gift Horace in the Mouth: Affective Poetics in the Middle Ages', *Litteraria Pragensia*, 10 (1995), 59–82.

was to produce wonder and pleasure and to trigger acts of imagination.[115] Moreover, both Avicenna and Al-Farabi claimed that metaphors and similes invited responses from audiences that were not mediated by the rational faculties but were more instinctive.[116] As Deborah Black explains, these devices encourage audiences to 'transfer to [one thing] the emotive attitude generally associated with [another]'.[117] The famous example which Avicenna gives to illustrate this transferal is 'honey is vomited bile': regardless of whether one likes honey or not, and regardless of whether one wishes to be affected by the image, one cannot help feeling disgusted when honey is described in this way.[118]

The theories of these Arabic thinkers were transmitted to the Latin West by translators such as Gerard of Cremona, John of Seville, and Hermann the German.[119] Consequently, similar ideas about physical and emotional transference appear in later writings: like Avicenna, Thomas Aquinas gives the example that a man can be persuaded to hate a food which is described to him in distasteful terms.[120] Such transferrals of corporeal and emotional responses are clearly relevant to the similes in medical texts where parts of ailing, wounded, and leaking bodies are described through more neutral or pleasant phenomena. Consider the following example from John Trevisa's fourteenth-century translation of Bartholomew the Englishman's description of *scabbe*, an unpleasant type of scurfy skin affliction. This comparison,

---

[115] Deborah Black, 'The Imaginative Syllogism in Arabic Philosophy: A Medieval Contribution to the Philosophical Study of Metaphor', *Medieval Studies*, 51 (1989), 242–67 (p. 245).

[116] Dahiyat, ed. and trans., *Avicenna's Commentary*, ch. 1.2, pp. 61–2: 'The imaginative is the speech to which the soul yields, accepting and rejecting matters without pondering, reason or choice. In brief, it responds psychologically rather than ratiocinatively, whether the utterance is demonstrative or not. The demonstrative is different from the imaginative, for an utterance may serve to prove the truth (of something) without exciting emotion. Yet if said again, in a different way, it may often affect emotion without conviction occurring as well, and [in this case] the soul responds in keeping with imaginative assent rather than with conviction.' See also Black, 'The Imaginative Syllogism', p. 246.

[117] Black, 'Imaginative Syllogism', pp. 256–7. The estimative faculty—which resides near the imagination—is considered responsible for these emotive attitudes: see E. Ruth Harvey, *The Inward Wits: Psychological Theory in the Middle Ages and Renaissance* (London, 1975), p. 45.

[118] Avicenna, *Kitāb al-Qiyās*, ed. by S. Zayed (Cairo, 1964), ch. 5.7, cited in Black, 'The Imaginative Syllogism', p. 257.

[119] *Medieval Literary Theory and Criticism c. 1100–c. 1375: The Commentary Tradition*, ed. by A.J. Minnis and A.B. Scott, rev. edn (Oxford, 1991), pp. 277–84. Hermann the German translated Averroes's commentary on the *Poetics*, which was heavily influenced by Avicenna's writings. On the earlier intermingling of poetic traditions and the presence of similar ideas in Horace's writings, see Gillespie, 'Never Look a Gift Horace in the Mouth', pp. 59–82.

[120] Minnis and Scott, eds, *Medieval Literary Theory*, p. 283.

which is taken directly from Bartholomew's Latin text, is a particularly apt example because it uses honey, one of the terms of Avicenna's metaphor:

> Þe heed is igreued specialliche wiþoute in þe skyn wiþ pymples and whelkes and scabbis, out of þe whiche comeþ quittir iliche hony. And þerfore Constantinus clepiþ suche scabbe *fauum* 'honycomb', for suche whelkes haue smale holes out of þe whiche quittir comeþ as hony out of þe honycombe.[121]

[*igreued* = troubled; *whelkes* = pustules; *quitter* = pus; *clepiþ* = calls]

Bartholomew's simile reverses Avicenna's metaphor: whereas Avicenna's comparison turns honey into the unpleasant bodily substance bile, Bartholomew's construction turns bodily pus into sweet and pleasant honey. Honey was, of course, one of the most common ingredients in medieval remedies and was traditionally associated with healthy nourishment: Trevisa's translation later claims that 'The honycombe hatte *fauus* and haþ þat name of *fouendo*, "norischinge and socourynge"... for þe honycombe conforteþ and socoureþ þe hony þerwiþinne.'[122] Because of this association with sweetness, nourishment, and health, honey was often used figuratively in both secular and spiritual writings to portray the object of earthly and sacred desires: the English visionary Richard Rolle proclaims, 'Swete Ihesu, þy bodi is like to a hony combe, for hit is in euche a way ful of cellis, and euch celle ful of hony.'[123] In creative play with this disturbingly microscopic compartmentalization of Christ's body, Rolle sets the reassuring image of plenteous honey. Bartholomew's comparison between pus-filled scabs and honeycomb may be less emotively charged than Rolle's comparison, but it is hard to imagine that the image of honey could there be entirely segregated from these widespread and densely layered positive cultural associations with pleasure, devotional fulfilment, and nourishment.

This image is testament, then, to the messy, fluid, and reciprocal associative networks in which medical language partook: the medical, amatory, and spiritual meanings of 'honey' are all folded inside one another. A substantial amount of critical attention has been paid in recent years to the

---

[121] Trevisa, *On the Properties of Things*, I, Bk 7, p. 344, lines 19–23. For the Latin, see Bartholomaeus Anglicus, *Tractatus de proprietatibus rerum* (Nuremberg, 1483), Bk 7, Section II.
[122] Trevisa, *On the Properties of Things*, II, Bk 19, p. 1320, lines 10–16.
[123] Richard Rolle, *Meditation B*, in *Richard Rolle: Prose and Verse*, ed. by S.J. Ogilvie-Thomson, EETS os 293 (Oxford, 1988), p. 74, lines 227–9.

importation of medical language into other kinds of discourse in order to represent diverse experiences metaphorically.[124] However, aside from Marie-Christine Pouchelle's exploration of the broader cultural and psychological significance of the metaphors used in Henri de Mondeville's surgical writings, far less attention has been paid to the reverse process: the representation of medical phenomena by more pleasant non-medical phenomena, such as spiders' webs, shields, raindrops, and honey.[125] The emotive transferrals that these comparisons invite are important, however, since they indicate that the similes might not only have helped practitioners and patients identify sickness, but also to *feel* better about it: emotions or passions were one of the non-natural aspects and activities of everyday life that, if not managed properly or allowed to stray into excess, could cause ill health.[126]

Moreover, as Joy Hawkins explains, sights were thought to have a direct impact upon health because the humoral qualities of the object being viewed were assimilated into the body of the viewer. Shocking images could disturb the workings of the animal and vital spirits. Thus, 'if the image in question was disgusting, such as a rotting carcass, a noisome dung heap or even an ugly, diseased person, it would have a detrimental effect, potentially destabilising the entire [bodily] system'.[127] By encouraging self-healing readers to transfer onto their ailing bodies the more pleasant feelings they had towards raindrops and spiders' webs, medical texts may have calmed some of these extreme feelings of disgust and fear and assisted, or been felt to assist, in the patient's easing.

Admittedly, the similes in medical writings occasionally prioritize finding an appropriate comparison for bodily ailments over making that ailment amenable: for instance, in Trevisa's translation of Bartholomew's encyclopaedia, the excrement produced by a patient with dysentery 'semiþ as it were waisschinge of fleisch' ('a flushing out of flesh').[128] Although the aptness of this simile may have produced pleasure in a reader, it leads him

---

[124] For further discussion, see the Introduction, note 81.
[125] Pouchelle, *The Body and Surgery*, pp. 91–205. Pouchelle sometimes psychologizes Mondeville's analogies too much, interpreting, for instance, Mondeville's comparison between a cook and the stomach as evidence of his attitude to the rising middle classes (p. 102). Nonetheless, her work is important in highlighting the need to pay closer attention to the extra-medical associations of medical analogies.
[126] On the non-naturals, see Horden, 'A Non-Natural Environment', pp. 133–45 and McCann, *Soul Health*, pp. 7–8.
[127] Joy Hawkins, 'Sights for Sore Eyes: Vision and Health in Medieval England', in *On Light*, ed. by K.P. Clarke and S. Baccianti (Oxford, 2014), pp. 137–56 (pp. 141–8).
[128] Trevisa, *On the Properties of Things*, I, Bk, 7, p. 403, lines 7–8.

or her straight back to the bodily.[129] Normally, though, the similes are not only more pleasant than the bodies they represent, but—just like the simile form itself—they also straddle the boundary between the aesthetic and the utilitarian. For example, in the comparisons examined earlier on in this chapter, the hairnet, shield, and broached doublet are all functional clothing items and accessories, but they are also aesthetic adornments to one's appearance. Similarly, when Gilbert the Englishman compares the faeces of a man with dysentery to the shavings of parchment, he refers to a material that could be used to record all kinds of useful information but was also the surface upon which painters and poets displayed their skills.[130] Even those images which seem more explicitly functional appear multivalent upon closer inspection: whilst the gutter in Gilbert's description of a man urinating is a functional device, the raindrops falling intermittently from it are beautiful and mesmerizing. Just like the simile form, then, these phenomena draw together the aesthetic and practical; they too are hybrids which contribute to the patchwork texture of remedy writing and its varied, fragmentary effects.

The Place of Puns

The final poetic fragment to be discussed is puns.[131] Puns not only provide another example of the interactions, fusions, and conflicts between the practical and poetic that can occur in recipes: they can also introduce a comic, playful thread into the texture of remedies which can be difficult for modern readers to know how to approach. Consider the phrase 'welle tham wele' ('boil them well') in the remedy quoted at the beginning of this chapter. That particular remedy book, which is Robert Thornton's copy of the *Liber de diversis medicinis*, contains at least sixteen variations of this sonic and visual echo.[132] 'Wele' is also attached to many other verbs in the

---

[129] Interestingly, similes in herbal texts also operate in this self-referential way, likening aspects of one herb to aspects of another. This, however, creates a less accessible, interlocking web of similes as the reader must already have some prior knowledge of the plants.

[130] For the Latin version of the parchment simile, see Gilbertus Anglicus, *Compendium medicine* (Lyon, 1510), f. 219r.

[131] Like similes, puns occur in verse and prose remedies, but, for no obvious reason, are more frequent in prose texts.

[132] Ogden, ed., *The 'Liber diversis medicinis'*, pp. 1, 7, 9, 12, 13, 32, 34, 35, 46, 54, 74, 77, and 78.

collection such as 'stampe' and 'boyle'. The latter is a synonym for 'welle'.[133] This range of verbs and synonyms might suggest that Thornton, or whoever was responsible for his exemplar, recognized the appropriateness of an unadorned, straightforward style for copying recipes, but could not resist—and did not deem inappropriate—the occasional indulgence in more playful language. Perhaps he thought that, like the rhyme and rhythm of charms, that sonic echo would bolster healing action through favourable occult powers.[134]

An appeal to the hidden forces of natural magic is certainly present in ingredients presented in recipes as homophonic doublets: two of the most common are the 'hertis herte'[135] or the 'hares here'.[136] Sometimes there is an obvious connection between the ailment and the ingredient: for instance, the hart's heart was recommended for strengthening the human heart, because the animal's long life and enduring heart were legendary.[137] In other instances, a specific kind of *verbal* homeopathy is at play, where 'the possession by one object of a name identical with or closely resembling that of another, even though there be little or no resemblance in function or appearance, enables it to exert some magic influence'.[138] For example, eggs—often spelt *ei*, *eye*, or *aye*—are frequently used to treat eye disorders.[139]

The relationship between puns, practicality, and efficacy is not, however, entirely straightforward. This system of correspondences and influences was increasingly challenged by late medieval philosophers as an accurate means of understanding the world.[140] Moreover, there was a long tradition of medieval thought, influenced by classical ideas, which argued that the

---

[133] Ibid., p. 34, line 31; p. 44, lines 20–1.
[134] See the earlier discussion of natural magic in this chapter.
[135] BodL, MS Laud misc. 553, f. 46r. See also BodL, MS Ashmole 1443, p. 239.
[136] TCC, MS O.1.65, f. 248v. This pun also occurs in BodL, MS Ashmole 1438, Part I, p. 23; BodL, MS Ashmole 1438, Part II, p. 14; BodL, MS Ashmole 1438, Part II, p. 102; BodL, MS Laud misc. 553, f. 72r; and BodL, MS Rawlinson C. 506, f. 95v.
[137] Getz, ed., *Healing and Society*, p. xix. See also BodL, MS Ashmole 1443, p. 239 where it is used in a remedy for 'þe cardyakyl' (heart pain and palpitations).
[138] Eugene S. McCartney, 'Verbal Homeopathy and the Etymological Story', *The American Journal of Philology*, 48 (1927), 326–43 (p. 326).
[139] E.g. BodL, MS Ashmole 1477, Part I, f. 36r; TCC, MS O.1.13, f. 71v; BodL, MS Laud misc. 553, f. 42r.
[140] On analogical thought, see Sheila Delaney, *Medieval Literary Politics: Shapes of Ideology* (Manchester, 1990), pp. 19–41; Stephen Penn, 'Literary Nominalism and Medieval Sign Theory', in *Nominalism and Literary Discourse: New Perspectives*, ed. by Christoph Bode, Hugo Keiper, and Richard J. Utz (Amsterdam, 1997), pp. 157–89 (pp. 182–7); John Henry, 'The Fragmentation of Renaissance Occultism and the Decline of Magic', in John Henry, *Religion, Magic and the Origins of Science in Early Modern England* (Farnham, 2012), pp. 1–48 (pp. 9–10).

relationship between words and things was arbitrary.[141] These competing and coexisting models mean that puns could have been poised for medieval readers between revealing fundamental cosmic connections and revealing the random, messy nature of human language. They may also have been poised between the serious and the playful. The following example of the eye/egg pun illustrates just how disorientating such pairings can be in remedies:

> For to mak an oygnement for þe eyen
>
> Tak an eye and roste it ryght harde or boyle it and kytte it in the myddylle and tak owte the ʒelke and þere as þe ʒelke was putt poudre of coporose whyle it is hotte but loke it be white coperose and panne it all to gedre in a lynnen clothe and presse it strongly bytwen thyn hondys so þat the ius of þe eye and coperose come owte togedre and with þat ius anoynte thyn eyne[142]
>
> [*eyen* = eyes; *eye* = egg; *ʒelke*= yolk; *coperose* = metallic sulphate]

The puns on 'eyen'/'eye' and 'eye'/'eyne' are chiastically arranged at the beginning and end of the recipe. This word play could convince a reader of the cure's homeopathic power. But it could also confuse and disturb: the pun momentarily invites a reader to imagine roasting, boiling, and cutting an eyeball. It therefore has the opposite effect to the similes, which, by comparing bodily ailments to natural and domestic phenomena, make the former *less* grotesque. Another remedy punning on the word *eye* is similarly disorientating:

> For red eyen tak an ey bolle and ful hit ful of red wyn and put þerto a peny wiʒt of salt and let hit stonde so vj daies in þe bolle after anoynte þyn eyen[143]
>
> [*ey bolle* = eggshell or eyeball]

---

[141] Howard Bloch, *Etymologies and Genealogies: A Literary Anthropology of the French Middle Ages* (Chicago, IL, 1983), pp. 44–54. On the Augustinian theory of conventional signs and perceived abuses of the arbitrary relationship between words and things in Chaucer's *Pardoner's Tale*, see Laila Abdalla, "'My body to warente...': Linguistic Corporeality in Chaucer's Pardoner', in *Rhetorics of Bodily Disease and Health in Medieval and Early Modern England*, ed. by Jennifer C. Vaught (Farnham, 2010), pp. 65–84.
[142] BodL, MS Ashmole 1477, Part I, f. 36r. [143] BodL, MS Laud misc. 553, f. 42r.

'Bolle' (eggshell) does not help to clarify things because it could also be used to refer to the eyeball or the white of the eye.[144] In fact, it only makes the play more noticeable and the sense of confusion greater.

Scribes clearly recognized this potential for confusion and some were troubled by it. In an early sixteenth-century eye remedy, the scribe has written 'eyren' before crossing it out and replacing it with the more unambiguous 'egg':

For þe syte of the Eyen

Tak wylde tansye and stampe it welle and mengle þe iuse with þe whyte of an <Eyren> ^Egg^ and laye it to the Eyes evine and mornyngs and wasshe þe Eyes with hotte whyte wyne and do so ofte for it proved[145]

The correction suggests that the scribe considered the near-pun inappropriate. Perhaps this was because it might distract a reader from following the recipe's instructions or perhaps it was because the word play seemed incongruous with the remedy's sparse, imperative tone. This correction, however, makes scribes' decision to keep the word play in other manuscripts even more striking.

Puns such as this suggest that creativity and humour could be deployed in remedies, even when there was a high chance that that creative play would actually impede the recipes' communicative purpose, rather than coexist with or fulfil that aim, as many of the other creative structures examined in this chapter seem to do. Sometimes, then, play took precedence over practicality. In these moments, genuine recipes do not seem at all far removed from Henryson's mock-remedy poetics, where he has amplified and exaggerated the imaginative tics of recipes to make play the governing principle of the text. Recipe collections afford no such consistency or predictability: as we have seen repeatedly, their poetics is of a more disorganized, fragmentary kind. Nevertheless, the syntactic structures, similes, and puns examined in this chapter show that writers and scribes of remedy collections were attentive to the smallest of details. Indeed, their use of puns suggests that attention to the smallest literary fragments could have

---

[144] *MED*, *eie*, n.1, entry 1(g).
[145] BodL, MS Radcliffe Trust e. 10, f. 8v. Normally in transcriptions I have decapitalized letters which are randomly capitalized; here, however, I have preserved the capital 'E' as it is only used to capitalize the words *eye* and *egg*. Perhaps it was used in the scribe's exemplar to draw attention to the sonic similarity or healing connection between these two words or things.

monumental effects, unlocking the occult correspondences structuring the cosmos. It follows, then, that we too should be paying these small fragments more attention. In Chapter 2, I continue to do so by exploring how particular kinds of verse fragment also encourage us to challenge unifying or reductive narratives of practicality.

2
Making Verse Remedies

The later Middle Ages were heir to a long tradition of writing instructional texts in verse: instructional poems were composed in classical Greece and Rome and many examples survive from medieval Arabic culture.[1] Western European scholasticism produced several notable works too: Gilles of Corbeil's Latin verse treatises on pulse and urine diagnostics, written in the late twelfth or early thirteenth century, were popular university teaching aids. Indeed, M. Teresa Tavormina describes Gilles's *Carmen de urinis* as 'the equivalent of a medical bestseller'.[2] Also influential was a verse herbal produced in Latin by an eleventh-century writer living in France, usually identified as Odo de Meung but known, pseudonymously, as Macer Floridus.[3] This poem inspired at least three extensive Middle English prose translations in the fourteenth and fifteenth centuries. Parts of an English verse herbal and parts of a fourth prose text also derive from versions of the Macer herbal.[4]

As these examples indicate, Latin medical verse continued to circulate in the later Middle Ages and new verse and prose translations started to be produced in the vernacular. This affirms the continual intertwining of past and present, Latin and English, verse and prose. However, fourteenth- and fifteenth-century Middle English medical verse had a slightly different role and status from earlier Latin verse because of the increasing popularity and ubiquity of prose during this period: although individual medical poems do survive in relatively high numbers of manuscripts, there was less renewal, adaptation, and composition of medical verse; the number of different prose

---

[1] See Rabie E. Abdel-Halim, 'Medicine and Health in Medieval Arabic Poetry: An Historical Review', *International Journal of the History and Philosophy of Medicine*, 3 (2013), 1–7; Peter Toohey, *Epic Lessons: An Introduction to Ancient Didactic Poetry* (London, 1996).

[2] M. Teresa Tavormina, 'Three Middle English Verse Uroscopies', *English Studies*, 91 (2010), 591–622 (p. 592).

[3] Odo was known by medieval readers pseudonymously as Macer Floridus, evoking the Roman didactic poet Aemilius Macer. See Frank J. Anderson, *An Illustrated History of the Herbals* (New York, 1977), pp. 30–2.

[4] On these translations, see George Keiser, 'Vernacular Herbals: A Growth Industry in Late Medieval England', in *Design and Distribution of Late Medieval Manuscripts in England*, ed. by Margaret Connolly and Linne R. Mooney (York, 2008), pp. 292–307 (p. 300).

adaptations of a text was often far greater than the number of different verse ones.[5] Scholars normally explain this disproportion through increased levels of literacy in the later Middle Ages: if one could read a written prose text, one had less need to commit a medical poem to memory through the mnemonic aid of verse.[6] However, despite emphasizing this decreased dependence on memory, critics continue to analyse surviving copies of verse medical texts in terms of memorability and accessibility, assuming that certain features of verse, such as end-rhyme, made the text easier for readers to remember.[7]

Clearly, there is value in this approach: past motives for composing medical verse would inevitably shape the stylistic choices of inheritors of that tradition, even if the motives were no longer so pressing. Moreover, the fact that scribes were writing medical poems down does not mean that those poems were not still being memorized by some: Mary Carruthers has shown that all kinds of mnemonic aids took written, diagrammatic form and she has emphasized the importance of the visual appearance of manuscript pages in the process of memorization.[8] The written poem could, then, be a prompt or starting point for memorization.

The stylistic choices made by late medieval writers and scribes of medical verse are, however, unlikely to have been wholly or perfectly shaped by that practical goal. Accordingly, this chapter aims to show that memorability and accessibility did not circumscribe what medical verse could signify for late medieval writers and readers: they framed the relationship between prose and verse in a *multitude* of ways, usually asserting the advantages of one form over the other in terms of comprehension, aesthetics, or truthfulness. In actuality, the experience of reading and writing medieval medical verse was likely to be one in which the advantages *and* limitations of writing in verse were being constantly negotiated—both from a practical and an aesthetic perspective.

This chapter examines evidence of that negotiation in verse remedy books, herbals, and other related kinds of medical verse such as bloodletting

---

[5] On prose recipes, see Chapter 1.
[6] E.g. George Keiser, 'Verse Introductions to Middle English Medical Treatises', *English Studies*, 84 (2003), 301–17. For an analogous discussion of the relationship between prose, verse, oral transmission, and memory in relation to romance, see Cooper, 'Prose Romances', p. 216.
[7] The views of these scholars are described in more detail later on in the chapter.
[8] Carruthers, *The Book of Memory*, pp. 103, 163, and 281; see also Michael Clanchy, *From Memory to Written Record: England 1066–1307*, 3rd edn (London, 2013), pp. 174–5.

texts and dietaries. It expands the focus of extant scholarship on end-rhyme to consider other 'literary fragments' that distinguish verse medical writings from their prose counterparts. These include manipulation of the relationship between rhyme and sense units, more concentrated and visually perceptible semantic and syntactic play, and greater experimentation with speaking voices. Just like the piecemeal poetic fragments of prose texts, these features can appear more or less carefully shaped. Consequently, some scholars—echoing the Host's condemnation of Chaucer's tail-rhymed *Sir Thopas*—have been quick to dismiss all medical verse as 'doggerel'.[9] In contrast, I argue that, whilst medical verse can appear crude and ill thought out, there are often moments where the spectre of a more artful, shaping hand is present. What is more, some of the evidence discussed below suggests that writing medical texts in verse did not always, or only, refocus writers' minds onto the real-world functionality of their texts: it could also encourage them to pay closer attention to the playful possibilities of language, form, and voice.

Medieval Conceptions of Medical Verse

One might assume that verse remedy books and herbals—written in the vernacular, easy to understand, and engaging—would have been widely copied by different kinds of readers: as Anke Timmermann remarks in relation to scientific verse in general, 'Science now spoke not just the language of the man outside the university, but also in a rhythmic, melodious voice'.[10] This is true for other branches of medieval science: vernacular alchemical poetry, for example, proliferated in the fifteenth century and brought that craft (or at least its textual description) out of clerical circles and into the public domain of lay literacy.[11] In medicine, though, there was less proliferation, with a smaller number of verse texts circulating.

---

[9] George Keiser, 'Rosemary: Not Just for Remembrance', in *Health and Healing from the Medieval Garden*, ed. by Peter Dendle and Alain Touwaide (Woodbridge, 2008), pp. 180–204 (pp. 185, 191).
[10] Anke Timmermann, 'Scientific and Encyclopaedic Verse', in *A Companion to Fifteenth-Century English Poetry*, ed. by Julia Boffey and A.S.G. Edwards (Woodbridge, 2013), pp. 199–211 (p. 199).
[11] Timmermann, 'Scientific and Encyclopaedic Verse', pp. 200–2; Michela Pereira, 'Alchemy and the Use of Vernacular Languages in the Late Middle Ages', *Speculum*, 74 (1999), 336–56.

The surviving late medieval verse medical corpus can be tentatively confined to the following texts.[12] These are: a rhymed dietary by the poet John Lydgate (*DIMEV* 1356, 2369),[13] a verse remedy book existing in multiple versions and sometimes intermingled with prose remedies and attached to a verse herbal (*DIMEV* 2343, 2519),[14] several individual or short sequences of rhymed remedies and diagnostic, prognostic, or gynaecological texts which are sometimes seen as part of the longer remedy book (*DIMEV* 1355, 4165, 5251 and *eVK2* 2576.00, 7969.00, 8145.00, 6399.00, 8105.00, 7012.00, 6969.00, 2757.00),[15] a substantial verse herbal (*DIMEV* 4171), two poems predominantly about rosemary (*DIMEV* 5977, *eVK2* 1321.00), five blood-letting texts containing verse (*DIMEV* 847, 1570, 5395, 6847 and *eVK2* 7463.00),[16] two verse plague treatises including Lydgate's 'A Doctrine for Pestilence' (*DIMEV* 6586, 1944), three uroscopy poems (*DIMEV* 1791, 1975 and *eVK2* 7757.00), several verse prologues and epilogues (*DIMEV* 438, 2687, 2688, 3527, 3808, 5390, 5458, 5656, 6710), several short verses on the humours, anatomy, or medicine in general (*DIMEV* 1142, 4168, 4926, 4367, 5650 and *eVK2* 0982.00), verses on lifestyle and diet (*DIMEV* 560, 6552, 6614), and multiple rhymed charms (for example, *DIMEV* 789, 1018, 2154, 4322, 4601, 6243 and *eVK2* 3274.00).[17] One might also count a prayer with medical intent (*DIMEV* 4327) or lines of medical verse embedded in larger prose works (*DIMEV* 5458, 6062 and *eVK2* 7426.00). In addition, lunaries and astrological verse texts often contain useful information about favourable times for medical treatment and recovery.[18]

---

[12] To produce this survey, I have used *DIMEV*, *eVK2*, and George Keiser's *Manual of the Writings in Middle English, 1050–1500: Works of Science and Information* (see List of Abbreviations and Bibliography for full details). Where possible, I have included the *DIMEV* number for the text. When the text is missing from *DIMEV*, I have used the number attached by *eVK2* to a specific version of the text; that database can be searched to find other versions.

[13] The second *DIMEV* number refers to a disordered version of 'The Dietary'.

[14] *DIMEV* lists these as separate items but they seem to be interrelated, sharing some of the same material with different additions and abridgements. These verse remedies are also often attached to the verse herbal, suggesting that the boundary between such texts was porous.

[15] I have not included *DIMEV* 5094 or 5114 here because I consider it part of an extended remedy book (*DIMEV* 2343). I have included *DIMEV* 5251 even though it often circulates with the remedy book because, as a longer text on dropsy, it may originally have circulated independently: see SKB, MS X.90, p. 43 where the text has a separate incipit.

[16] *DIMEV* 6847 can be seen as a variant version of *DIMEV* 5395.

[17] One might also include *DIMEV* 5379, a text explaining the different effects that parts of the body have on man's physical, emotional, and cognitive capacities; it is not rhymed and is written in irregular lines but has been set out as verse (see CMC, MS Pepys 1236, f. 91r).

[18] On this corpus, see Irma Taavitsainen, 'The Identification of Middle English Lunary MSS', *Neuphilologische Mitteilungen*, 88 (1987), 18–26.

Out of the above texts, Lydgate's 'The Dietary', partly based on the widely copied, twelfth-century Latin poem *Regimen sanitatis Salernitanum*, survives in the highest number of copies, appearing in at least fifty-nine manuscripts.[19] Only a few Middle English poems—including Chaucer's *Canterbury Tales*, Gower's *Confessio Amantis*, Langland's *Piers Plowman*, and the *Prick of Conscience*—survive in comparable numbers.[20] Sometimes 'The Dietary' occurs with other scientific texts, but sometimes it occurs alongside quite different kinds of verse.[21] In twenty-seven of the medieval witnesses listed in *DIMEV*, 'The Dietary' circulates with other poems by, or attributed to, Lydgate. Some of the compilers and scribes of these manuscripts may have copied the poem simply because it was by Lydgate (and merited a place in an anthology of his writings) or because it occurred in a ready-made anthology. And yet Lydgate was such a prolific writer that it seems likely that at least some of these scribes would have been able to pick and choose which of his writings they included. 'The Dietary' may have been selected because it was considered medically or morally useful, pleasingly crafted, or, as Jake Walsh Morrissey has suggested, because it addressed a broad non-specialist audience, contained orthodox and familiar medical advice, and could be easily excerpted or expanded to suit a reader's purpose.[22] None of these reasons precludes the others.

The popularity of Lydgate's poem shows that verse *did* retain its appeal for some late medieval vernacular readers as a mode of instruction. Although the number of extant witnesses is exceptionally high for 'The Dietary', a few other extended verse writings also survive in reasonably high numbers of manuscripts. For instance, a bloodletting poem (*DIMEV* 5395, 6847) survives in at least thirty manuscripts in two versions.[23] The next highest text is the verse herbal mentioned in the introduction to this chapter; versions, adaptations, and fragments of this poem have been identified in at least twenty-four late medieval or early sixteenth-century manuscripts.[24] Many of the other poems listed above, however, survive in fewer

---

[19] Jake Walsh Morrissey, '"To al Indifferent": The Virtues of Lydgate's "Dietary"', *Medium Aevum*, 84 (2015), 258–78 (p. 258).

[20] Derek Pearsall, *John Lydgate* (London, 1970), p. 219.

[21] On the varied manuscript contexts of 'The Dietary', see Orlemanski, 'Thornton's Remedies', pp. 251–5.

[22] Walsh Morrissey, '"To al Indifferent"'.

[23] Together, *eVK2*, *DIMEV*, *NIMEV*, and Keiser's *Manual* list thirty late medieval manuscripts. On these versions, see Tony Hunt, 'The Poetic Vein: Phlebotomy in Middle English Verse', *English Studies*, 77 (1996), 311–22.

[24] In Lincoln, Lincoln Cathedral Library, MS 91, ff. 317r–321v (included in my total) most of the text is torn away. Another manuscript, linked to Uppington School and not included in

than ten copies.[25] These numbers are not particularly remarkable when compared to the survival rates of other Middle English poems: Chaucer's *Troilus and Criseyde* survives in sixteen copies and his *House of Fame* survives in only three manuscripts.[26] But what is significant is that, for many genres of medical writing, the total number of copies of verse (ignoring how many copies survive of individual texts) is significantly lower than the total number of copies of their prose counterparts.

Medical recipes provide the starkest contrast: as the above count shows, only a handful of individual vernacular verse remedies and one substantial verse remedy book survive and each text only seems to survive in single figures.[27] In comparison, thousands of vernacular prose remedies survive: Voigts and Kurtz's database yields 1,861 results when searched for fourteenth- and fifteenth-century medical recipes and only twenty-three of these are listed as verse.[28] Of course, some of these results are copies or variations of the same prose recipes; the task of mapping the relations between all of the extant texts is such a large one that it has not yet been attempted. In other medical genres, though, the number of *different* texts is easier to compare. For instance, whilst only one verse herbal and two poems about rosemary survive, at least ten prose herbals exist: these include *Agnus Castus*, *Circa Instans*, Henry Daniel's prose *Herbal*, at least three Middle English translations of Odo de Meung's *De virtutibus herbarum*, a more partial adaptation commonly known as *Here Men May See the Virtues of Herbs*, a text on the virtues of betony, and two prose tracts on the virtues

---

my total, is listed in *DIMEV* 4171 as missing. Of the surviving twenty-four copies, I have been able to consult nineteen versions in manuscripts or editions; these are marked in my Bibliography by an asterisk.

Some versions of this verse herbal contain bits of other verse herbal texts embedded within them, suggesting that the boundaries between texts were fluid: for instance, the copy of *DIMEV* 4171 in New Haven, Beinecke Rare Book and Manuscript Library [hereafter BRB], MS Takamiya 46, ff. 3r–14v contains an excerpt listed as part of *DIMEV* 5977 on f. 14r.

[25] E.g. *DIMEV* 2343, 4165, 5977, 847, 1570, 1944, 1791, 1975, 1142, 4168, 4926, 4367, 5650, 6552, 6614.

[26] Benson, ed., *Riverside*, pp. 1161 and 1139, respectively.

[27] The verse remedy book survives in at least eight copies in seven manuscripts: BRB, MS Takamiya 46, ff. 14v–20v; HEHL, MS HM 64, ff. 114r–120r and 143v–176r (the recipes are intermingled amongst prose remedies); SKB, MS X.90, pp. 36–47, 78–80 (copied twice); BL, MS Additional 17866, ff. 16r–21v; PML, MS Bühler 21, ff. 45r–49v; TCC MS R.14.39, f. 1v; TCC MS R.14.51, ff. 1r–18r.

[28] See Introduction, note 4 on my arrival at this figure. The database only includes groups of three recipes or more and individual recipes of interest; on Voigts and Kurtz's selection principles, see Kari Anne Rand Schmidt, 'The Index of Middle English Prose and Late Medieval English Recipes', *English Studies*, 75 (1994), 423–9 (p. 428).

of rosemary. This suggests that more adaptation and renewal of prose texts took place.

What affected verse texts' regeneration? The few medical genres that did produce large numbers of *different* verse texts—such as bloodletting texts and charms—may have done so because of their performative element: charms could be incorporated into more impressive and convincing performances if recited from memory.[29] Similarly, bloodletting texts could be helpfully recited aloud as the practitioner navigated the patient's network of veins.[30] In contrast, texts such as recipes could often be just as conveniently consulted as written texts in manuscript compendiums: as George Keiser argues, increased literacy and the production of increasingly cheap paper books in the fifteenth century made such manuscripts more accessible to the urban and upper classes and made more people less dependent on the oral transmission of medical writings and the mnemonic aid of rhyme.[31] To support this theory, Keiser points to the fact (confirmed by the above count) that, aside from charms, the type of verse medical text for which the greatest number of different examples exist is the verse prologue or epilogue. He argues that, because there would be no practical benefit in memorizing these introductions and conclusions, verse must have served a 'primarily ornamental' role in late Middle English medical writing, adorning the beginnings and endings of texts.[32] Keiser's theory helpfully shifts attention away from the mnemonic purpose of verse. After all, the fact that individual medical poems (such as Lydgate's 'Dietary' and the verse herbal) survive in higher numbers of manuscripts than many other Middle English poems could suggest that they were *not* always memorized and orally transmitted; people needed to write them down.

In spite of this, the mnemonic aspect of medical verse is often discussed to the exclusion of—and in isolation from—its other qualities.[33] For example, Linda E. Voigts claims that 'it is artificial to separate prose from verse in considering Middle English medical writings', contending that verse

---

[29] On the mnemonic elements of charms, see Lea T. Olsan, 'Charms in Medieval Memory', in *Charms and Charming in Europe*, ed. by Jonathan Roper (Basingstoke, 2004), pp. 59–88.
[30] As the above count shows, five different bloodletting poems survive (though one may be a variant version of another).
[31] Keiser, 'Verse Introductions', pp. 301–17.   [32] Keiser, 'Verse Introductions', p. 316.
[33] An exception is Jessica Brantley's recent claim that some versified calendars do not 'serve...a purely mnemonic purpose' but 'begin to capitalize, in fact, on the aesthetic possibilities suggested by versification'. See Jessica Brantley, 'Forms of the Hours in Late Medieval England', in *The Medieval Literary Beyond Form*, ed. by Meyer-Lee and Sanok, pp. 61–84 (p. 68).

was only considered different from prose because it was 'mnemonic'.[34] In his study of versified Latin adaptations of Constantine the African's *Liber graduum*, Winston Black adopts a more nuanced perspective, claiming that 'verse herbals were not simply mnemonic repositories of ancient pharmacological knowledge' or 'frivolous adaptations of prose works' but 'can be seen as independent medical treatises with their own view and presentation of medicinal ingredients, their qualities and applications'.[35] This aligns with my view that verse shapes medical content in distinctive ways from prose. Like many commentators, though, Black segregates literary effects from utilitarian purposes, returning to the claim that, though medical verse may be 'charming' and 'artful', 'originality was not the goal of composing [it], but accessibility and memorability'.[36] The precise means by which aesthetic effects help to fulfil—or supplement, transcend, and impede—utilitarian functions remain to be explored.

Medieval writers and readers of medical verse also subordinated the aesthetic to the practical. But, in the process, they *did* dwell upon the sensual and cognitive effects involved in the experience of writing and reading medical poems. An example is Gilles of Corbeil's comparison of verse and prose in the prologue to his late twelfth- or early thirteenth-century verse uroscopy, *Carmen de Urinis*:

> In hoc autem opere metrice describuntur urinarum praeceptorum traditiones. Metrica autem oratio succincta brevitate discurrens definitis specificata terminis alligata est certitudini; ideoque confirmat memoriam, corroborat doctrinam. Prosaica vero oratio propria subterfugiens libertate turbat memoriam, ignorantiae parit confusionem. Unde, quae certa ratione debent censeri et expresso commemorationis charactere sigillari, potius metricae brevitatis affectantur compendium, quam prosaicae prolixitatis dispendium.[37]

---

[34] Voigts, 'Medical Prose', p. 317.

[35] Winston Black, '"I will add what the Arab once taught"': Constantine the African in Northern European Medical Verse', in *Herbs and Healers from the Ancient Mediterranean through the Medieval West: Essays in Honor of John M. Riddle* (Farnham, 2012), pp. 153–85 (pp. 155–7).

[36] Black, '"I will add what the Arab once taught"', p. 157. See also Linne Mooney, 'A Middle English Compendium of Astrological Medicine', *Medical History*, 28 (1984), 406–19 (p. 411) and, for a similar point about alchemical verse, see Timmermann, *Verse and Transmutation*, pp. 18, 20, and 21–2.

[37] Aegidii Corboliensis, *Carmina Medica*, ed. by Ludovicus Choulant (Leipzig, 1826), p. 3, lines 6–14.

Now in this work, the traditions of the teachers of urines are described. For verse, which takes its path with succinct brevity and is made precise with well-defined terms, is bound to certainty; and thus it strengthens memory and reinforces instruction. But prose, slippery through its very freedom, disrupts the memory and gives birth to the confusion of ignorance. Therefore, the things that should be judged with solid reasoning and sealed with the sharp imprint of recognition strive more for the economy of metrical brevity than the extravagance of prosaic prolixity.[38]

The mnemonic advantages of verse over prose are forcefully asserted by Gilles: verse encourages brevity, succinctness, and precision. Recent scholarship by Daniel Wakelin has partly corroborated Gilles's assertions, demonstrating through manuscript evidence that verse could encourage scribal attentiveness and accuracy (as well as inhibit it).[39] In the process of describing these practical advantages, however, Gilles also emphasizes their aesthetic qualities: verse moderation and clarity are juxtaposed favourably against prosaic extravagance and disruption. Moreover, the language of sealing ('siligari'), binding ('alligato'), and strengthening ('confirmat') which Gilles uses to describe the enforcing and empowering effects of medical verse is pleasantly visceral, suggesting that verse intertwines the cognitive and somatic more emphatically than prose, rejuvenating the body through its formal properties.[40]

Other medieval accounts also dwell upon the agreeable sensual effects serving pedagogical ends. The following extract is from a thirty-five-line prologue, which is lineated like verse. This prologue survives in only one manuscript and introduces a short Middle English medical treatise given the Latin title *Manuale de Phisica et Cirurgica* by its fifteenth-century scribe:

> Þerfore in þis tretys þat namely is of vrynes
> I wole trete togydere boþe theorik and practyk
> Namely of phisyk and sumwhat of surgery
> So liȝtlyere man to draw in to hem boþe.
> And in metir I it make raþer þan in prose
> Þat it be lustiere to lere & liȝtere to kunne[41]

---

[38] Tavormina, 'Three Middle English Verse Uroscopies', p. 591.
[39] Wakelin, *Scribal Correction*, pp. 220–7. Brantley, 'Forms of the Hours', p. 77 also shows scribes and readers extending and modifying verse calendars with different information.
[40] On connections between memory and binding in other kinds of medieval writing, see Anke Bernau, 'Figuring with Knots', *Digital Philology: A Journal of Medieval Cultures*, 10 (2021), 13–38.
[41] BL, MS Sloane 340, ff. 65v–66r.

This part of the prologue asserts the practical and cognitive advantages of verse: it makes material 'liȝtere', or easier to comprehend, and 'lustiere', more enjoyable and pleasant to learn. Once again, these advantages are described in aesthetic terms: the word 'lustiere', itself artfully connected to 'lere' and 'liȝtere' by alliteration, does not only declare the experience of reading medical poetry pleasant, but, because in Middle English it literally means 'brighter', it also evokes more formal medieval discussions of aesthetic experience. Light was central to medieval ideas of beauty and these theories frequently connect sensual and cognitive experience: Thomas Aquinas argued that for something to be beautiful it needed to possess *claritas* or radiance.[42] This connection was also embedded in the meanings of *illuminen* or, in Latin, *illuminare*, meaning 'to brighten' *and* 'to enlighten morally or intellectually'.[43] By combining pleasure with enlightenment in this way, the prologue evokes the Horatian dictum that poetry should teach *and* delight, as well as the medieval reinterpretation of this formula which claimed that poetry should delight the reader *in order* to make him or her more inclined to learn its lessons.[44]

A sense of irony, though, underpins this prologue's account of the advantages of verse. Neither the prologue nor the text of the *Manuale* are actually written in verse, despite the prologue's layout.[45] Tavormina has suggested that the prologue's composer wrote it out in these unrhymed lines with the intention of rhyming it at a later date.[46] In the above passage, the half-rhyme of 'prose' and 'boþe' in the very lines where the composer is discussing the text's 'metir' perhaps suggests that he was already pondering how that rhyme might work.[47] For whatever reason, though, the composer never did

---

[42] Umberto Eco, *The Aesthetics of Thomas Aquinas* (London, 1988), pp. 102–21; see also Knapp, *Chaucerian Aesthetics*, pp. 36–9.

[43] *MED*, illuminen, v., entries 1, 2; *DMLBS*, illuminare, v., entries 1, 5, 6.

[44] On the popularity of this dictum, see Olson, *Literature as Recreation*, pp. 20–38.

[45] The prologue has irregular line lengths, though *pairs* of lines often have a similar syllable count. The lines, each beginning with a majuscule, do not usually rhyme or alliterate and only a few have a medial point like that in alliterative poetry. Ink braces join pairs of lines together, but sometimes they also draw groups of three lines into a visual pattern on the page: on BL, MS Sloane 340, f. 65v, two short lines and a long line are bracketed together before two sets of two long lines and a short line are bracketed together (length here is measured visually). Much of the main text is written in this style and is frequently disrupted by diagrams and lists not in verse. See CMC, MS Pepys 1236, f. 91r for a medical text with similarly ambiguous verse status.

[46] Tavormina, 'Three Middle English Verse Uroscopies', p. 594.

[47] For another passage from the main text in which the composer experiments with rhyme, see BL, MS Sloane 340, f. 68r: 'Colre is row and gyleful. wraþing hardy and wastful | Sotil. smal and wakful. drie. lusty. and salowe coloured.'

transform the treatise into rhymed or syllabic verse, meaning that the prologue's claim that the text is written 'in metir' seems oddly inaccurate. A similar irony is detectable in Gilles's prologue: although it explains the merits of verse, the prologue is itself written in prose. Perhaps Gilles considered it a useful meta-discursive mode: by virtue of its difference, prose could introduce and defer the effects it discusses, meaning that, when those effects are eventually felt in the main poem, they are felt even more keenly. Alternatively, both ironies might suggest that the advantages of verse over prose were more rhetorical than actual; asserting them was a convention and not a real-world reality. In other words, the prologues were required to train a reader's mind to perceive or—in the prologue to the *Manuale*—imagine from the visual cue of verse lineation, advantages that were not otherwise obvious or palpable. There are clear parallels here with the way in which some of the repetitive prose syntax examined in Chapter 1 worked to simulate—rather than stimulate—the feeling of acquiring new medical knowledge.

This tension between clear-cut rhetoric and complicated practice can be observed in many late medieval meditations on didactic prose and verse. Influential upon them was, of course, Boethius's prosimetric Latin text *De consolatione philosophiae*. In this work, Lady Philosophy suggests that verse and prose perform different roles in Boethius's ethical and spiritual education: prose is the medium used to communicate rational thought, whilst verse is the medium which, through its pleasant sensual qualities, prepares readers for, and relieves them from, the hard, rational work of prose.[48] However, in practice, things are not this straightforward: as scholars have demonstrated, the metrical passages in Boethius's text also perform rational work and the prose passages are aesthetically crafted in the sense that they are 'designed by their style to be sense perceptible'.[49] Eleanor Johnson and Christopher Cannon have shown that this blurring also characterizes late medieval adaptations of *De consolatione*. For instance, in his all-prose translation, Chaucer creates a sensual prose style in which rhetorical prose schemes are used to make the logic of *both* Boethius's prose and verse

---

[48] Boethius, *Anicii Manlii Severini Boethi Philosophiae consolatio*, ed. by Ludwig Bieler (Turnhout, 1957), Bk 1, pr. 1, sent. 7; Bk 1, pr. 5, sent. 11–12; Bk 4, pr. 6, sent 5–7. For discussion of these passages, see Eleanor Johnson, *Practicing Literary Theory in the Middle Ages: Ethics and the Mixed Form in Chaucer, Gower, Usk and Hoccleve* (Chicago, IL, 2013), pp. 19–25.

[49] Johnson, *Practicing Literary Theory*, pp. 25–37.

passages perceptible.[50] Other writers chose to translate the entirety of the prosimetric treatise into verse.[51]

These examples demonstrate that the relationship between verse and prose could be formulated in a great variety of ways in the later Middle Ages: verse could signify much more than memorability and accessibility and, even when those characteristics were explicitly flagged in metatextual prologues, the poems themselves could point towards a multitude of other possible effects—including the cognitive, affective, and aesthetic. Poems could also problematize such claims by showing the qualities of verse ringfenced in prologues to be rhetorical rather than actual and palpable. This capaciousness seems to threaten any rigid prose/verse distinction: both forms could be manipulated for similarly wide-ranging goals and effects. However, because of the distinctive formal properties of prose and verse, those manipulations were of a different kind. The rest of this chapter will demonstrate that medieval writers were sensitive to the distinctive *formal* opportunities that verse offered, even in the humblest, most unassuming medical poems.

Formal Distinctions

The headache remedy below is extracted from a substantial, late fifteenth-century remedy book, which contains a mixture of verse and prose remedies intermingled with one another:

> A medycyn here I have in mynde. For hedde werke to telle as I fynde. To take ayeselle and puliolle ryalle. And camamylle and seethe hit withe alle. And[52] that iouce anoynte thy nassethrellis welle. And make a plaster of that othere deele. And doo hit in a goode grete clowte. . And wynd the hedde therewithe abowte. So sone as hit is layde thereon. Alle the hedde werke awaye schalle gon.[53]

---

[50] Johnson, *Practicing Literary Theory*, pp. 37–91; Christopher Cannon, *The Making of Chaucer's English: A Study of Words* (Cambridge, 1998), pp. 22–31.

[51] Consider, for example, John Walton's ornate verse translation in John Walton, *Boethius: De Consolatione Philosophiae*, ed. by Mark Science, EETS os 170 (London, 1927); for further discussion of Walton's translation process, see Daniel Wakelin, 'Classical and Humanist Translations', in *A Companion to Fifteenth-Century English Poetry*, ed. by Boffey and Edwards, pp. 171–85 (pp. 174–6).

[52] The word 'with' may have been missed here by the scribe.

[53] HEHL, MS HM 64, f. 113va.

[*ayeselle* = vinegar; *puliole ryalle* = pennyroyal (plant) or wild thyme; *nassethrellis* = nostrils; *clowte* = piece of cloth]

The intermingling of prose and verse recipes in this manuscript suggests that the scribe saw the remedies as compatible—connected through subject matter and genre. The fact that the verse remedies are lineated like prose—a common technique for saving space in medieval scribal practice—might also suggest an obliviousness to, or disinterest in, their formal differences. However, this scribe was clearly aware that he was copying verse: he marks each line of verse (except for one) with a rubricated capital at its beginning (marked above in bold) and a punctus at its end.[54] These visual markers clarify the text's form for the reader. The couplets themselves also seem designed to serve a clarifying function: in his analysis of rhyme in late medieval devotional poetry—another kind of practical verse—Daniel Sawyer emphasizes how the alignment of rhyme units with sense units helps to 'emphasize meaning, ease the reading process, and aid memory'.[55] The above passage bears testimony to this: each couplet contains within it one or two stages within the recipe. A stage may be straddled across a couplet, as in the list of ingredients in the second couplet, but it never exceeds the couplet. This alignment breaks the recipe into easily processed chunks and means that, as one moves through the couplets, one experiences a satisfying sense of progress. Indeed, some medieval writers and readers were sensitive to the distinctive clarifying potential of the couplet: in the introduction to his fourteenth-century *Chronicle*, Robert Mannyng claims that if he had written the poem in 'ryme couwee' ('tail-rhyme') or 'enterlace' ('intricate rhymes'), or another 'strangere' form than the couplet, 'som [readers] suld haf ben fordon'.[56]

---

[54] This parallels the blue and red rubrication used to mark verse divisions in Bibles lineated as prose from the thirteenth century onwards: see Carruthers, *The Book of Memory*, pp. 121–2. Daniel Sawyer, *Reading English Verse in Manuscript, c. 1350–1500* (Oxford, 2020), p. 118 notes that 'most examples of verse copied in non-standard lineation are the work of scribes who knew their business and who were careful to punctuate verse as verse'.

[55] Sawyer, *Reading English Verse*, pp. 110, 113–17.

[56] Prologue to Robert Mannyng's *Chronicle*, in *The Idea of the Vernacular: An Anthology of Middle English Literary Theory*, ed. by Jocelyn Wogan Browne (Exeter, 1995), p. 21, lines 45–54. Mannyng does, however, include some tail-rhyme songs within his *Chronicle*, perhaps leading us to question just how absolute a barrier to comprehension he considered more intricate verse forms to be; this is another example of how the perceived advantages and disadvantages of verse forms could be rhetorical rather than actual. On the layout of these forms in one manuscript, see Sawyer, *Reading English Verse*, p. 118.

Further evidence of authorial and scribal sensitivity to form can be found in a verse prologue which appears in at least three manuscripts before a prose remedy book.[57] In one of these manuscripts it is paired with another prologue in prose. The verse prologue is copied after the prose one without any gap in between:

> Here bygynneth gode medecyns for alle manere euel / that any man hath in hys body / that gode leches haue ydrawe out of here bokes / that Balent / Archipeus / Ipocras and galyen / For the were the beste leches / that wern in the worlde / And therfore hoso wylle do as thys bok wyl teche / he may be syker . forto haue help of alle eueles / and woundes // Ipocras made thys bok / hoso wylle ther inne loke / goud hyt wyl hym teche / yf he wyl ther inne rede / the ry3te way hyt wyl hym lede And yf he wyl be a leche / the fyrste way ate the hed he moste begynne / and afterward atte alle othere lymmys //[58]

[*Ipocras* = Hippocrates]

The fact that the scribe of this manuscript includes both a prose and a verse prologue suggests that he saw them serving different functions. In content, the prologues are very similar: both attribute the collection to esteemed medical authorities and assure the reader that the following collection will help him or her to practise medicine. For the scribe, then, the difference must have been formal. This is reinforced by the fact that, despite writing both prologues out in lines like prose, the scribe separates the prose and verse with a double virgule and uses virgules to punctuate each text differently: in the prose prologue he uses virgules to mark main and subordinate clauses as well as items in a list, but in the verse prologue, he uses them to separate individual lines of verse.

The scribe's virgules highlight to a reader the poem's end-rhymes. They do not, however, draw attention to another kind of formal patterning embedded in the poem by its original author. This patterning is better observed by lineating the poem as verse:

> Ipocras made thys bok
> Hoso wylle ther inne loke
> Goud hyt wyl hym teche

---

[57] The other two manuscripts are BL, MS Sloane 3160, f. 153r and BL, MS Sloane 3466, f. 6r.
[58] BodL, MS Laud misc. 685, f. 72v.

Yf he wyl ther inne rede
The ry3te way hyt wyl hym lede
And yf he wyl be a leche
The fyrste way ate the hed he moste begynne
And afterward atte alle othere lymmys

In addition to end-rhyme, the composer of the poem makes heavy use of internal rhyme and parallelism: lines 2 and 4 are syntactically parallel and contain autorhyme and lines 2, 3, 4, 5, and 6 all contain a construction with the verb *will* at its centre. The fact that the prose prologue beforehand also includes a construction containing *hoso* and parallel *will* constructions ('hoso wylle do as thys bok wyl teche') suggests that one prologue was composed in relation to the other. This comparison points to the different formal choices encouraged by verse and prose: a single instance of parallelism in the prose prologue is repeated across five lines in the verse prologue and combined with other internal patterns. Such concentrated internal patterning is a feature of other verse prologues too. For example, a verse introduction written out like prose, and appended to medical writings in at least nine manuscripts, contains this internal, chiastic rhyme: 'wytyþ wel þat þys boke ys gode leche al thyng hit doþ teche.' and do also þis boke þe byt hit techeþ lechys al here wyt' ('know well that this book is a good physician; it teaches all things. And do as this book commands you; it teaches physicians all their wit').[59] The tongue-twisting rhyme ('leche'/'teche'/'techeþ'/'lechys') again suggests that verse encouraged denser, more concentrated syntactic play: this might have been because of the shortness of the line (in contrast to what Gilles of Corbeil calls the 'prolixity' of prose lines) or it might have been because of the opportunity offered by consecutive lines of verse to engage in visual patterning.

In these verse introductions, this blatant sonic and visual patterning performs the 'ornamental' and 'rhetorical' functions that George Keiser associates with medical prologues. But it can also function in longer medical poems as an important cognitive aid. In fact, Derek Pearsall isolates concentrated syntactic play within the unit of the line as a defining feature of didactic poetry; the verse of 'literary' authors such as Chaucer is, he argues, more often characterized by prolixity and syntactic diffuseness.[60] A stanza

---

[59] BodL, MS Laud misc. 553, f. 30v. For a full list of versions, see Keiser, 'Verse Introductions', p. 310.
[60] Pearsall, *Lydgate*, p. 9.

from John Lydgate's 'The Dietary' demonstrates how this patterning can be used to communicate and clarify practical content:

> And yiff so be leechis doth the faile,
> Than take good heed to vse thynges thre,
> Temperat diet, temperat travaile,
> Nat malencolius for non adversite,
> Meeke in trouble, glad in pouerte,
> Riche with litel, content with suffisaunce,
> Nevir grucchyng, mery lik thi degre,
> Yiff phisik lak, make this thi gouernance.[61]

This stanza contains numbered lists (98), parallelism (99, 101, 102), and antithesis (102), all of which might make the verse more memorable. It is also given a satisfying circularity and coherence by the parallel 'Yiff...' constructions in the first and final lines. All of these constructions might be considered 'clarifying', as they are both aesthetically gratifying and cognitively useful, illuminating, underlining, and imprinting upon a reader's mind the sense of the passage.[62]

These examples affirm that, in medical writing, verse was more than prose put into lines that rhyme at their end: more thought was invested in the poems' form. This thoughtfulness can range from the simple (but significant) aligning of rhyme units with sense units to bolder, more brazen displays of crafting, such as internal patterning and syntactic play. Such features, however unsubtle, demonstrate that medical writers were aware of—and exploited—the different expressive possibilities that verse offered from prose.

Tensions

In the headache recipe and Lydgate's 'The Dietary', the meanings produced by the poem's formal features appear to be in harmony with their content, with their proclaimed instructional goal. That relationship, however, is not

---

[61] John Lydgate, 'The Dietary', in *The Minor Poems of John Lydgate: Part II*, ed. by Henry Noble MacCracken, EETS os 192 (London, 1934), p. 705, lines 97–104.

[62] In relation to devotional verse, Sawyer, *Reading English Verse*, p. 110 similarly notes that rhyme can be 'both enjoyable and mnemonically and rhetorically useful—useful because it is enjoyed, and perhaps sometimes enjoyed in part because it is useful'.

always so straightforward in medical writing and this throws up some problems for traditional modes of literary analysis: Derek Attridge notes that the work of modern literary critics, influenced by New Critical and early formalist schools of thought, often follows an analytical model in which form and content are distinct but complementary. He writes, 'it is difficult to verbalize a positive response to the formal features of a [literary] work without using some version of the scheme whereby sound echoes sense, form enacts meaning'.[63] Attridge argues, however, that we should see form as a more active and unpredictable producer of meaning: 'instead of being opposed to content, then, form...includes the mobilization of meanings, or rather of the events of meanings'.[64]

This formal capacity to generate unpredictable meanings is highly relevant to verse recipes and other kinds of anonymous medical poetry where unexpected generations of meaning and tensions between form and content often appear as side-effects of writing in verse that were encountered and negotiated by medical writers, but not deliberately cultivated or fully controlled. Consider, for instance, the vague filler phrases that are frequently employed to complete couplets: after a list of ingredients, a verse headache remedy contains this instruction, 'And menge thes togeders sannes delaye. Al so welle as euer ye maye' ('And mix these together without delay | As well as ever you may').[65] A sense of irony is created because, after recommending urgency in the first line of the couplet, the poet delays the reader's progress through the text with a second line that is, in terms of practical information, meaningless. The formal requirement to complete the couplet stands in tension with the urgency of the medical action.

Ironically, the vague filler phrases completing couplets are often concerned with time. Another rhymed cure for headaches in the same remedy book contains these lines:

> If man or woman more or lesse. In his hedde have grete sickenes.
> Or any grevaunce or any wirkynge. Averuayne he take witheout lettynge.[66]

> [*wirkynge* = pain; *averuayne* = southernwood; *lettynge* = delay]

---

[63] Derek Attridge, *The Singularity of Literature* (London, 2004), p. 108.
[64] Ibid., p. 109.   [65] HEHL, MS HM 64, f. 113vb.
[66] Ibid., f. 113va.

The phrase 'withowte lettyng', though providing a convenient half-rhyme for the tricky 'werkyng', delays readers in their completion of the recommended action, even as it urges haste. Read as circumlocution, these fillers undercut Gilles of Corbeil's claim that brevity is one of verse's distinctive features.

Similar tensions are also produced by a verse bloodletting text copied earlier in the same manuscript and by the same hand as the remedy book. This verse, copied in lines like prose, describes the dangers of letting blood when the moon is in the astrological sign of Aries:

> Biware howe thou the body keytte. For the blode may not to faste out fleitte. Iffe the mone in Ariete be. Kutte not the hed and thou do byme.[67] And in euery leme of the body also Kut not the place the signe longithe to. When that euer the mone <in> that sine be. Kutte not that place and ye do byme. If in alle thes thou be hurte. From dethe thou mayste not lightly sturte. Dayes there bethe and howris also. That causithe men to have moche woo. An eville daye and an eville howre. And the signe that dothe no socowre[68]

[*fleitte* = flow; *leme* = limb; *sturte* = escape]

These rhymed lines, which only survive in this manuscript, may have been excerpted from a longer poem, dealing with more of the zodiac. Alternatively, they may have been intended as a supplement or complement to the more comprehensive Latin astrological prose material in the manuscript.[69] They may actually have been based upon the paragraph in Latin prose that immediately precedes them:

> Caueatis quando luna est in aliquo signno Respondenti membro malum est et maximum periculum ledi in isto membro vt quando est in Ariete malum est ledi in capite et sic de ceteris membris Et eciam (etiam) eadem die ut in die lune et in hora eius ut in prima hora diei et octauo et sic de

---

[67] *Byme* does not appear in the *MED*, but it seems to denote harm and may derive from *bimenen*, to lament or complain (*MED*, *bimenen*, v., entry 1).
[68] HEHL, MS HM 64, f. 13v.
[69] Astrological texts and tables, including information on the astrological positioning of the moon and the sun, occupy ff. 1r–17v. On the folio before the above English verse text (and covering very similar content in a more complete and robust way) is a zodiac man accompanied by an explanatory text in Latin prose: see HEHL, MS HM 64, f. 12v. The text accompanying the zodiac man seems to have been based on a version of John Somer's fourteenth-century *Kalendarium*: see John Somer, *The Kalendarium of John Somer*, ed. by Linne R. Mooney (Athens, GA, 1998), pp. 148–9.

ceteris Respice infra de luna quando est in signis Caueatis a Merte et a Saturno et de horis eorundem.[70]

The first part of this prose text ('Caueatis...et sic de ceteris membris') corresponds very roughly to the first eight lines of the English verse: both instruct the reader in general terms not to cut or injure the body part corresponding to a particular astrological sign when the moon is in that sign. More specifically, both texts warn the reader against cutting the head and the limbs when the moon is in the sign of Aries. After this point, however, the texts diverge: the prose Latin text offers readers slightly more specific advice about dangerous hours and reminds them to beware of the influences of Mars and Saturn too. In contrast, the content of the verse text becomes diluted: lines 9 to 14 read as vague, generic truisms ('Dayes there bethe and howris also. That causithe men to have moche woo. An evill daye and an evill howre. And the signe that dothe no socowre'). These lines are void of any specific instructional content. The compulsion to rhyme seems to have taken priority over the obligation to provide any useful information. The poem's refrain ('Kutte not...')—which could have functioned as a mnemonic aid—only increases this sense of frustrating circularity, of failing to progress towards new knowledge. Perhaps this feeling that the text's verse form had overshadowed and diluted its content was why the scribe only copied (or composed) rhymed lines for Aries, leaving the preceding Latin prose texts and a diagram of a vein man on the following page to explain the rest of the zodiac. This sense of disappointment is heightened by the fact that the subject of the verse is, once again, time: the focus on 'dayes' and 'howris' draws a reader's attention to the time being wasted through empty rhymes.

These examples open up the possibility that ambiguities and disjunctions in the relationship between practical content and impractical form could be a palpable part of the experience of reading instructional verse. That aspect of reading experiences is neglected in accounts of the poems which assume that medieval writers and readers had a fixed set of ideas about the poems' instructional and mnemonic function that was not in any way thwarted, challenged, altered, or adjusted by the actual practice of writing or reading an instructional poem. Medieval readers were clearly sensitive to such frictions between form and content because they noted similar conflicts in other kinds of verse. *The Canterbury Tales* makes this clear when the Host

[70] HEHL, MS HM 64, f. 13v.

responds to the Chaucer Pilgrim's *Tale of Sir Thopas*, a parodic tail-rhyme romance:

> Thou doost noght elles but despendest tyme.
> Sire, at o word, thou shalt no lenger ryme.[71]

[*despendest* = waste]

The Host makes the same connection between rhyme and time-wasting that is evoked by the empty, time-based rhymes in the medical verse above. He then commands the Chaucer Pilgrim to use prose or another type of verse to tell a story that has either 'murthe' or 'doctryne' in it (935). The Host implies that, as a highly structured, repetitive verse form, tail-rhyme can deprive a work of useful or thought-provoking meaning.[72] It is, of course, significant that, in the *Tale of Sir Thopas*, Chaucer ridicules tail-rhyme and not couplets, the latter being a form he adopted in many of his other, more serious works. Nonetheless, his comments are still relevant to the couplet poems I am examining: the filler phrases Chaucer uses in *Sir Thopas*, such as 'as it was Goddes grace' (723) and 'For sothe, as I yow telle may' (749), clearly resemble the empty lines completing the couplets in the medical verse. By using these phrases more frequently in *Sir Thopas* than in his other writings, Chaucer self-consciously highlights the constraints under which verse forms can place writers. Scholars discussing medieval instructional verse in isolation from verse such as Chaucer's tend to forget, however, that all writers were working within similar constraints: even if they wanted to, writers of instructional verse could not invent a new form that would *only* communicate practical 'doctryne', without any accidental circumlocution, dilution of content, and time-wasting. Chaucer recognized this potential friction between 'ryme', 'doctryne', and 'tyme', between verse form and useful content. So why should we assume that readers of instructional poems did not?

---

[71] Geoffrey Chaucer, *The Tale of Sir Thopas*, in *Riverside*, ed. by Benson, lines 931–2. Future line references are within the text.

[72] His comments resemble the argument of modern detractors of rhyme that rhyme, and other rigid verse forms, can constrain thought and perpetuate fixed, narrow ways of seeing the world, some of which are ideologically or politically conservative. For summaries of these views see J. Paul Hunter, 'Formalism and History: Binarism and the Anglophone Couplet', in *Reading for Form*, ed. by Wolfson and Brown, pp. 129–49 (pp. 129–33) and Simon Jarvis, 'Why Rhyme Pleases', *Thinking Verse*, 1 (2011), 17–43.

Artfulness

From the above analysis, one might construct an image of medical versifiers as limited in skill and agency, as individuals incapable of negotiating in creative ways the constraints placed upon them by the couplet form. Consequently, they were compelled to deploy conventional filler phrases that were not their own responses to the formal constraints they were confronting but a response supplied to them by a long verse tradition; these filler phrases in turn opened them up to mockery such as that represented in Chaucer's *Sir Thopas*. But this account of limitation, ridicule, and substandard verse is not the whole story. There are moments in medical poems which suggest more active and thoughtful crafting, even if those moments do not raise the question of agency in any straightforward, answerable way. It is important, however, that we wrestle with these questions and try to develop a critical idiom responsive to the poem's ambiguities and to the kind of appeal they retained for those medieval readers—not insignificant in number—who owned and copied them. Otherwise, our literary canons risk distorting medieval textual culture. As Lisa Cooper writes in relation to Lydgate's more practical, mundane, and material poetry:

> We...continue to privilege some of the tallest trees (Chaucer, Langland, the *Pearl*-Poet) at the expense of the forest, that vast body of material that sits somewhere in between the plainly poetic and the insistently instructional...we continue to give rather short shrift to the many texts whose 'literariness' falls below the high standard we continue to set for medieval writing, the texts that survive in numerous and as-yet-not-fully-documented compilations, the texts that late medieval readers seemed actually eager to be reading, if numbers of surviving manuscripts are any evidence.[73]

Cooper's summary applies not only to Lydgate but also to instructional poems like the verse remedies and the verse herbal. To be sure, it might be anachronistic to consider these as having the same relationship to the 'tallest trees' as a poet such as Lydgate: as already noted, Lydgate's instructional verse intersects closely with practical poetry *and* more explicitly wrought literary works by virtue of its ballade forms, practical subject matter, and

---

[73] Cooper, 'Recipes for the Realm', p. 200.

mixed manuscript context. In contrast, the verse remedy book appears in manuscripts containing verse of a scientific and medical nature. This suggests that the rhymed recipe book was not thought of as possessing the same modal and formal flexibility as Lydgate's works or the same poetic potential. It might thus be thought of as existing in a slightly different compartment of medieval textual culture from the writings of the 'tallest trees'. However, these compartments should not be thought of as absolute or the boundaries between them completely impermeable: instructional poems like the remedy book and verse herbal were sometimes sites of stylistic and modal experimentation, even if it is often difficult to detect a distinctive or consistent shaping hand, mind, and voice behind those moments.

One example of such sporadic crafting is afforded by the different versions of the verse herbal, as changes have been made between versions which subtly alter the style of the text. In most versions that I have consulted, a description of the virtues of betony is recorded (with minor variations) as 'For the hede ake it abriggith and the bytternes | And castith to the eye bryghtnes' ('For it reduces the severity of the headache and the suffering | And lends brightness to the eyes').[74] In another manuscript, though, this couplet is written as: 'It brekis þe hede werke | And gifis bryghtnes to þe syth derke'.[75] Such variations undermine the insistence of Gilles of Corbeil, and more modern commentators, that verse imprints matter upon the memory more emphatically than prose; in practice, verse cannot prevent changes or errors in oral and written transmission, even when, as in the copying of texts, only a short-term kind of memory is required. This is again affirmed by another manuscript witness where a scribe has copied the first version of the couplet as 'Off þe hede ake yt abreggyth þe bytternesse | Also castyþ to þe eye bryȝt <sygt> nesse'.[76] The conventionality and memorability of the rhyme 'bryȝt/sygt' actually misleads the scribe here, again showing that rhyme could be a hindrance to accuracy and retention as much as a help.[77]

The two versions of the couplet are also of interest, though, because they both display signs of more deliberate and thoughtful crafting than the couplets surrounding them: both contain internal half-rhyme ('abriggith'/'castith',

---

[74] TCC, MS R.14.32, f. 136r. Nine out of nineteen manuscripts consulted contained a variation of this version; three contained alternative versions, and seven do not contain these lines on betony at all.
[75] BL, MS Sloane 147, f. 96r.   [76] BL, MS Sloane 1571, f. 20r.
[77] For other instances where verse promotes inaccuracy, see Wakelin, *Scribal Correction*, pp. 220–7.

'brekis'/'gifis') and end-rhyme. They are also stylistically cohesive: the first version is characterized by polysyllabic fullness, whilst the second is characterized by monosyllabic clarity.

Another layer of thoughtfulness is suggested by the possibility that one version may be a conscious rewriting of the other, rather than an error or misremembering: the fact that the couplets are structurally similar but stylistically opposite may suggest that the variation came about because a scribe adapted what he remembered, heard, or found before him in an exemplar regardless of whether or not his source was corrupt. Perhaps this individual found the polysyllabism of 'abriggith' and 'bytternes' out of place in a herbal characterized by simple, accessible English and chose to rewrite it. So, although neither of the versions can be compared to the sophisticated couplets of poets such as Chaucer and Gower, they (and their possible connection to one another) suggest that instructional poets could think actively about stylistic cohesiveness within the unit of the couplet, and could set themselves formal challenges beyond end-rhyme. They also show, once again, that an important part of understanding the artfulness of these texts is comprehending the sporadic, fragmentary, and whimsical nature of that artfulness. There is no clear reason why one couplet in a practical text should be more palpably crafted or densely patterned than another, but this is sometimes the case.

Often, however, medical poems contain aesthetic effects that cannot confidently be proclaimed the products of active craftsmanship *or* the unintended products of formal constraints. Instead, they appear poised between the two. For instance, the verse remedy book frequently contains simple monosyllabic rhymes such as: 'So sone as hit is layde there on. Alle the hedde werke aweye schalle gon'.[78] Elsewhere, however, rhymes seem to work in more sophisticated ways: 'And this dryngke lete hym fastynge dryngke . And alle his heddewerke aweye schalle syngke'.[79] 'Syngke' is far more specific, somatic, and evocative than 'gon'. The same can be said of another couplet that occurs later in the poem: 'And alle the hed werke and the acke. In a litille throwe hit schalle a slacke'.[80] *Slacken*, meaning to end or relieve, also has a strongly somatic edge, often being used in Middle English to refer to the loosening of some kind of constraint.[81]

These rhymes pose and evade the question of agency in several ways. On the one hand, the more evocative and vivid verbs 'syngke' and 'slacke' could

---

[78] HEHL, MS HM 64, f. 113va.   [79] Ibid.
[80] Ibid., f. 113vb.   [81] See *MED*, *slaken*, v., entry 1(a).

be evidence that the limited choice of synonyms afforded by the couplet form compelled writers to select less literal and more polysemous or semantically suggestive words than they would in prose. The couplet form is here the generator of an accidental artfulness. On the other hand, the poem's author might here have asserted his agency over the constraints of the rhyme scheme, by refusing to indulge in vagueness, circumlocution, or triteness for the sake of an easy rhyme; instead he might have carefully negotiated the limited choices afforded by the rhyme scheme in order to select a word that was still appropriate, precise, and evocative. In support of this view is the fact that *sinken* is medically appropriate in this headache remedy: medieval medical theory taught that some headaches were caused by excess humours which produced vapours in the body that then rose up to the head.[82] The headache could be treated by expelling these through openings lower down in the body: in another remedy collection it is written, 'Hit beoueþ þat whan ache lasteþ long in þe heued for to draw matere out be þe mouþ or be þe nose þrilles.'[83] Others recommended diuretics, emetics, laxatives, and bloodletting.[84] Describing the relief of a headache as a downward, sinking movement may, then, have been an attempt to recreate readers' somatic experience accurately. In this interpretation, the author chooses a word that, like most poetic language, exceeds the basic referential function of language, in order to describe and evoke a phenomenon more vividly and create a closer affective relationship with the bodies of readers.

The 'dryngke'/'syngke' rhyme also foregrounds the tension between agency and compulsion because *sinken* and *drinken* are often rhymed together in Middle English poetry. Indeed, their meanings became intwined: as well as the obvious meanings of downward movement and disappearance, *sinken* could be used in Middle English to describe the way impressions are made on the mind and senses, the way alcohol enters the brain, and the movement by which food, drink, and medicine are taken into the body.[85] This semantic interplay between sinking and drinking may be why Chaucer used the rhyme in Book II of *Troilus and Criseyde* when

---

[82] In Trevisa's fourteenth-century translation of Bartholomew the Englishman's *De proprietatibus rerum*, it is written 'Constantinus [seiþ] þat it is good to garse þe legges byneþe, þat þe humours, fumosite, and spiritis þat beþ cause of þe hedeache may be drawe fram þe heed donward to þe neþir parties': Trevisa, *On the Properties of Things*, I, Bk 7, p. 346, lines 10–13.

[83] BL, MS Additional 34111, f. 40v.

[84] Luke Demaitre, *Medieval Medicine: The Art of Healing from Head to Toe* (Santa Barbara, CA, 2013), p. 124.

[85] *MED*, sinken, v., entry 1(a) and 3(b), (c).

Criseyde, feeling the first signs of love, asks herself whether she has been intoxicated:

> Criseÿda gan al his chere aspien,
> And leet it so softe in hire herte synke,
> That to hireself she seyde, 'Who yaf me drynke?'
>
> (II. 649–51)

'Synke' initially refers to the forming of an impression in Criseyde's heart. However, the appearance of 'drynke' in the next line retrospectively draws out *sinken*'s association with absorption and intoxication. A more direct connection between 'syngke', sickness, and absorption occurs in a version of the romance *Guy of Warwick*: 'Thre dayes myȝt he nodur ete nor drynke/ Hyt wolde not in hys body synke'.[86] The verse remedy book offers readers a similar effect: whilst evoking the downward movement of the headache, 'syngke' also interacts semantically with 'dryngke' to recreate the means by which the medical drink will be absorbed into the patient's body. Consequently, the rhyme is at once technical and playful in tone.

Did the author intend all these associations or were they the unforeseen effects of a common rhyme? We cannot know. Ambiguity over whether such interplay was intentional does not, though, prevent a reader from experiencing its effects: the rhyme assists—through sonic and semantic interplay—in the practical tasks of comprehension and recall, but it is also aesthetically pleasing because the separate lines of the couplet are brought into balance, harmony, and intersection in multiple ways simultaneously. In an essay on Alexander Pope's eighteenth-century couplets, Simon Jarvis argues that we must stop reducing rhyme to a two-dimensional trifle, or careless automatism that 'cannot itself be admitted to be a kind of thinking or involved in noticing'.[87] Rather, rhyme's effects are 'indissociably ideal, conceptual, semantic, syntactic, phonological, phonetic, material, contingent...Rhyme sounds on all these instruments at once'.[88] This is not only true of the 'great rhyming authorship[s]' but can also apply, at times, to those practical verses which modern literary canons have marginalized as

---

[86] *The Romance of Guy of Warwick: The Second or Fifteenth-Century Version—Part One*, ed. by Julius Zupitza, EETS es 25 (London, 1875), p. 284, lines 9901–2.
[87] Jarvis, 'Why Rhyme Pleases', p. 24.   [88] Ibid., pp. 19–20.

poems of the least aesthetically appealing or cognitively challenging kind.[89] Medieval medical verse was not always, only, or consistently 'doggerel'.

Literary Voices and Intertextual Experimentation

The final literary fragment of medical verse to be explored in this chapter is voice, because it offers the clearest evidence of deliberate stylistic and modal experimentation. To a far greater extent than prose, verse seems to have encouraged writers to experiment with the assumption of different kinds of voice. Consider this prologue which is attached, alongside other verse and prose prologues, to a large collection of medical recipes written in English prose, copied in the fifteenth century, and entitled *Speculum medicorum*:

> Mislike it noght to þe þo I be of litel bodi
> For þis litel short begynnyng bereþ profitable þinges
> Many iproued bien here of wisemen befor tyme
> Gladly tak þow here þe þenges þat þou seest best
> Doyng sheweþ where of þe medicines bien
> Draw þo to þe and þat mislykeþ þow fle
> ʒif þow be riche seke þo þat be most worþe
> And ʒif þow wanteþ auer chese þat þou may
> No dispise vs noʒt for foule whan þou seest herbes
> þe leche of heuene whose hond ʒiffiþ alle þing
> Sheweþ wonders in herbes þo it be noʒt so to þe[90]

[*iproued* = proved; *doyng* = putting (the recipes) into practice; *þat mislykeþ* = that which displeases; *wanteþ auer* = lack wealth; *chese* = choose]

This English prologue—unrhymed but lineated in the surviving manuscript as verse—is a translation of the pseudo-Ovidian Latin verse prologue in elegiac couplets which immediately precedes it in the manuscript and which had circulated separately alongside Latin medical treatises since the twelfth century.[91] What is remarkable about this prologue and its Latin verse source

---

[89] Ibid., p. 19.   [90] BL, MS Additional 34111, f. 40r.
[91] On the twelfth-century circulation of the Latin prologue alongside a variety of earlier Latin medical treatises, see Klaus-Dietrich Fischer, 'A Mirror for Deaf Ears? A Medieval Mystery', *The Electronic British Library Journal* (2008), 1–16. Fischer shows that the

is the use of prosopopoeia: the verse prologues examined earlier personified remedy books as physicians and teachers ('þys boke ys gode leche al thyng hit doþ teche'), but in this introduction the 'boke' or prologue speaks for itself, commanding the reader not to dislike its 'bodi', its shape and size. The playful aptness of a medical prologue describing itself as a body is clear. In Old English riddles inanimate objects are often made to speak and, in later medieval literary writings, prosopopoeia (understood in the broad medieval sense of an imagined or absent person, abstract concept, or inanimate object speaking) is also common, appearing frequently in allegorical writings such as *Le Roman de la Rose*.[92] Several examples of narrators *imagining* what rings or books might say to patrons and loved ones also occur in late medieval verse.[93] However, very few depictions of books actually speaking survive before the establishment of print.[94]

Listening again to the above prologue, one might also detect other poetic voices. The prologue instructs the reader not to 'mislike' its brevity and, a few lines later, to avoid any remedies that 'mislykeþ' (or displease) him or her, producing an alliterative pattern not present in the Latin original. The verbs are both in prominent positions, drawing the reader's attention to them: one is the first word of the prologue and the other occurs near the centre of the prologue's central line. Because of such explicit patterning, it is possible to hear echoes of the stanza at the end of *Troilus and Criseyde* in which Chaucer addresses his 'litel boke' with the words, 'So prey I God that non myswrite the, | Ne the mysmetre for defaute of tonge' (V. 1795–6).[95]

---

fifteenth-century remedy collection to which this English prologue is attached is a translation of one of these earlier Latin treatises. He also traces the Latin source of the prose prologue that appears in the manuscript. As far as is known, this manuscript contains the only surviving witnesses of these English prologues, and as George Keiser suggests, they may well be the scribe's own translations. Keiser argues, however, that the above English prologue—though a translation of verse and lineated as verse—should not be considered as verse itself. See Keiser, 'Verse Introductions', pp. 305–6.

[92] *DLMBS, prosopopoeia*, n., entries 1, 2.

[93] E.g. *Secular Lyrics of the XIV*[th] *and XV*[th] *Centuries*, ed. by Rossell Hope Robbins, 2nd edn (Oxford, 1964), pp. 87, 92.

[94] A Latin ownership note in which a book 'speaks' is discussed in *A Middle English Translation from Petrarch's Secretum*, ed. by Edward Wilson with an introduction by Daniel Wakelin, EETS os 351 (Oxford, 2018), pp. xviii–xix.

[95] As Wakelin, *Scribal Correction*, p. 30 points out, the scribe of a set of ordinances for London's Mercers' Company between 1442 and 1443 composes a rime royale stanza in imitation of Chaucer's, which jokingly compares the scribe's civic production to Chaucer's poetic creation: 'Go litel boke go litel tregedie | The lowly submitting to al correccioun'. This suggests that scribes of many different kinds of 'practical' text could be interested in stylistic exchanges and experimentation. The stanza is transcribed in full in P.R. Robinson, ed., *Catalogue of Dated and Datable Manuscripts*, 2 vols (London, 2003), I, 58.

Perhaps the translator of the medical prologue recalled this stanza not only because Chaucer addresses another 'litel boke', a modesty topos with a long history, but also because he uses apostrophe, a trope which is the opposite of prosopopoeia since it can involve speaking to, rather than speaking as, an inanimate object.

Evidence that medical writers and scribes experimented with the importation of different literary voices also appears in a copy of the verse herbal discussed earlier. In a manuscript copied in the late fourteenth or early fifteenth century, the verse herbal is copied after a poem on bloodletting. The two are connected by the rubricated lines: 'And now and ȝe wollen dwelle | The uirtues of the lylye I schal ȝow telle' ('And now, if you will dwell | The virtues of the lily I will you tell').[96] In these added lines, the two poems are reimagined on the page as oral performances within a physical space where an audience might 'dwelle'. Similar rubricated links have also been written by the scribe of this manuscript between discussions of different herbs. A selection of these are transcribed below:

> And now and ernest and an game
> I schal telle the virtues of henbane
>
> ...
>
> Withouten any envie
> Y schal telle of astrologye
>
> ...
>
> Do now and ful the bolle
> And ȝe schal here of pympurnolle
>
> ...
>
> And now ȝong and also holde
> Takeþ hede of the uirtues of marigolde[97]

[*and ernest and an game* = in seriousness and in play; *astrologye* = a medicinal plant of various kinds, perhaps galingale; *pympurnolle* = variety of pimpernel or burnet plant]

These links—which do not appear in other versions of the herbal that I have examined—extend the oral element already present in other copies of the

---

[96] BL, MS Sloane 2457/2458, f. 2r–v.
[97] BL, MS Sloane 2457/2458, ff. 4r–6v. In the nineteen manuscripts I have consulted this is the only copy containing these links.

poem: we now not only have a speaking 'I', but an 'I' who makes reference to props such as a drinking bowl ('bolle') and an in-house audience ('ʒong and al so holde').[98] These links might be rare evidence that the herbal was intended to be performed aloud from the codex for the entertainment or edification of an audience; they might thereby return us to the common critical conception of verse medical texts as poems to be memorized and orally transmitted.[99] And yet, in the late medieval period, this oral framing could function as a stylistic convention of romances, chronicles, and lyrics, rather than as evidence of, or stimulus for, a real-world performance.[100] The insertions could, then, have appeared to some readers as a conscious creative adornment, diversifying the rhetorical texture of the herbal by drawing it closer to other types of verse writing. The rubrication of the additions certainly functions as a visual embellishment, reframing and adorning the text on the page.

It is easy to see why writing in verse—a form that is explicitly musical and invites voicing, whether orally or internally—may have sensitized poets' minds to the possibilities of this kind of vocal play: verse, more than prose, invites one to consider (and manipulate) *who* is speaking and to whom. Such manipulations not only shape how something is being said but also *what* is being said. For instance, in medical verse, vocal play can encourage a particular kind of uncertain and doubting voice. The following lines appear in at least two copies of the verse herbal under the section on rose. Within them, a writer (and reader) has versified his uncertain response to his source material and incorporated it into his copy of the herbal:[101]

> Wheþer it is soth or it ne is
> I seye noʒt but as þe bok me wys.

---

[98] Although these links have (to my knowledge) received no literary critical attention, Jake Walsh Morrissey, 'Unpublished Verse Rubrics in a Middle English *Receptarium*' (British Library, MS Sloane 2457/2458)', *Notes and Queries*, 61 (2014), 13–15, has noted a few similar verse rubrics later in the manuscript which introduce individual recipes.

[99] On evidence for public readings in late medieval England, see Joyce Coleman, *Public Reading and the Reading Public in Late Medieval England and France* (Cambridge, 1996).

[100] E.g. see 'Fill the boll, butler', in *Medieval English Lyrics: A Critical Anthology*, ed. by R.T. Davis (London, 1963), pp. 276–7. See also Robert Mannyng's fourteenth-century *Chronicle*, in *The Idea of the Vernacular*, ed. by Wogan Browne, p. 20, lines 3–6.

[101] In the nineteen manuscripts I have consulted, this version only appears in SKB, MS X90, pp. 49–78 (consulted in Stephens, ed., *Extracts in Prose and Verse*, pp. 364–93) and CMC, MS 1661, pp. 288–309. Some of the other versions do not contain this section on rose at all or only contain an abridged version: for examples of the rose section without these lines see BL, MS Sloane 147, ff. 103v–104v and BRB, MS Takamiya 46, ff. 8v–9v.

> Þe autowurs name þat þis wroth
> Þe bok wythnessit ryth noth.[102]

These lines might reflect the anxiety of a real scribe and reader, but the 'I' which speaks them is also a construct, a product of the verse medium and its connections to orality: hence the construction 'I seye noȝt' rather than 'I write not'. It is possible that this explicit declaration of uncertainty, which is not paralleled in the confident, third-person attributions to medical authorities found in prose herbals, was facilitated and partly encouraged by verse's self-conscious oral style, as that first-person framing immediately encourages a writer to consider his or her own relationship with, and attitude to, the knowledge he or she has received: it frames that knowledge as mediated, transmissible, and potentially corruptible. A similar uncertainty is also detectable in other parts of the verse herbal. After a list of the various medical and miscellaneous virtues of henbane, the following lines are sometimes copied:[103]

> But of henbane be kendes thre
> I am in dowte qwich he schulde be
> For ther is of hem rede . yelwe . and blake
> And alle bene wykkyd of odour and smake[104]
>
> [smake = taste or smell]

The uncertainty in this passage contrasts with the precise, detailed, or certain descriptions of plant varieties that one finds in other sections of the herbal and in prose herbals. It is understandable why the author of these lines may have been wary: black henbane, which has toxic and narcotic properties, was treated with caution in many Middle English herbal writings. In the fourteenth-century English translation of Bartholomew the

---

[102] Stephens, ed., *Extracts in Prose and Verse*, p. 378, lines 951–4.
[103] On sources for the miscellaneous tricks using henbane, see Jake Walsh Morrissey, 'An Unnoticed Fragment of *A Tretys of Diverse Herbis* in British Library, MS Sloane 2460, and the Middle English Career of Pseudo-Albertus Magnus' *De Virtutibus Herbarum*', *Neuphilologische Mitteilungen*, 115 (2014), 153–61.
[104] TCC, MS R.14.32, f. 139v. See also BL, MS Additional 17866, f. 12r; BL, MS Sloane 1571, f. 28r; BL, MS Sloane 2457/2458, f. 4v; TCC, MS R.14.51, f. 41v; CMC, MS Pepys 1661, p. 303 (variant phrasing); BRB, MS Takamiya 46, f. 10v. A similar expression of uncertainty occurs on SKB, MS X. 90, p. 67, edited in Stephens, ed., *Extracts in Prose and Verse*, p. 382, lines 1065–9: 'Of hennebane arn spycys iij. | I schal ȝow telle whyche it be, | There is red ȝelw and blac... No ferþere tellyth þe bok of here kende'.

Englishman's *De proprietatibus rerum*, it is proclaimed 'venemous'.[105] However, it is still significant that, instead of glossing over this uncertainty or omitting the passage entirely, the writer draws explicit attention to it with the line 'I am in dowte qwich he schulde be'. This voice parallels that of the kind of 'dull' narrator which David Lawton claims characterizes late medieval poetry: he describes this narrator as '"lewed", "rude", lacking in "cunnyng"... in a word dull'.[106]

We see different versions of this kind of bumbling, uncertain narrator in the writings of many fourteenth- and fifteenth-century European writers, such as Chaucer, Machaut, and Hoccleve. One particularly close parallel for the above passage occurs in Chaucer's *House of Fame*, where the narrator, paraphrasing contemporary scientific writings on dream lore, recounts different types of dream:

> Why that is an avision
> And why this a revelacion,
> Why this a drem, why that a sweven,
> And noght to every man lyche even;
> Why this a fantome, why these oracles,
> I not; but whoso of these miracles
> The causes knoweth bet then I,
> Devyne he; for I certeinly
> Ne can hem noght...[107]

Just as the flowers of henbane can be red, yellow, and black, a dream can be a vision, a revelation, or a phantom. In both instances, explicit attention is drawn to the narrator's uncertainty or 'dowte', to his inability to sort, process, and apply the information he receives.

Lawton claims that Chaucer uses such dullness as 'a playful means of making authorship and authority... problematic', and this reading is certainly applicable to the *House of Fame*: the narrator's uncertainty shows that the scientific theories of *auctores* do not always fit the experience of the layman.[108] In contrast, the author of the passage on henbane probably did not

---

[105] Trevisa, *On the Properties of Things*, II, Bk 17, p. 977, line 11. See also *A Middle English Translation of Macer Floridus de viribus herbarum*, ed. by Gösta Frisk (Uppsala, 1949), p. 173, lines 9–14.
[106] David Lawton, 'Dullness and the Fifteenth Century', *ELH*, 54 (1987), 761–99 (p. 762).
[107] Geoffrey Chaucer, *The House of Fame*, in *Riverside*, ed. by Benson, lines 7–15.
[108] Lawton, 'Dullness', pp. 762–4.

wish to make authority problematic as part of a rhetorical point; if he was genuinely unsure about the three varieties of henbane and unable to consult another source, he perhaps considered it safer to communicate uncertainty to his readers than simply to omit the material. Nonetheless, it seems plausible that he was encouraged to include such uncertainty within his herbal, a genre that, in its prose form, usually dealt with certainties, because the speaking 'I' encouraged by verse's musicality immediately framed such knowledge as mediated and uncertain, and because a voice characterized by doubt and struggling with questions of textual integrity was already widespread in late medieval literary verse. This was one of the many voices in medieval literary culture which, as Lawton's work has shown, were ripe for assumption, inhabitation, and reinvention.[109] There is, of course, a neat irony here: composers of medical verse are usually thought of as genuine, unknowing versions of Lawton's dull narrator, having the same 'limited competence in feeling and in poetry, in rhetoric and in rhyme'.[110] This reading raises the possibility, however, that those authors have deployed that 'dull' voice in a creative and resourceful way to negotiate the tensions between uncertainty and instruction.

The distinctive modes of communicating medical content which verse promoted are not, then, superficial or inconsequential, as they shaped how that content, and the authority behind it, were understood by readers. But many of the examples of artistic shaping that I have examined in this chapter have hovered between, on the one hand, conscious craft and witty play and, on the other, a less thoughtful and less skilful deployment of conventional verse tics; even the deployment of an uncertain, doubting voice may have been the result of unconscious osmosis rather than conscious importation. I have tried to remain sensitive to that tension and to remain alert to the temptation verse presents to overread a text: the smallest hint of (re)arranging language to produce rhyme and rhythm is liable to make a close reader see the evidence and effects of crafting everywhere. Consequently, this chapter has consistently acknowledged the 'simplicity' of the poems, recognizing that the formal patterning they contain is sometimes less subtle, intricate, or consistent than that in other literary works.

Such simplicity is not, though, incompatible with complexity: the tensions and shifting dynamics often palpable between the avowedly practical

---

[109] See David Lawton, *Voice in Later Medieval English Literature: Public Interiorities* (Oxford, 2017).
[110] Lawton, *Voice*, p. 162.

content of the verse and its crafted forms mean that the writing, copying, reading, memorizing, and performing of the poems should not automatically be considered straightforward or one-dimensional acts. Sometimes the form will assist in communicating and clarifying content, but at other times it will impede or distract from that content, or supplement its communication with added entertainment and pleasure. This may seem obvious: forms, literary or otherwise, never just fulfil a single purpose. But when it comes to didactic verse, we must not overlook this, distorting the complex ways in which a seemingly simple form can work in practice in favour of an established, but unnuanced, mnemonic model. Writing about late medieval spiritual miscellanies, Vincent Gillespie has commented that 'many religious texts in the vernacular, and particularly those in verse, seem uneasy about the conditions or use for which they are designed'.[111] A similar uncertainty characterizes verse medical texts: the evidence amassed in this chapter indicates that they could simultaneously have seemed outdated *and* up to date, popular in some contexts *and* decreasing in circulation in others, useful *and* whimsical, conventional *and* adaptable, crudely crafted *and* playfully experimental. Chapter 3 continues to attend to this uncertainty and to the multiple, polysemous ways in which forms can function, but—rather than focusing on literary fragments—it turns its attention to the cumulative, compilatory nature of remedy books.

---

[111] Vincent Gillespie, *Looking in Holy Books: Essays in Late Medieval Religious Writing in England* (Turnhout, 2011), p. 129.

PART II
COLLECTING FRAGMENTS

3
The Idea of the Remedy Collection

In her exploration of the 'psychopathology' of writing, Juliet Fleming offers an escape from the functional:

> A woman may pen a novel, fill out a form, or sign her name, not for an instrumental reason but because she wants to write...Now our woman writes to fill a gap or dominate an environment, or because she has an impulse to measure, stretch, cover, cut, fit, join, contain, open, close, begin, end, or repeat...nothing can close this list.[1]

Writing can have a multitude of motives besides promoting and facilitating action in the world. Of course, many authors, scribes, and compilers of medieval remedy collections probably did intend their books to facilitate healing action: a sixteenth-century reader seems to testify to this when he or she writes 'vse' next to a remedy from the previous century for the scab.[2] However, there is something ironically *im*practical about the act of writing that verb: it defers the practical action it simultaneously records. The example thus anticipates in miniature an argument that this chapter will make about various features of manuscript remedy books: a complex combination of motives often seem to lie behind a simple, physical act of mark-making.

So far, this study has focused on the plurality of effects that individual recipes and parts of recipes could have had on readers. In this chapter, I turn my attention to material acts of collecting, copying, arranging, and navigating large numbers of recipes, shifting my emphasis from fragments to patchwork accumulations, from a smaller scale to a larger one. Furthermore, whilst remaining sensitive to the diverse interpretations particular textual manipulations could invite from readers, I pay more explicit attention to the *motivations* driving those acts of writing, compiling, and reading. This chapter contends that, as cumulative texts, copied and arranged

---

[1] Juliet Fleming, *Cultural Graphology: Writing After Derrida* (Chicago, IL, 2016), p. 31.
[2] BodL, MS Ashmole 1477, Part I, f. 35v.

in manuscripts, recipe collections are more opaque and polysemous than scholars have appreciated: frequently, the tangible form and visual layout of remedy books suggest that the needs and motivations driving the emergence of the collection were multiple, mixed, contradictory, or changing.

The evidence for these divergent motivations resides in textual, formal, palaeographical, and codicological features such as the script deployed, the presence or absence of finding aids, the presentation, ordering, arrangement, and accrual of recipes, and readers' annotations. In recent years, there have been calls for literary critics to pay more attention to these material or paratextual features and to understand them as opaque signs that lend themselves to close reading and interpretation. For example, Arthur Bahr and Alexandra Gillespie have called for a new type of formalism that incorporates, instead of opposing, book history, and which requires 'more discussion of the forms of books in literary criticism, and yet more imaginative, critical approaches to those forms'.[3] Daniel Wakelin has echoed this, calling for analysis of 'the forms and aesthetics of books in a literary-critical vein'.[4]

Until now, such attention has often been directed onto manuscripts transmitting literary writings. Bahr and Gillespie raise 'a question that has been important to work on medieval English manuscripts for some time, *especially those bearing literary texts*: what is the relationship between the study of medieval books and the study of medieval literature?'[5] Helen Marshall and Peter Buchanan's essay on the relationship between book history and formalist criticism—'New Formalism and the Forms of Middle English Literary Texts'—has a similar focus upon the literary.[6] Consider too the substantial amount of critical attention devoted to compilations, anthologies, and miscellanies. Whilst some studies have focused on the ways different kinds of text—literary, practical, and devotional—come together to form household compilations, many have focused specifically on how such compilations shape the experience of reading *literary* texts.[7] For

---

[3] Bahr and Gillespie, 'Medieval English Manuscripts', p. 360.
[4] Wakelin, *Scribal Correction*, p. 15. See also Marshall and Buchanan, 'New Formalism' and Caroline Levine, *Forms: Whole, Rhythm, Hierarchy, Network* (Princeton, NJ, 2015), where a more creative literary-critical approach to textual, social, and political forms is advocated.
[5] Bahr and Gillespie, 'Medieval English Manuscripts', p. 346.
[6] Marshall and Buchanan, 'New Formalism'.
[7] On compilations see Seth Lerer, 'Medieval English Literature and the Idea of the Anthology', *PMLA*, 118 (2003), 1251–67; Ralph Hanna, 'Miscellaneity and Vernacularity: Conditions of Literary Production in Late Medieval England', in *The Whole Book: Cultural Perspectives on the Medieval Miscellany*, ed. by Stephen G. Nichols and Siegfried Wenzel (Ann Arbor, MI, 1996), pp. 37–51; Boffey, 'Bodleian Library, MS Arch Selden B.24'; Julia Boffey and A.S.G. Edwards, 'Towards a Taxonomy of Middle English Manuscript Assemblages', in *Insular*

instance, Arthur Bahr's concept of 'compilational reading', which will be extremely helpful in the final three chapters of this study, offers a means of thinking about how readers can 'bring comparable interpretive strategies to bear on the formal characteristics of both physical manuscripts and literary works', detecting in both the same 'discontinuities and excesses, multiple and shifting meanings...and openness to re-reading'.[8] Working on a smaller scale, Ingrid Nelson has explored the connection between literary form and compilational practice across versions of the Middle English poem 'Erthe toc of erthe': breaking down any fixed opposition between form and practice, text and material manifestation, Nelson considers the 'practice of dilation'— the way in which writers expand and clarify existing forms—as integral to literary effects.[9]

Both of these studies have informed my response to remedy books' ambiguous textual and material forms because recipe collections frequently appear as expansive and incomplete (or incomple*table*) compilations of knowledge. However, in extending the reach of this literary-critical analysis to the textual and material features of such 'practical' compilations, I have had a much smaller, but still highly illuminating, circle of studies to draw upon.[10] These include Sarah Star's analysis of the polyvocal, compilatory style of the uroscopy writer Henry Daniel and Chiara Crisciani's examination of the different attitudes found in scholastic medical genres to novelty, progress, and the accretion of new knowledge.[11] Furthermore, by examining the intermingling of genres in encyclopaedic compendiums, Emily Steiner has highlighted the craftsmanship that can be born from compendiousness, claiming that it is the encyclopaedias' 'very drive to compendiousness' that generates lyrical additions, 'producing language and form in excess of what use requires'.[12] Finally, in the more material, cumulative terrain of recipes,

---

Books: Vernacular Manuscript Miscellanies in Late Medieval Britain, ed. by Margaret Connolly and Raluca Radulescu (Oxford, 2015), pp. 263–80.

[8] Bahr, *Fragments and Assemblages*, p. 10.

[9] Ingrid Nelson, 'Form's Practice: Lyrics, Grammars, and the Medieval Idea of the Literary', in *The Medieval Literary Beyond Form*, ed. by Meyer-Lee and Sanok, pp. 35–60.

[10] Useful studies concerned with early modern scientific material include Mari-Liisa Varila, 'In Search of Textual Boundaries: A Case Study on the Transmission of Scientific Writing in 16th-Century England' (unpublished doctoral thesis, University of Turku, 2016) and Ann Blair, *Too Much to Know: Managing Scholarly Information Before the Modern Age* (New Haven, CT, 2010).

[11] Star, 'Textual Worlds', pp. 191–216; Chiara Crisciani, 'History, Novelty and Progress in Scholastic Medicine', *Osiris*, 6 (1990), 118–39.

[12] Steiner, 'Compendious Genres', p. 87. See also Brantley, 'Forms of the Hours', pp. 61–84, which argues that the calendars in medieval books of hours focus readers' attention on their crafting through the juxtaposition of different material forms, such as text and image.

Peter Murray Jones has observed that collections of *experimenta* (medical remedies, practical jokes, optical illusions, and household tips) often occur in codicologically complex experimental books in which a particular 'starter' text from the book-of-secrets tradition has encouraged the subsequent accumulation of other recipes.[13] Here, recipe collections almost appear self-generating: the ownership and preservation of one recipe seems to stimulate the copying of others.

Building upon the specific focuses of these articles, this chapter attempts to show that *many* material and paratextual features of remedy compilations are best illuminated through close literary-critical analysis. After all, remedy books' visible and tangible collectiveness immediately raises formal questions for modern readers: why are there this number of recipes? Why are these recipes copied in the order that they are? How does the collection's organization or *mise-en-page* suggest that a reader was expected to engage with it in a particular way? The fact that the same recipes reappear from manuscript to manuscript in different orders, scripts, and navigational systems is a reminder that, in each collection, a specific formal decision was made from a multitude of choices.

My argument, therefore, is paradoxical. I contend that remedy collections are unusual because they draw a reader's attention to these formal questions so explicitly. And yet they need not always be discussed in isolation from other text-types.[14] Instead, they can contribute to broader discussions about medieval conceptions of order, textual integrity, and aesthetic experience. Paying closer attention to remedy books' material forms also allows modern readers to speculate more about the links between book, body, and mind. Personal notebooks and household compilations often appear to have been produced by an individual or group over extensive periods of time. Consequently, although they cannot be thought of as unmediated or uncomplicated channels for self-expression, they might be linked to medieval ideas of 'affect' as delineated by Holly Crocker: best compared to the modern term 'structures of feeling', affects 'organized abstract categories or...[the] nodes of subjectivity that intersected to form personal identity'; although affects were 'larger, longer-worn circuits of identity formation' than emotions, they still enveloped experiences of hope, fear,

---

[13] Peter Murray Jones, '*Experimenta*, Compilation and Construction in Two Medieval Books', *Poetica*, 91 and 92 (2019), 61–80.
[14] This is the case in studies such as Mooney, 'Manuscript Evidence' and Voigts, 'Scientific and Medical Books'.

despair, and resolution, which need not interact in the subject in consistent or coherent ways.[15] Affects therefore provide a useful lens for thinking about unwieldy and expansive remedy books which display organizational features and navigational systems that were sustained over time, but were also inconsistent and changing. Perhaps their inconsistent, opaque, and polysemous nature was not only the result of varying material circumstances and shifting practical priorities, but also of changing interactions between hope, fear, impatience, and resolution.

Opaque Signs

The narrative generally accepted in medieval scholarship—and testified to by many different kinds of manuscript—is that navigational aids designed to help readers locate particular material within a text or codex became increasingly sophisticated and commonplace between the twelfth and fifteenth centuries.[16] Tables of contents were regularly deployed from the thirteenth century onwards and compiling indexes became more popular in the fourteenth and fifteenth centuries.[17] The manuscript organization and *mise-en-page* of a large number of late medieval remedy books affirm that these finding aids were being deployed in vernacular books, of both an intellectual and domestic bent, and in those with uncertain or ambiguous links to academic learning environments. Consider the manuscript Oxford, Bodleian Library, MS Ashmole 1443, in which a single fifteenth-century hand has copied the majority of the following texts: a text describing place value in decimals; a short, informal collection of medical recipes; *The Wise Book of Philosophy and Astronomy*, which contains information about human complexions and celestial influences upon them; an English version of the Latin herbal *Circa instans*; a medical treatise composed of large numbers of recipes organized by ailment and preceded by short, theoretically inflected paragraphs of aetiological, diagnostic, and prognostic information;

---

[15] Holly Crocker, 'Medieval Affects Now', *Exemplaria*, 29 (2017), 82–98 (p. 84).

[16] The most influential account remains Parkes, *Scribes, Scripts and Readers*, pp. 35–70. For a summary of the debates and defences Parkes's argument has provoked see A.J. Minnis, 'Nolens Auctor Sed Compilator Reputari: The Late Medieval Discourse of Compilatio', in *La méthode critique au Moyen Âge*, ed. by Mireille Chazan and Gilbert Dahan (Turnhout, 2006), pp. 47–63. See also Sawyer, *Reading English Verse*, pp. 52–80 for an account of different kinds of discontinuous reading, which nuances the idea that 'the history of reading is...a teleological narrative of ever-increasing sophistication' (p. 53).

[17] Parkes, *Scribes, Scripts and Readers*, pp. 53–4, 62–3.

a Latin plague tract by John of Burgundy as well as an English translation; an additional note on treating the plague; and a large collection of surgical recipes.[18]

This selection is already revealing. *The Wise Book of Philosophy and Astronomy* is a vernacular encyclopaedic text which was owned, read, and used by people from different social and intellectual circles.[19] Similarly, the herbal *Circa Instans*, which in its original Latin form is believed to have been written by a Salernitan physician, was translated into multiple vernaculars; it has attracted critical comment for its user-friendliness and accessibility to a broad, non-specialist audience.[20] The presence of Latin and English versions of John of Burgundy's plague tract might also suggest a reader not fully comfortable with Latin or an awareness on the part of the compiler that the book was going to be used by individuals (perhaps students, apprentices, friends, or family members) with limited Latin literacy.

What more can we deduce about the owner of this manuscript or the original author(s) of the remedy collections within it? The two large recipe collections suggest that whoever originally wrote or compiled them (either in this manuscript or an earlier source manuscript) was a medical practitioner, operating within the community and wide-ranging in his expertise: in the medical treatise composed of recipes and short theoretical explanations, a first-person 'I' not only claims to have witnessed, read, or heard cures by learned 'doctours', but also frequently claims that he has proved the efficacy of cures, with impressive affirmations such as 'þus curyd y a gentil woman of dyuers euelis in eyne' and this eye remedy was 'by þe duces of ȝork preuid'.[21] A first-person voice also appears in the surgical remedy collection, which includes phrases such as 'myne mastir put þer to... and fond hit gode'.[22] The appearance of this first-person voice in both substantial remedy collections makes it possible that—either in this manuscript or its exemplar—a practitioner with wide-ranging expertise wrote, or at least

---

[18] For the contents, see *A Handlist of Manuscripts Containing Middle English Prose in the Ashmole Collection, Bodleian Library*, ed. by L.M. Eldredge (Cambridge, 1992), pp. 72–4. The original manuscript pages, heavily damaged and incomplete in places, have been pasted onto new leaves.

[19] *The Middle English Wise Book of Philosophy and Astronomy: A Parallel Text Edition— Edited from London, British Library, MS Sloane 2453 with a Parallel Text from New York, Columbia University, MS Plimpton 260*, ed. by Carrie Griffin (Heidelberg, 2013), pp. lv–lxv.

[20] Iolanda Ventura, 'Il "Circa instans" attribuito a Platearius: trasmissione manoscritta, redazioni, criteri di costruzione di un'edizione critica', *Revue d'Histoire des Textes*, 10 (2015), 249–362.

[21] BodL, MS Ashmole 1443, pp. 197, 210, and 214.   [22] Ibid., pp. 422–3.

adapted, *both* recipe collections and incorporated into them examples from personal experience.

There are some ambiguous clues to the kind of practitioner he may have been: the first-person 'I' not only refers to 'myne mastir' but also refers frequently to other masters in the medical and surgical collections, including a 'Mastir Rychard Salysbery'.[23] References in surviving records to a physician of this name refer to a well-connected practitioner of the late fourteenth century who seems to have treated the diplomat and poet John Clanvowe.[24] At one point the scribe writes, 'þis wastir (sic. watir?) was mastir mastir Richardys drynk þat he vsyd in wowndyd men'.[25] Later on in the manuscript, certain recipes—still written by the same scribal hand—are accompanied by initials that look like 'R SY': these attributions read 'þes beþe expert and proud pro[26] R SY' and 'this goode and ypreuid by me R SY'.[27] The scribe shifts here between referring to Richard in the third and first person, but the personal attribution 'by me' in the last example could have been copied wholesale from another source; it may not mean that the original author or compiler of the two recipe collections (in this manuscript or its exemplar) was himself Master Richard.[28]

---

[23] Ibid., p. 435; for other references in the manuscript to Richard Salisbury, see notes 25 and 27 in this chapter.

[24] There is a reference to a fourteenth-century Salisbury surgeon called Richard Le Leche in C.H. Talbot and Eugene Ashby Hammond, *The Medical Practitioners in Medieval England: A Biographical Register* (London, 1985), pp. 280–1. In 1382, this surgeon was exempted for life 'from being put on assizes, juries, inquisitions or recognizances, or from being made sheriff, escheator, mayor, bailiff, collector of tenths or fifteenths or other minister of the King against his will in consideration of his services in surgery to John Clanevou, knight of the King's Chamber'. John Clanvowe was a courtier, poet, and diplomat closely connected to Chaucer (see Nigel Saul, 'Sir John Clanvow', in the *Oxford Dictionary of National Biography*, accessed online at https://doi.org/10.1093/ref:odnb/37286). In *The First General Entry Book of the City of Salisbury 1387–1452*, ed. by David R. Carr (Trowbridge, 2001), p. xxxiv a Richard Leche is also listed as Mayor of Salisbury in the year 1400.

It is, of course, entirely uncertain whether the Richard mentioned in the recipe collections in MS Ashmole 1443 is this Richard, but it is interesting that the 'I' of those remedy collections makes reference to cures of knights, ladies, duchesses, and squires, suggesting an upper-class milieu of associates like Clanvowe's and (possibly) Richard's (see BodL, MS Ashmole 1443, pp. 214, 317, 350, and 443).

[25] BodL, MS Ashmole 1443, p. 404.   [26] This is perhaps an abbreviation error for 'per'.

[27] BodL, MS Ashmole 1443, p. 443. Other references in the manuscript to Richard Salisbury occur on BodL, MS Ashmole 1443, pp. 264, 295, 333, and 433b (two pages have been paginated the same but an attempt has been made to turn the '3' into a '5'), and (possibly) on p. 249 where an abbreviated form of the name seems to be present.

[28] Of course, this fifteenth-century manuscript was produced some years after Clanvowe and Richard Le Leche are known to have been active: the slightly jerky, calligraphic secretary letter forms, e.g. 'w', 'g', and 'a' (and two-compartment 'a' in some initial positions); the use of unlooped 'd', and the long ascenders and descenders could push the manuscript into the second half of the fifteenth century. This means that—if the recipe collections within MS Ashmole

Nevertheless, the repeated references to these 'masters' can still function as ambiguous indicators of the remedy collections' social milieu. The word could refer to a master craftsman or head of a guild, which would be in keeping with the apprenticeship training surgeons received. However, it could also refer to a clerical or university-educated physician or be used of less formally educated medical practitioners as a more general mark of respect and authority.[29] The original author or compiler of these recipe collections (if a single individual) certainly seems to have had a wide sphere of contacts and influences: as well as referring to these remedies 'moche vsyd among folke', among 'gret surgiens', and among masters and 'doctours', he also includes precise references to learned texts and authorities such as Galen and Avicenna.[30] Furthermore, he distinguishes between cures that work through empirical means rather than established medical theories and he uses (and explains) technical words such as 'mundifier' along with basic medical theory.[31] This could suggest that he had some connection to clerical medical practice and bookish culture.[32] But, at the same time, the use of the vernacular, of terminological explanations, and of abbreviated theoretical passages in the remedy collections suggests that he was writing or compiling for an audience with slightly different needs and priorities than those associated with Latin academic learning. The same is implied by the context of the recipe collections in this particular manuscript: as noted earlier, in MS Ashmole 1443 the collections are accompanied by vernacular translations of Latin herbals and plague treatises. Perhaps, then, the manuscript was meant to function as a quick-reference guide for an educated practitioner, his family members, students, or colleagues (inside or outside of a clerical community).[33] The showy, often rubricated first-person references

---

1443 are referring to Talbot and Hammond's Richard of Salisbury—MS Ashmole 1443 would probably be a copy of an earlier manuscript compiled by Richard and in close proximity to him.

[29] *MED, maister*, n., entries 3(a), 5(a). On this terminology, see also Nancy Siraisi, *Medieval and Early Renaissance Medicine: An Introduction to Knowledge and Practice* (Chicago, IL, 1990), pp. 20–1.

[30] BodL, MS Ashmole 1443, pp. 403, 197. For references to learned Latin, Greek, and Arabic authorities see BodL, MS Ashmole 1443, p. 193 (Avicenna), p. 216 (Hippocrates and Constantine the African), p. 219 (Galen and Avicenna), p. 411 (Macer), p. 425 (Galen), and p. 427 (Avicenna).

[31] For descriptions of cures as 'emperyk', see BodL, MS Ashmole 1443, pp. 211, 219. (See *MED, emperik*, adj., entries 1 and 2.) For 'mundifier' see p. 403 and for a basic explanation of humoral opposites see p. 438.

[32] On clerical medical practitioners, see Getz, *Medicine in the English Middle Ages*, pp. 6–7, 13–19.

[33] Notes and colophons in manuscripts demonstrate that Latin-speaking practitioners did sometimes acquire vernacular translations and simpler texts alongside densely theoretical

to successful cures certainly imply that the manuscript was meant to be seen by others.

All of this helps—albeit in an ambiguous and tentative way—to contextualize the finding aids in MS Ashmole 1443: like many learned compilations, the remedy collection that is more concerned with physic than surgery is arranged from head to toe and it contains cross-references between sections, allowing easy navigation back and forth.[34] Both this collection and the extensive collection of surgical recipes contain running titles, another useful finding device. There is also a table of contents at the beginning of the first collection; this contents page is largely copied by the main hand of the manuscript but, perhaps on account of an unexpected change in ownership of the book, the list of contents is completed by a later fifteenth- or early sixteenth-century hand; this same hand has also added a table of contents to the collection of surgical recipes.[35] These aids add weight to the speculation that MS Ashmole 1443 may have been used by one or more persons in a professional or semi-academic context where ease of accessibility for practical healing purposes was vital. The large margins and the space afforded by beginning entries for new ailments on new leaves might also suggest that the scribe of these recipe collections anticipated that helpful annotations or additional recipes accrued later on would need to be added to the manuscript, either by himself or by future readers.

Not all surviving recipe books are so well organized: in other manuscripts, no attempt at a contents page or index by the original scribe survives and finding aids have had to be added by later fifteenth-, sixteenth-, and seventeenth-century hands.[36] Indeed, in a sample of forty-six vernacular medical collections each containing over seventy-five remedies, only thirteen had a complete table of contents or an index page.[37] Eight of these were

---

works: see Robbins, 'Medical Manuscripts', pp. 408, 410 and Voigts, 'Scientific and Medical Books', pp. 383–4.

[34] E.g. in the section on toothache on BodL, MS Ashmole 1443, p. 218, it is written 'þe grete charm ywrit in þe chaptir of þe mygrem ys ful gode þer fore'.

[35] Ibid., pp. 191–2, 399.

[36] E.g. BL, MS Sloane 468, ff. 2–6r; BodL, MS Radcliffe e. 10, ff. 55r–56r; TCC, MS R.14.51, ff. iv–v.

[37] Eleven manuscripts had contents pages and two had indices, suggesting that the former finding aid was more popular. See Appendix 1 for details of the collections sampled. There is, of course, always a degree of subjectivity involved in deciding what counts as *one* collection, which is why I have included very little of this kind of quantitative analysis in this study. Are multiple stints of recipes intermingled with other texts in a manuscript to be counted as one or more collections? In the above sample, I have tended to treat these as distinct collections if they are clearly written in a different hand or if the organizing principle or topic of the collection

in the same hand as the main collection but five were added by a later reader. Such additions suggest that those later readers found a lack of order or navigational assistance in medieval remedy collections which they felt compelled to redress if the collections were to be made usable. It is easy to see why they may have felt this way. One of the most obvious internal finding aids for modern readers, alphabetical order, did not become commonplace in practical writings and reference works until the late sixteenth and early seventeenth centuries: in the above sample of forty-six collections, only two were alphabetically organized.[38] Eleven other collections displayed no obvious ordering principle that would help a reader navigate the collection and find a particular remedy for a particular affliction.[39]

Even systems which appear to cajole the recipes into a navigable order become more problematic—or opaque—on closer inspection. For example, thirty-one of the forty-six late medieval collections sampled were ordered partly or entirely from head to toe. This structure had long been deployed in learned medicine and occurs in Old English recipe collections based on Roman and Greek sources, as well as twelfth- and thirteenth-century academic medical treatises.[40] But it is not always synonymous with order. Consider London, British Library, MS Lansdowne 680, a fifteenth-century manuscript which appears, from superficial evidence, to have been designed with a practical healing purpose in mind: its small dimensions (115 mm in width by 142 mm in length) would make it portable for a travelling practitioner. Helpfully, the remedy collection, which is copied after a herbal, begins with remedies for the head.[41] After the head-to-toe order is complete,

---

changes in such a way as to suggest a new exemplar—for example, if one collection is for all kinds of remedies and the other is for preparing medical waters only.

[38] Blair, *Too Much to Know*, pp. 117–18, 121. For alphabetically ordered collections, see BodL, MS Ashmole 750, ff. 184r–194r and WT, MS London Medical Society 136, ff. 1r–95v. This latter collection opens with a head-to-toe structure, beginning with remedies for head-, eye-, and toothaches; some of the recipes are similar to those in other head-to-toe orders (compare the head and ear recipes on YM, MS XVI, E.32, ff. 15r and 18v–19r). However, after remedies for toothache on WT, MS London Medical Society 136, f. 3r, the compiler starts listing remedies for all kinds of 'ache', in line with the alphabetical system he has adopted. A large initial 'B' starting a new section on f. 6r is the first explicit sign of the ordering system, which continues until f. 88v (though initials are not always used to signal new sections).

[39] E.g. HEHL, MS HM 1336, ff. 2v–18v, 29r–34v; HEHL, MS HM 64, ff. 104r–113r, 143v–153v, 156v–176r; BL, MS Harley 2378, ff. 17r–61v. Some collections, such as YM, MS XVI, E.32, ff. 82r–109r, contain an ordering principle in the sense that all the recipes are for waters or ointments, but it is still not apparent how readers would find a particular treatment.

[40] On an Old English head-to-toe ordering system, see Debby Banham, 'Dun, Oxa and Pliny the Great Physician: Attribution and Authority in Old English Medical Texts', *Social History of Medicine*, 24 (2011), 57–73 (p. 59).

[41] BL, MS Lansdowne 680, ff. 22r–73r.

the scribe copies recipes for all-over-body afflictions, such as *jaundise, morphea*, and *wilde fire* (erysipelas).[42] These all-over afflictions frequently occur at the end of head-to-toe structures and so, in itself, this addition is not a problem. What is problematic, though, is that copied amongst these all-over afflictions are slightly more specific recipes that might have been more appropriately placed earlier in the collection, such as cures for a tick in the ear and for swollen knees, and a remedy for a headache mixed among the gout remedies.[43] (This is perhaps because gout can cause pain in the head, although this logic is never articulated in this manuscript.) Potential confusion is also generated by the fact that, shortly after, a new head-to-toe cycle begins with eye and head recipes.[44] Towards the end of the manuscript, a possible third short cycle begins.[45] *Within* these cycles, a significant degree of disorder is also present: for example, remedies for *gout festre* (festered swelling) are interspersed in the second cycle between remedies for other ailments.[46] A reader searching for a cure for *gout festre* may easily have overlooked some of these.

One experiences disruption to the head-to-toe order in most manuscripts. Such disorder may have been an unavoidable consequence of the piecemeal process by which scribes accessed different exemplars; the recipes had to be bolted onto one another rather than integrated. However, even if such disorder was unavoidable, other evidence in MS Lansdowne 680 suggests that its scribe did not actively *prioritize* navigability: there is no evidence that a contents page ever accompanied the manuscript and the herbal copied before the remedy collection (a version of the text known as *Here Men May See the Virtues of Herbes*) is not organized through any consistent finding aids or through internal alphabetical order (such as the herbal *Agnus Castus*).[47] Furthermore, the inclusion of rubricated titles for each recipe stops intermittently for a few pages partway through the remedy collection and blank spaces are left where the titles should be.[48] This cessation coincides with the beginning of a new head-to-toe order which may suggest

---

[42] All-over afflictions begin on BL, MS Lansdowne 680, f. 28v.
[43] Respectively see BL, MS Lansdowne 680, ff. 30v, 31r–v. In the contents page on WT, MS Wellcome 5262, f. 6r, a manuscript containing many of the same remedies as MS Lansdowne 680, the connection between gout and head pain is made explicit by the title 'For þe gout þat nemeþ mon in þe hed'.
[44] BL, MS Lansdowne 680, f. 33v.
[45] On BL, MS Lansdowne 680, f. 72r–v, headache, migraine, and toothache recipes are copied before other more random ailments.
[46] BL, MS Lansdowne 680, ff. 57v–58r, 62r, 63v–64r.
[47] Instead, later readers seem to have added their own marginal notes and finding aids.
[48] BL, MS Lansdowne 680, ff. 33v–39v.

that the exemplar the scribe used for this part of the remedy book was faulty or that he did not have ink for rubrication at hand. Although the scribe could have worked out what many of the remedies were for from their contents, he never returns to fill the majority of the spaces in; instead, it usually falls to a later reader to add recipe titles to the manuscript margins.[49]

In this example, then, the size, organization, and annotation of the collection function as opaque signs which—especially when considered in conjunction with one another—give ambiguous (and sometimes contradictory) clues about whether the scribe or compiler of the collection intended it to be fit for practical use. Two small notebook collections provide the most emphatic examples of the way in which the practical intentions of a scribe or reader can be manifest and yet simultaneously opaque. Each of these informally executed manuscripts, which both contain hundreds of recipes, seem to have been copied predominantly by single scribes, who were probably also the manuscripts' first owners. Judging by the frequent changes in ink and script style, this copying was done over a long period of time, with the scribes copying recipes whenever they came across exempla, tried out a cure, or heard of one. The majority of one of them, Oxford, Bodleian Library, MS Rawlinson C.506, is copied by a mid- to late fifteenth-century secretary hand, and contains a large number of medical, herbal, gynaecological, astrological, and necromantic texts in both Latin and English; some of these—such as the recipes and herb glossary—seem like they could be accessible to a reader without a formal medical education but others, such as a bloodletting poem and an abbreviated English translation of Lanfranc of Milan's *Antidotarium* (part of the *Chirurgia parva*), suggest that the scribe or initial owner was a practising medic with a reasonable degree of learning, training, and expertise. Later medieval and early modern owners, however, have added to blank folios extra recipes along with advice texts on horse care, veterinary medicine, fishing, gardening, dye-making, and care of hawks. This suggests that the manuscript evolved to suit the needs of a more domestic readership.[50]

---

[49] An exception is BL, MS Lansdowne 680, f. 35r where the scribe does seem to have written the title 'for hede ache' in black (rather than red) ink; another title may have been erased from f. 34v.

[50] The manuscript is discussed briefly in Mooney, 'Manuscript Evidence', pp. 196–9, where Mooney notes that it was associated with a 'Humphridus Harrison, capellanus' in the late fifteenth century.

THE IDEA OF THE REMEDY COLLECTION   119

As it stands today, the part of the manuscript written by the main (and initial) hand fills over 250 folios, and clusters of recipes (predominantly medical but occasionally culinary) in English or Latin occur throughout these leaves, often interspersed between other texts. No contents or index page survives. Recipes are distinguished from one another by rubricated titles and readers' marginal crosses. Although some of the mini-collections contain head-to-toe orders (or at least parts or beginnings of them), others do not. As in MS Lansdowne 680, the restarting and disturbing of this order negates its usefulness as a navigational aid.

There is some evidence, though, that the scribe initially intended the manuscript to be usable: in some of the clusters of recipes, a number has been written next to each recipe and these numbers might have corresponded to a contents page that no longer survives. (The manuscript begins with a recipe for the falling evil—rather than a head recipe—which could suggest that it is acephalous).[51] The numbering seems to have been written in the same ink as the once red, now faded rubrication highlighting the recipes' titles (see Figure 3.1) and it looks as though it was completed by the collection's scribe as the form of the numbers is similar to those within the text.[52] Interestingly, these recipe clusters are almost the only texts in the manuscript to be included within the numbering system: the great majority of the other longer medical, astronomical, and necromantic texts have no such markings.[53] Other recipe clusters also go unnumbered.[54] In the first one hundred folios of the manuscript, this lack of consistent numbering can probably be explained by the fact that the manuscript seems to have been compiled from texts copied separately on different quires by one scribe and later assembled; recipes accompanied by numbers are thus interspersed with texts without them. For instance, on folio 39r, a series of texts beginning with necromantic conjurations appears between numbered recipe collections; the necromantic writings start on a new quire which bears signs of

---

[51] The numbering begins at '2' with the Latin recipes on f. 15r. The loss of f. 14 probably accounts for the absence of an item numbered '1'. The beginning of this numbering here indicates that the unnumbered English recipes copied between ff. 1r and 13v were copied on a separate quire by the same hand and added onto the beginning of the book after the numbering of items had already commenced on f. 14.
[52] The numbers in the table on f. 30v provide a helpful means of comparing number forms in the text to those forms in the marginal numbering system and foliation system.
[53] An exception is the bloodletting verse numbered on BodL, MS Rawlinson C.506, f. 27r.
[54] Clusters of recipes go unnumbered on ff. 1r–13v; 62v–69v; 70r–82v (Latin); 101v–116r; 117v–119v; 120v; 131r–147v (Latin); 148r–169v (mixed Latin and English); 230r–231v (Latin and English); 261r–265v.

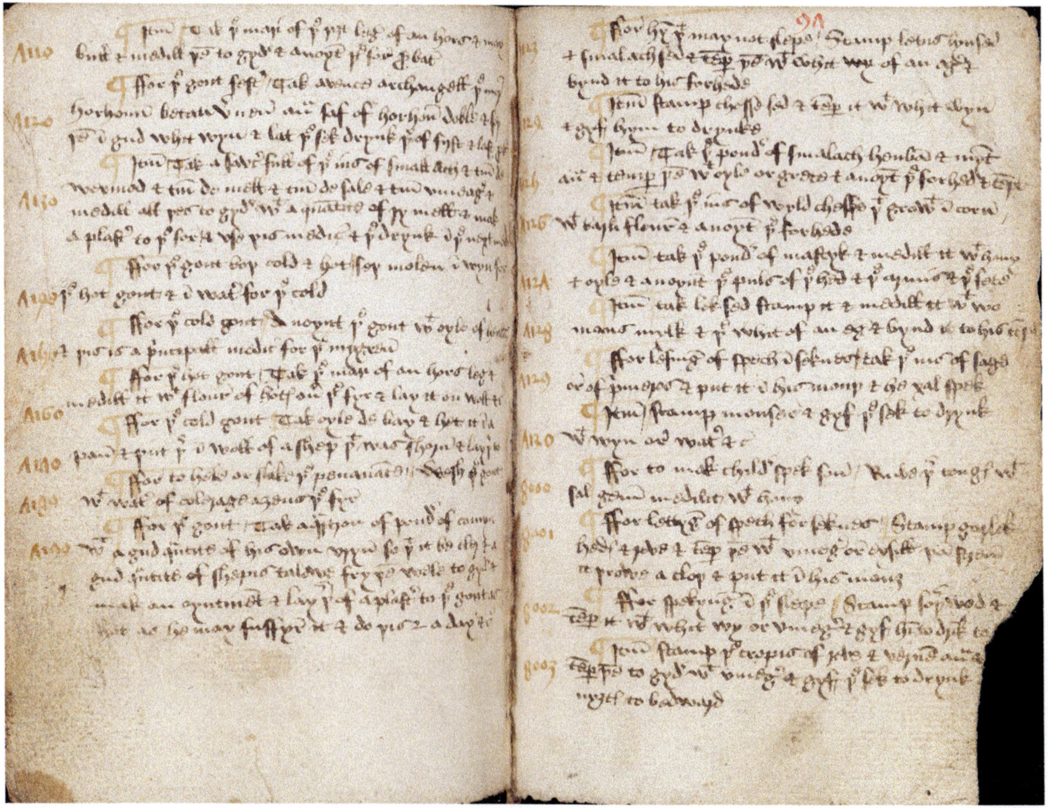

Figure 3.1 A numbered recipe collection. The Bodleian Libraries, University of Oxford, MS Rawlinson C.506, ff. 96v–97r. Reproduced with kind permission from the Bodleian Libraries, University of Oxford through the Creative Commons licence CC-BY-NC 4.

THE IDEA OF THE REMEDY COLLECTION   121

a former pagination system, suggesting that it was placed in between recipe clusters initially conceived of as part of a larger sequence.[55]

Later in the manuscript, though, the reason for the incompleteness of the numbering system seems different. In the middle of the largest, continually numbered recipe collection in the manuscript, the numbering suddenly ceases, six recipes after the scribe (who—struggling with an unfamiliar Arabic number system—counts incorrectly) seems to think he has reached 10,000 recipes.[56] Perhaps the annotator grew tired of numbering; counting the recipes may have drawn his attention to just how many recipes he had numbered and copied. The fact that no table of contents survives also casts doubt over whether the scribe's organizational task was ever fulfilled. But the page numbers, apparently copied by the same hand in a much brighter red ink at the top of the folios and consistent throughout the entire manuscript, might suggest that he later returned to the task of organizing the codex, attempting to make it in some way consistent throughout even if the individual recipes were never numbered or organized.

All of this evidence leaves us with conflicting impressions. On the one hand, the size of the manuscript (150 mm in height by 105 mm in width) could suggest that it was intended, at least at the beginning of the copying process, to be portable and consultable on the go.[57] Linne Mooney has also argued that material evidence within the manuscript, such as herb fragments and splashes of liquid, illustrates that it was actually used in medical encounters.[58] And yet, because it is inconveniently thick (62 mm) and

---

[55] The recipes copied between ff. 1r and 13v also seem to have been written separately and added onto the beginning of the numbered collection: see note 51 of this chapter.

[56] BodL, MS Rawlinson C.506, f. 101v. On BodL, MS Rawlinson C.506, f. 101r, the scribe reaches 9190 and he (it seems) then begins numbering again from 1 in a different-colour ink; he reaches number 5 before ceasing on f. 101v. The scribe may have decided to begin numbering from 1 again because he thought he had reached 10,000. On multiple occasions the scribe's numbering suggests that he was not confident using Hindu-Arabic numerals, which only started to become standard in the fifteenth century: on f. 99v, for example, he makes the same error, proceeding straight from 8190 to 9000; elsewhere he proceeds from 100 to 110, 120, 130; from 1009 to 2000, from 2009 to 3000, etc. On the difficulties that Hindu-Arabic numerals presented, see John N. Crossley, 'Old-Fashioned versus Newfangled: Reading and Writing Numbers, 1200–1500', *Studies in Medieval and Renaissance History*, 3rd series, 10 (2013), 79–109.

The practice of restarting from 1 when a certain number has been reached can also be observed in WT, MS Wellcome 5262, f. 6v, where numbering of recipes in a table of contents stops at 99 and begins again at 1.

[57] On the relationship between portability and the size, shape, and weight of codices in relation to practical devotional manuscripts see Sawyer, *Reading English Verse*, pp. 81–109. Sawyer suggests that all of these pieces of evidence needed to be considered together when speculating about the uses of a codex.

[58] Mooney, 'Manuscript Evidence', pp. 196–9.

because its finding aids are sporadic and incomplete, it is unclear how readers could handle or navigate it with ease or make full use of the individual remedies contained within it. The desire to accumulate more recipes seems to have outweighed the ability or desire of the scribe to catalogue them appropriately. Perhaps the scribe's satisfaction derived, then, from the process of ordering rather than its result: after all, ordering can—with its emphasis on patterns, neatness, and propriety—be a very therapeutic and aesthetically satisfying act.

An early Tudor recipe collection, Oxford, Bodleian Library, MS Ashmole 1389, has similarly small dimensions (156 mm in height by 100–105 mm in width) but it is far thinner than MS Rawlinson C.506 (measuring approximately 25 mm). This could suggest that it was copied with portable use in mind. Indeed, a pox remedy within the collection ends 'probatum est per me w aderston' and this has led several commentators to speculate that the copier and compiler of the collection was William Altoftes of Atherstone, practising surgeon to Henry VII.[59] As Juhani Norri notes, though, this attribution could simply have been copied wholesale from another source.[60]

The manuscript's finding aids offer more ambiguous evidence about whether it served a practical purpose. The remedy collection is preceded by the beginning of a contents page copied in the same hand.[61] This contents page seems designed to counter the fact that the collection is not structured by any ordering principle: occasionally afflictions for the same ailment are grouped together, but this is not the norm, and there is no obvious logic behind the order in which the ailments are discussed.[62] Furthermore, throughout the collection, the recipes are written one after the other with nothing to separate them aside from their titles and a few horizontal lines. The contents page is necessary, therefore, to make the collection navigable. And yet it cannot perform this function because it is incomplete: only fifteen of the recipes in the manuscript are listed in the contents page; the rest of the eight-leaf quire is left blank. No pages seem to be missing and so the rest of the contents page does not seem to have been lost. It seems more likely that the scribe left those leaves vacant in order to finish the contents page at a later date. Unforeseen circumstances may have prevented this or

---

[59] BodL, MS Ashmole 1389, p. 28. For this identification, see Talbot and Hammond, *The Medical Practitioners*, pp. 380–1.
[60] Juhani Norri, 'Entrances and Exits in English Medical Vocabulary, 1400–1550', in *Medical and Scientific Writing*, ed. by Taavitsainen and Pahta, pp. 100–43 (p. 103).
[61] BodL, MS Ashmole 1389, p. 2.
[62] E.g. in BodL, MS Ashmole 1389, pp. 26–9, six remedies for the pox are copied together.

perhaps the scribe felt that the task of inventorying the many recipes he had accumulated was too great.

All three of these manuscripts, then, contain finding aids which imply that scribes and readers intended the recipes—at some point in time or at one level of consciousness—to be conveniently consultable and deployable. However, an unwillingness to undertake the time-consuming task of inventorying them, a privileging of the appearance of order over actual order, unforeseen disruptions, or a temptation to accrue more recipes than could be catalogued seems to have overpowered or thwarted that intention. Other kinds of medieval compilation present similar enigmas. Describing a late medieval spiritual miscellany composed of texts copied in a variety of hands, Vincent Gillespie notes that 'although [it is] a carefully produced book, that care has not been extended to facilitate access or reference'.[63] He observes that, because there is no contents page and an inconsistent approach to introducing and demarcating texts, 'intimate knowledge would be required to locate a specific text', raising the possibility that 'it was the product of a closed society, either lay or clerical'.[64] MS Rawlinson C.506 and MS Ashmole 1389 might also have been used in an insular household or circle but, because recipes are much shorter than the texts in a spiritual miscellany and because there are so many recipes in these volumes, it seems unlikely that even the original scribe or compiler of the text would be able to remember exactly where he had copied a particular remedy.

Perhaps, then, 'intimate' knowledge of a more bodily kind would have been deployed to locate recipes: readers might not only have used their visual memory of what a particular page looked like to help locate a specific remedy when flicking through the book's many pages, but may also have relied on tangible clues such as the natural parting of the leaves at a particularly well-thumbed cure. An instinctive 'muscle memory' may have guided a reader's hands to the rough area of the book that a recipe resided in. Once again, then, we can see how the body could be intimately involved in its own healing. Indeed, in the end, merely possessing an extensive, all-encompassing book of medical recipes may have been enough of a comfort for owners and scribes: knowing one had cures at one's fingertips, even if one could not easily find them, may have felt like a reassuring initial defence against future illness or professional inadequacy. The manuscript here takes

---

[63] Vincent Gillespie, 'Lukynge in haly bukes: Lectio in some Late Medieval Spiritual Miscellanies', in Vincent Gillespie, *Looking in Holy Books*, pp. 113–44 (p. 136).

[64] Gillespie, 'Lukynge in haly bukes', p. 136.

on its own talismanic quality. We can begin to see, then, how affective dispositions and emotions, such as hope, fear, and impatience, could have shaped the acts of accumulation and organization defining remedy books' forms.

Accrual

This model of the medical book as talisman offers one possible motivation for a reader's decision to accumulate large numbers of recipes. However, like the presence or absence of finding aids, the accrual of multiple remedies is itself an opaque sign, an arrangement or structure that could have been motivated by a variety of reasons and could, in turn, have stimulated a variety of different interpretations from subsequent readers. The interplay of these motivations and interpretations is the subject of the remainder of this chapter.

Extensive accumulation of recipes occurs at two levels: as we have seen, the collection as a whole can be extensive, containing many individual recipes for different ailments. Accumulation can also occur at the level of the individual affliction. In the example below from a large fifteenth-century collection, multiple recipes for removing hair are listed. Bold type represents rubrication (see Figure 3.2 for a photo of the original):

> To don her to go awey
>
> Tak and mak leyȝe of otestraw askes and wasche þe hed þerwiþ ofte **Anoþer** for contrarious heere take þe iuys of yuyleues and when þe heer is pulled away anoynte the stede þerwiþ // **Anoþer** tak þe askes of holmen barkes and vnslekked lyne orpyment and welle water and do þer on // **Anoþer** tak þe leuys of wodebynde stamp hem wel þan tempre hem vpp wiþ vynegre than ley it on þe hery place // **Anoþer** tak amtys eroun and þe blode of a remows þat is to say of a bakke and þe gumme of yuy orpyment and aysel and stamp hem wel togeder wiþ vnslekked lyme frote þe place ofte þerwiþ þis is good but it is violent. // **Anoþer** tak nettel seed and stamp it wiþ vynegre and aftur gret hete anoynte þerwiþ // **Anoþer** tak moure eroyne ymeyd wiþ oille þat an yrchon hatte be soþen þan do þer on // **Anoþer** tak and do awey þe heer ferst than tak þe blood of a remows

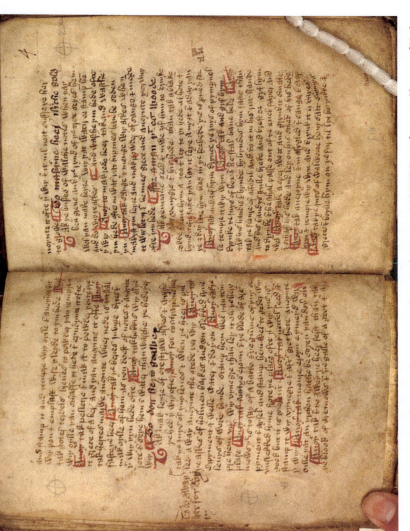

Figure 3.2 Accumulated recipes for removing hair. York Minster, MS XVI.E.32, f. 17v. © Chapter of York: reproduced by kind permission.

and þe galle of a goot and anoynte it ofte þerwiþ and it nil no3t suffre þe here to growe⁶⁵

[*ley3e* = alkaline mixture formed through the leaching of ashes; *otestraw askes* = burnt ashes of oats; *yuy* = ivy, buck's horn plantain, or the European ground pine;⁶⁶ *stede* = place; *askes of holmen barkes* = ashes of the bark of the evergreen oak; *vnslekked lyne* = unslaked lime, calcium oxide; *orpiment* = arsenic trisulphide; *amtys eroun (ampte eiren)* = pupae of ants; *remows* = bat; *bakke* = bat; *aysel* = vinegar; *frote* = rub; *moure eroyne* = pupae of ants; yrchon = hedgehog; *goot* = goat]

Eight recipes for removing hair are given and this is typical for many of the ailments listed in the collection. The same compulsion to keep adding and connecting recipes can also be observed in manuscripts where later readers have copied recipes, sometimes linked to those already written and sometimes not, in the blank spaces of leaves.⁶⁷ There seems to be a recurrent compulsion amongst the scribes and readers of these texts to add, supplement, and complete. However, as in the recipes for hair removal quoted above, the paratactic construction 'another...another...another' frequently implies that the list can never reach completion—that there is always room for one more remedy to be added. To deploy Juliet Fleming's words, it seems as though 'nothing can close this list'.

Acts of adding, combining, and completing are not unique to manuscripts containing remedies, encyclopaedic texts, or other practical writings. In fact, this action might be seen as one of the defining features of medieval and early modern aesthetic practices: as Ingrid Nelson has shown through the various (expanded and contracted) versions of the lyric 'Erthe toc of erthe', dilation is integral to medieval acts of interpretation and creation; medieval literary form is not static or stable, but open to change and expansion.⁶⁸ On a larger scale, this is also evident in the way that writers such as Jean de Meun and Robert Henryson continue poems by previous writers, the way that compilers add and connect texts to one another in literary miscellanies, and the way that poets such as Boccaccio, Chaucer, and Gower create miscellaneous tale collections by adding texts (which, in Chaucer's case, we now speak of as 'fragments') to one another. Indeed, Chaucer may

---

⁶⁵ YM, MS XVI.E.32, ff. 17v–18r.
⁶⁶ *MED, ivi*, n., entry 1(a) and *MED, herbe-ive*, n., entry 1.
⁶⁷ E.g. BodL, MS Ashmole 1443, pp. 6–11; BodL, MS Laud misc. 685, f. 86r; TCC, MS R.14.32, ff. 94r–95r.
⁶⁸ Nelson, 'Form's Practice'.

have left poems such as *The House of Fame*, *The Legend of Good Women*, and *The Canterbury Tales* deliberately unfinished, incorporating into the poems a comment upon the difficulty of finishing an artwork; there are always more tales that could be told. Subsequent readers certainly recognized—and responded to—a challenge in Chaucer's writing, composing and adding their own tales to Chaucer's Canterbury structure.[69]

This tendency to add, however, seems *especially* notable in recipe collections. Lots of people today still paste recipes together in scrapbooks. Perhaps it is the small, self-contained nature of many recipes and the consequent ease with which they can be excerpted and reassembled that creates the compulsion to collect them. Medieval scribes and readers certainly seem to have been conscious of this impulse: in MS Ashmole 1389, the early Tudor collection discussed above, the scribe copies two recipes for *saucefleume* before writing 'thes suffysyth for thys dysease'.[70] This declaration of sufficiency reads as a recognition of the temptation to keep on acquiring remedies and the need to impose an end on that potentially end*less* process.

A similar temptation can be observed in a collection of surgical recipes copied predominantly by a fifteenth-century hand onto a quire now incorporated into the composite manuscript, Oxford, Bodleian Library, MS Ashmole 1438.[71] The hand copying these recipes—which display linguistic and orthographical features associated with Lincolnshire—possibly belonged to 'Nicholas Neesbett', whose name is written at the top of the collection.[72] Although this name is not recorded in Talbot and Hammond's register of medical practitioners in medieval England, several notes embedded amongst the recipes suggest that the scribe practised surgery and that he copied the recipe collection with the intention of sending it to another

---

[69] The most frequently discussed continuations of the *Canterbury Tales* are John Lydgate's prologue to *The Siege of Thebes* and the anonymous *Canterbury Interlude* and *Merchant's Tale of Beryn*.

[70] BodL, Ashmole 1389, pp. 205–7.

[71] The recipes by this hand are copied in BodL, MS Ashmole 1438, Part I, pp. 57–71, with recipes by later hands inserted into blank spaces at a later date. There is some evidence, however, that the main hand collaborated with another writer (possibly the addressee): the recipe at the top of p. 63 looks like it may have been copied by another hand, but the title of the recipe and the correction in the final line have been written by the main hand of the collection, perhaps suggesting the main writer invited another individual to copy this particular remedy into a space he had left for it. That second hand also seems to have been responsible for the recipe for sciatica copied at the bottom of p. 60.

[72] This collection comprises profile 908 in the *Linguistic Atlas of Late Medieval English*. See M. Benskin and others, *An Electronic Version of A Linguistic Atlas of Late Medieval English*, accessed online at www.lel.ed.ac.uk/ihd/elalme/elalme_frames.html [accessed 02/04/2018]. For further discussion of the manuscript, see the Introduction.

practitioner. The second note begins by proclaiming 'whatt mysters me to wryte ʒow mo [remedies] when þ^i^se er sufficient'.⁷³ Sufficiency is again declared, but straight after the scribe proclaims 'neuer þe lesse one schalle ʒe haue þat is general'.⁷⁴ The temptation to add another remedy is too great. Similarly, in the third note in this collection, the scribe declares 'Me mystyrs noʒt to sett ʒow in powders for corvasyse⁷⁵ for þe oyntmentes aforesayd er gude enawgh for syche maters and þerfore I wryte none to ʒow at þis tyme'.⁷⁶ The final phrase, 'I wryte none to ʒow *at þis tyme*', anticipates another instalment of recipes and undoes the earlier declaration of sufficiency.

The scribe of this collection in MS Ashmole 1438 seems to have imagined the textual exchange with his addressee as an ongoing one.⁷⁷ Here we see how the accumulation of recipes might function as a way of maintaining personal and professional relationships. But that accumulation also shapes the power dynamic in such relationships: simultaneously flaunting and withholding knowledge allows one to cultivate authority for oneself and render oneself, as the possessor of withheld knowledge, a desirable person to know.⁷⁸

Consequently, one might compare these moments in recipe collections to the rhetorical manoeuvre of *occupatio*: this device, frequently deployed by Chaucer, involves denying one's intention to narrate something before proceeding to do exactly that. For instance, Chaucer's Knight opens his tale by proclaiming:

> And certes, if it nere to long to heere
> I wolde have toold yow fully the manere
> How wonnen was the regne of Femenye
> By Theseus and by his chivalrye;

---

⁷³ BodL, MS Ashmole 1438, Part I, p. 67.   ⁷⁴ Ibid.

⁷⁵ This is an unusual spelling of *corrosif* ('corrosive', a noun and adjective) which is not listed in the *MED* or Norri, *Dictionary of Medical Vocabulary*. However, the word's meaning is confirmed by a recipe on BodL, MS Ashmole 1438, Part I, p. 64 for 'anoþer oyntment þat is coruasy', which involves removing dead flesh, a typical property of corrosives. See *MED*, *corrosif*, adj. and n., entry 2(a), (b).

⁷⁶ BodL, MS Ashmole 1438, Part I, p. 68.

⁷⁷ Although the recipes in the collection are all copied on one quire, which suggests that they were sent and received at the same time, they are copied with different inks and nibs, which suggests that they were written in several stints. The quire extends from BodL, MS Ashmole 1438, Part I, pp. 57–80. Originally composed of twelve leaves, a page appears to have been removed between pp. 62 and 63. A parchment page containing a diagram of a vein man has also been inserted between pp. 76 and 79.

⁷⁸ On secrecy in medieval relationships, see Karma Lochrie, *Covert Operations: The Medieval Uses of Secrecy* (Philadelphia, PA, 1999).

> And of the grete bataille for the nones
> Bitwixen Atthenes and Amazones;
> And how asseged was Ypolita
>
> ...
>
> And of the feste that was at hir weddynge,
> And of the tempest at hir hoom-comynge[79]

After denying the possibility of narrating these events, the Knight does narrate them, just as the denial of the scribe of the above recipe collection contains within it an affirmation of further recipes. What is more, the Knight's speech displays a similar paratactic, polysyndetic structure ('And...And...And') to the recipe collections ('Another...Another...Another'), which serves in both cases to emphasize the process of accumulation taking place. This rhetorical accrual emphasizes the power that the Knight and the scribes have by drawing attention to the extent of their privileged knowledge about medicine and Theban history. It also showcases their *rhetorical* power: their capacity to manipulate discourse in order to provoke a desire for further information in their readers or listeners.

Accumulation, though, was not limited to signifying power and rhetorical control; in manuscripts without any commentating scribal voice, it could suggest a variety of motivations and invite a wealth of interpretations. For instance, there is an obvious practical justification for offering multiple remedies for one affliction: if readers were unable, for financial or geographical reasons, to procure the ingredients one recipe required, they could turn to another. This explanation alone, however, was not sufficient for medieval readers, who often offered more sceptical interpretations. Consider the response of the fifteenth-century Scottish poet Robert Henryson in his set of parodic remedies, 'Sum Practysis of Medecyne', discussed in Chapter 1: there, Henryson dismisses the 'saying' (spoken or written discourse) of an inept medical practitioner as 'geir of all gaddering, glaikit, nocht gude' ('borrowed and accumulative stuff which is foolish and not good').[80] Although almost all medical writings were compilations of earlier Latin and Greek writings, Henryson identifies the practitioner's thoughtless 'gaddering' of recipes from other sources as a sign of his *lack* of expertise.

---

[79] Geoffrey Chaucer, *The Knight's Tale*, in *Riverside*, ed. by Benson, lines 875–84.
[80] Robert Henryson, 'Sum Practysis of Medecyne', line 6. The translation is my own. See *DOST*, *saying*, n. 2.

Chiara Crisciani argues that scholastic authors of pharmacological medical writings were themselves often distrustful of the mass of ancient and modern knowledge that they had accrued, some of which was conflicting: 'their very manner of writing betrays the scholars' uncertainty, their sense of insecurity and alarm: lists of opinions ("some...others...I") proliferate, or series of contrasting views about a drug or a cure are simply reported and not resolved'.[81] Accumulation is here associated with panic, uncertainty, and fear of inefficacy. In a more explicitly polemical way, accumulation is also connected to inefficacy by the fourteenth-century Italian poet Petrarch, whose writings often express hostility towards physicians.[82] In a private letter to the famous Paduan physician Giovanni de' Dondi, he interpreted accumulation of cures as a sign of physicians' corruption or ineptitude:

> We must suspect that either this thing called medicine, whatever it may be itself, among men is still some kind of deceptive art thought up to the vast peril and loss of mortals, whereby a few become rich but many are imperiled, or that it is a true art, usefully devised but least understood by our fellow men and least applicable to the natures of men, of which the variety is inestimable. For what other conclusion remains when *out of a thousand remedies* not one helps us, many do harm and often kill?[83]

Petrarch reaffirms the opaque, polysemous capacity of accumulated remedies by depicting them as stunning and dividing his interpretative abilities: on the one hand, the proliferation of cures could point to physicians' eagerness to dupe prospective customers out of their money by offering them an endless string of remedies to try. On the other hand, physicians could propose hundreds of unsuccessful cures for one ailment because they have no complete (or completable) understanding of the way human bodies work: academic medical writings constantly emphasized that individual bodies

---

[81] Crisciani, 'History, Novelty and Progress', p. 137.
[82] See the *Invective contra medicum*, in Petrarch, *Invectives*, pp. 2–79.
[83] Francesco Petrarch, *Letters of Old Age: Rerum senilium libri*, trans. by Aldo S. Bernardo, Saul Levin, and Reta A. Bernardo, 2 vols (Baltimore, MD, 1992), II, Letter XII.2, p. 459, italics mine. For the Latin, see Francesco Petrarch, *Res seniles: Libri IX–XII*, ed. by Silvia Rizzo and Monica Berté (Firenze, 2014), Letter XII.2, p. 382: 'suspicari liceat aut hanc ipsam que medicina dicitur, qualiscunque sit in se, inter homines tamen artem quandam esse fallendi damno ingenti ac periculo mortalium adinventam, qua pauci ditarentur, multi periclitarentur, aut esse artem veram et utiliter excogitatem sed a nostris minime intellectam vel, si hoc tolerabilius dicitur, intellectam quidem sed naturis hominum, quarum est inextimabilis et infinita varietas, minime applicabilem. Quid enim aliud relinquitur, dum de mille medicinis una non proficit, multe officiunt et sepe conficiunt?'

varied according to a great number of factors (including humoral complexion, age, environment, and planetary influence) and that medicines needed to be tailor-made to these. Petrarch suggests, however, that this great variety of human constitutions will always exceed the physician's capacity to generate remedies. In his reading, then, the human capacity to accumulate becomes insufficient *and* overwhelming simultaneously.

Other interpreters of cumulative forms took a more neutral or positive approach. Consider the late medieval verse remedy book discussed in more depth in Chapter 2. Playfully imitating the anaphoric beginnings of remedy collections' cumulative structures ('Another... Another...'), the poet writes after a recipe for swollen testicles:

> Anodire and þat helpe nowth
> Anodire medysyn must be sowth[84]
>
> [*sowth* = sought]

The poet acknowledges that multiple recipes must be given because individual ones may prove inefficacious. In contrast to Petrarch, he does not seem troubled by this trial-and-error approach but accepts it as part of the natural course of medical treatment, as many medieval patients seeking expertise from different kinds of medical practitioner in quick succession seem to have done.[85] Other medical writers were actually excited by the capacity of the body to provoke proliferation. For example, in the prologue to his *Breviarium Bartholomei*, a Latin medical treatise probably intended for use at St Bartholomew's Hospital, the cleric John of Mirfield (d. 1407) justifies his inclusion of multiple remedies for one ailment with this explanation:

> I propose, in a good many cases, to set down in this compilation several medicines for one and the same disease; since it is a peculiarity of medicaments that at one time they are beneficial, and at other times they are not—a fact which is a matter for wonder! The diversity of effect is perhaps due to the influence of a man's natal planet[86]

---

[84] TCC, MS R.14.39, f. 1v.
[85] On these 'itineraries of care', see Orlemanski, *Symptomatic Subjects*, p. 52. On the comparable way that medieval writings invite selective itineraries of reading in healing contexts, see Joe Stadolnik, 'Gower's Bedside Manner', *New Medieval Literatures*, 17 (2017), 150–74.
[86] *Johannes de Mirfield of St Bartholomew's, Smithfield: His Life and Works*, ed. and trans. by Harold Richard Aldridge and Percival Horton-Smith Hartley (Cambridge, 1936), pp. 50–1:

Like Petrarch, Mirfield gestures to the 'inestimable' variety of human bodies by positing the changing interactions between those bodies and the influences of the planets as one reason why remedies were not consistently successful. But he puts forward this explanation tentatively, using the Latin 'forte' ('perhaps') to preserve a sense of mysterious wonder. What is more, for Mirfield, the marvellous inexplicability of the body's workings does not negate or overwhelm the medical practitioner's attempt to provide a remedy. It simply demands greater resourcefulness and flexibility in thinking.

In my final example, accumulation is also interpreted as a positive, practically minded response to inevitable circumstances. In the Middle English translation of Guy de Chauliac's fourteenth-century surgical treatise, *Chirurgia Magna*, Guy's treatise is described as 'a gadryng togedre of þe crafte of cirurgye', recalling Robert Henryson's description of patchwork knowledge as 'gaddering'.[87] A more positive justification is, however, offered in the *Chirurgia* for this accumulative form:

> In construcciouns alway bettre þinges comeþ. Conynges forsoþe beþ imade by putttyng to. It is not forsoþe possible to begynne þe same and ende it. We bene forsoþe children in þe nekke of a geaunt; neuerþelatter we may see als mykel as þe geaunt and somewhat more. Therfore þere is in construcciouns and gadryng onehede and profit.[88]
>
> [*conynge*s = knowledge; *onehede* = unity]

The image of a child or dwarf standing on the shoulders of giants seems to have been a commonplace metaphor for compilational practice.[89] The comparison suggests that, because each person only has a finite time on earth to further human knowledge, we can never begin and end a work, but only add to what has gone before. The process of accumulation is thus endless and incompletable but it is prevented in this translation from becoming chaotic and overwhelming by the assertion that each accumulated piece of wisdom is tending towards 'onehede and profit', towards a unified and complete body of knowledge, rather than a conflicted and uncertain one. Even though this desire for unity may have been continually challenged by the

---

'Propterea multas medicinas pro vna et eadem infirmitate ponere propono in multis locis istius compilacionis. Quoniam de proprietate medicaminum est quod iuuabunt vno tempore et non alio. Et hoc est mirabile. Et forte facit hoc varietas proprietatis adquisite ex influencia orbis alicuius.'

[87] See Ogden, ed., *Cyrurgie of Guy de Chauliac*, p. 1, line 13.
[88] Ibid., p. 1, lines 24–9.   [89] See Steiner, 'Compendious Genres', p. 77.

experiences of practice, it is clear that accumulative forms could signify as positive signs of intellectual collaboration.[90] There is no reason why readers of domestic remedy books might not also have seen the mass of recipes and knowledge fragments before them as part of a journey towards fullness and completion.

These responses demonstrate that the accumulation of recipes—a seemingly straightforward formal feature of remedy collections—was itself generative, accumulating before readers a multitude of interpretative choices. Crucially, the collections' practicality is foregrounded by these readings as a matter of interpretation: the accrual of recipes as a response to the changing nature of human bodies and human circumstances testifies to the collections' practical usefulness. However, when accrual is conceived of as a pre-empting of inefficacy, it testifies to remedy books' uselessness. Because many of the collections examined in this study, trimmed of theory and commentating voices, rarely state what the impulse behind such accrual is, it is left entirely to the reader to interpret these polyvalent structures. Each reader is thus invited to become a formalist critic in his or her own right, interpreting the forms of recipes rather than merely translating the texts' instructions into action.

Distinctions: Textual and Social

There is, however, a small minority of manuscripts where compilers and copiers of recipes *are* more explicit about why they have chosen to collect multiple cures for one affliction. These comments reveal yet more ways of interpreting accrual, as they normally compare particular qualities of different cures. For instance, in a large remedy collection in a late fourteenth- or early fifteenth-century collection, a remedy for burns concludes 'þys fayrest helyng þat ys of alle þe oþer but not þe hastyest' ('This is the fairest healing out of all the others but not the quickest'). The next remedy, for the same affliction, ends 'þys ys þe raþest helyng for soþe' ('this is the quickest healing truly').[91] Here, the reader is asked to choose between aesthetic and practical concerns, between a remedy that will heal the burn best and, as the adjective

---

[90] A similar point about the necessity of building on past discoveries is also made in Henry Daniel, *Liber Uricrisiarum*, p. 37, lines 70–82; he in turn cites the arguments of Aristotle: see Aristotle, *On Sophistical Refutations; On Coming to Be; On Passing Away; On the Cosmos*, trans. by E.S. Forster and D.J. Furley (London, 1955), pp. 152–3.
[91] BL, MS Additional 33996, f. 129v.

'fayre' implies, create the best cosmetic appearance, and a remedy that works more efficiently. In a similar way, a few recipe collections give the reader a helpful choice between expensive and cheap remedies. For example, one fifteenth-century collection contains fourteen successive remedies for gout.[92] Amongst them, one remedy finishes with the claim 'þis ys excelent and expert and preuid þing', and yet the next opens by proclaiming, 'But for lordis and ladys...'.[93] Social degree and cost decide the type of medicine that should be used. In these examples, the factors differentiating the remedies are made clear and the choice offered is, in terms of real-world practice, a useful one.

Sometimes, though, marks by writers and readers that appear to create distinctions between accumulated remedies actually confuse them further. For example, in a late fourteenth- or early fifteenth-century collection, there are seven recipes for the same eye afflictions.[94] Some of these are drawn into a hierarchical structure: the second remedy begins 'Item et melius' ('another and it is better'), suggesting that this remedy is more effective than the first. A third remedy is then copied without comment before a fourth remedy begins 'Item optimum' (another that is best); this remedy ends with the English claim 'þys ys souereyne'. Glossed by the preceding Latin word *optimus*, the adjective *soverain* functions here superlatively to mean 'foremost of its kind'.[95] This hierarchy, apart from the odd third recipe inserted between the better and best remedies, is easy to comprehend. However, the next remedy in the sequence begins 'Item þe moyst souereyn' ('another that is the most best'). This construction—adding the superlative 'moyst' to the already positive 'souereyn'—seems problematically tautological. The creator of this hierarchy, having used too many positive constructions, now seems to be straining to differentiate between the accumulated remedies, and one can imagine that a reader would have difficulty knowing how to distinguish between them too. Moreover, the decision to copy another two cures after this hierarchal structure is odd; like the third recipe, they are unmarked. Why would one choose these three unmarked cures over the avowedly 'better' and 'best' ones? The insatiable impulse amongst compilers to keep on accruing recipes is again demonstrated. That accrual may have been

---

[92] BodL, MS Ashmole 1443, pp. 312–15. Additional remedies seem, though, originally to have been present on damaged leaves. Four more recipes for gout (including one by a later hand) occur on p. 317. Remedies for epilepsy, which was sometimes considered a type of gout, appear in between on p. 316.
[93] Ibid., p. 313.   [94] BL, MS Additional 33996, f. 131r–v.
[95] MED, *soverain*, adj., entry 1(b).

motivated by the factors discussed earlier in this chapter. But it may also have been motivated by a desire to showcase social status and financial success: placing unremarkable cures next to superior ones affirms the ability of the collection's owner to choose the superior over the inferior, regardless of the extra cost and effort involved.

Such ostentatiousness may also be detected in other recipes made to stand out within collections.[96] The remedy below, which is for the skin affliction *saucefleume*, occurs in a short collection of recipes and charms copied by a fifteenth-century mixed hand and intermingled with other Latin and English scientific texts by other hands. It is entitled 'A souereyne medcyne for the sausflewme provid in hye and lowe', suggesting that it was intended to seem affordable to all levels of society. One would not expect such a catch-all remedy to be of the finest quality. Consequently, there is a peculiar disjunction between the recipe's title and its insistence that only the best ingredients be used:

> Take the fayrest baroweys grece þat ȝe can gete and newyst slayne of the flathys þan boyle hit fayre and white // than take þe fayryst and þe whytest brymston þat ȝe can gete[97]

> [*baroweys grece* = boar's fat; *flathys* = skate, a type of fish; *brymston* = a substance containing sulphur]

Although the recipe writer strives through multiple superlatives to convey quality, he or she does recognize through the phrase 'þat ȝe can gete' the limitations—be those geographical or financial—constraining some readers. It is possible, then, that the writer's concern was less with ostentation and more with best practice or with maximizing the chances of the remedy's effectiveness: one of the meanings of the adjective or adverb *fair*, used three times in the recipe, is 'suitable' or 'fitting' and it is logical to assume that using the most suitable type of an ingredient and boiling it for the most appropriate amount of time would produce the most effective, and therefore most useful, remedy.[98]

---

[96] Griffin, 'Reconsidering the Recipe', p. 148 makes a similar point in relation to culinary recipes.
[97] CUL, MS Ee.1.15, f. 15r. A later hand has crossed out this remedy and others on ff. 14v, 15r, 16v, 17r, 18r, 78r–v, 93r, and 94r–v. The majority of these are charms and, since the above recipe is followed by a crossed-out charm, it may have been crossed out by mistake.
[98] *MED, fair*, adj., entry 9.

Through this association with proper practice, though, the word 'fair' still evokes aesthetic concepts and particularly that of *decorum*: that term only began to be used and theorized in sixteenth-century discussions of literary practice, but the idea of fittingness was already integral to classical and medieval poetic handbooks.[99] For instance, a mid-twelfth-century commentary upon Horace's *Ars poetica* includes in a list of faults in poetic composition the incongruous arrangement of the parts of a work ('partium incongrua positio').[100] The commentator explains, 'Parts are placed incongruously when the beginning is discordant with the middle, and the middle is discordant with the end' ('Que utique incongrue ponuntur "Cum primum medio, medium quoque discrepat imo"').[101] This suggests that performing something in the correct, ordered, and proper manner can produce aesthetic pleasure—whether that be the writing of a poem, copying of a recipe, or preparation of an ointment.

The remedy's ostentatious demand for the 'fayryst' and 'whytest' kind of sulphur also evokes western European ideals of human, and particularly female, beauty.[102] These frequently centred around paleness.[103] For instance, a cosmetic recipe, copied by English landowner Robert Thornton amongst large numbers of medical remedies, contains instructions 'for to mak a woman white & softe'.[104] The application of this same aesthetic discourse in the above remedy to substances such as brimstone and boar's fat suggests that medical texts constituted a craft discourse both connected to, and distinct from, other accounts of aesthetic experience: medical writings are based upon the same aesthetic principles, but they apply these principles to the most unlikely of things, encouraging modern readers to diversify and expand their concept of what counted as 'aesthetic' in the Middle Ages.

Particular remedies, then, can be made to stand out in a collection in ways that envelop the practical and the aesthetic inside of one another. But,

---

[99] Copeland and Sluiter, eds, *Medieval Grammar and Rhetoric*, p. 41.

[100] Karsten Friis-Jensten, 'The *Ars poetica* in Twelfth-Century France: The Horace of Matthew of Vendôme, Geoffrey of Vinsauf and John of Garland', in *The Medieval Horace*, ed. by Karsten Friis-Jensen and others (Rome, 2015), pp. 51–99 (pp. 62–3).

[101] Latin quoted from Friis-Jensten, 'The *Ars poetica* in Twelfth-Century France', p. 62. Translation from Copeland and Sluiter, eds, *Medieval Grammar and Rhetoric*, p. 553.

[102] See also BodL, MS Rawlinson C.506, f. 115v for a recipe for *chare de quince* which claims that the medically useful preserve it produces is 'þe whitest of all'.

[103] Geraldine Heng, *The Invention of Race in the European Middle Ages* (Cambridge, 2018), pp. 181–4. Other ways of constructing colour and race of course also existed, including those in which black or non-Christian bodies are idealized: see Heng, *Invention of Race*, pp. 184–256; Cohen, 'On Saracen Enjoyment', pp. 119–20.

[104] Ogden, ed., *The "Liber de diversis medicinis"*, p. 58.

more often than not, there is no straightforward or obvious way of distinguishing between multiple remedies for the same affliction, just as there is no straightforward way of interpreting the act of accrual itself: as we have seen, large numbers of remedies could—and did—signify practical resourcefulness, intellectual and domestic collaboration, the necessity of trial and error, reassurance, and hope for medieval readers. But they could also signify information overload, the unmanageable variety of human bodies, false hope, and failure. The cumulative forms of many medieval remedy books are, therefore, opaque marks driven by a multitude of possible motivations and—to redeploy Bahr's terms—they are just as capable as any literary text or manuscript of generating 'discontinuities and excesses, multiple and shifting meanings...and openness to re-reading'.[105] In Chapters 4 and 5, these slippery and changeable acts of interpretation are foregrounded even more as we move to consider the consequences of compilatory forms and fragmentary arrangements in particular thematic contexts: how do such forms continually resituate the body in time? How do those forms repeatedly erect and erase boundaries for readers—be those boundaries bodily, sacred, or social? Such considerations inevitably foreground ideas of play, probing the particular kinds of imaginative and perspectival mobility that those compilations encouraged.

[105] Bahr, *Fragments and Assemblages*, p. 10.

PART III
FRAGMENTS IN PLAY

4
Recipe Time
(Re)Imagining Bodies

> All this processe concludith vp[on] time[1]
>
> John Lydgate, 'The Dietary'

This line only appears in two of the extant manuscript copies of Lydgate's 'Dietary'.[2] It is part of an eight-stanza sequence which, though written in Lydgate's characteristic style, does not always seem to have been considered part of the regimen. However, the line sums up much of the poem's advice: all versions of 'The Dietary' stress the importance of waking, eating, drinking, and sleeping at the optimum time and for the optimum amount of time: 'vse nevir late for to suppe' (32), 'bit agid men betymes go to rest' (56), and 'suffre no surfetis in thyn hous at nyht' (137). In all regimens, it is imagined that such advice will be put into practice by the reader throughout the course of his or her life: the recommendations are not just one-off, quick-fix cures, but rituals to be internalized and repeated *through* time.

Practising, writing, and reading about medicine usually necessitated careful attention to time: medicines had to be administered for certain durations and at particular hours; diagnostic and prognostic judgements required practitioners to look back and forward in time, and the patient's age and life circumstances (past and present) informed their individual bodily complexion and the kind of treatment they received. What is more, bodies—with their pulses, heartbeats, progressively wrinkled skin, and changing shapes—functioned as constant reminders of the passing of the years. This relationship between time and change has long been theorized: in a formulation that would influence many medieval thinkers, Aristotle

---

[1] Lydgate, 'The Dietary', in *The Minor Poems*, ed. by MacCracken, p. 704, line 89. Subsequent references within this chapter are included within the text.

[2] Walsh Morrissey, '"To al Indifferent"', p. 260.

suggested that without perception of change, we would not perceive time.[3] Echoing this, St Augustine defined 'mutability' as 'the means by which we are aware of time and measure it'.[4]

Bodily transformations, however, are not just indications of time's passing; those changes—understood (in part) through culturally constructed interpretive lenses—can also *shape* how individual bodies experience time.[5] Recently, scholars have tried to tease out, theorize, and increase the visibility of certain communities' temporal experiences; such experiences have traditionally been overlooked by modern cultures focused on normative, sequential time. For instance, scholars working within the field of disability studies have tried to build up a more nuanced idea of 'crip time' which, without being reductive, can encompass the unpredictable, non-linear, asynchronous temporalities that people with disabilities and chronic illnesses can experience. As Ellen Samuels writes:

> Crip time is time travel. Disability and illness have the power to extract us from linear, progressive time with its normative life stages and cast us into a wormhole of backward and forward acceleration, jerky stops and starts, tedious intervals, and abrupt endings.[6]

In a similar way, Carolyn Dinshaw's recent study of medieval texts and their reception by various modern 'queer' readers has explored 'forms of desirous, embodied being that are out of sync with the ordinary linear measurements of everyday life, that engage heterogenous temporalities or that precipitate out of time altogether', and she concludes that 'time itself is wondrous, marvelous, full of queer potential'.[7] Dinshaw moves between specific and capacious meanings of 'queer', using it to refer to a variety of temporal

---

[3] Aristotle, *The Physics*, trans. by Philip Wicksteed and Francis Cornford, 2 vols (London, 1929), vol. I, Bk IV.11, p. 383. For further discussion of Aristotelian and Augustinian conceptions of time, see Carolyn Dinshaw, *How Soon Is Now? Medieval Texts, Amateur Readers, and the Queerness of Time* (Durham, NC, 2012), pp. 1–16.

[4] Augustine, *Confessions: Books 9–13*, ed. and trans. by Carolyn J.B. Hammond (Cambridge, MA, 2016), pp. 272–3.

[5] On the relationship between biology and culture, see discussion of the distinction between impairment (an anatomical and biological condition) and disability (a social construct), and the limitations of both models, in Joshua R. Eyler, 'Introduction: Breaking Boundaries, Building Bridges', in *Disability in the Middle Ages: Reconsiderations and Reverberations*, ed. by Joshua R. Eyler (Farnham, 2010), pp. 1–8.

[6] Ellen Samuels, 'Six Ways of Looking at Crip Time', *Disability Studies Quarterly*, 37 (2017), n.p.

[7] Dinshaw, *How Soon Is Now?*, pp. 4, 130.

experiences, often informed by embodied desire, that do not fit normative, sequential constructions of time.[8] Most of us, studies such as Dinshaw's suggest, experience embodied varieties of non-linear, disrupted, and plural time at particular points in our lives. These flexible conceptions of time—with the somatic at their heart—are thus vital to this chapter's exploration of embodied being in health, sickness, and all the states in between.

Medieval writings offer many opportunities for exploring non-linear time in relation to illness and disability. Until now, critical attention has focused predominantly on canonical, literary writings. Consider, for example, chapter 56 of *The Boke of Margery Kempe*, where Margery's sequential succession of different sicknesses is recorded. Readers are told that Margery endured one of these ailments—a pain 'in hir ryth syde'—intermittently over a number of weeks: 'Sumtyme sche had it onys in a weke contunyng, sumtyme xxx owrys, sumtyme xx, sumtyme x, sumtyme viii, sumtyme iiii, and sumtyme ii...'.[9] The illness is irregular and unpredictable, disrupting any routine or order. However, there is a clear attempt to cajole the experience of illness *into* an order of descending frequency. In relation to a very similar passage, which records the irregular and intermittent nature of Margery's fervent crying, Dinshaw notes that, through that 'careful count', a 'strange commensurability is imposed on... explosive incommensurability'.[10]

Canonical literary writings like this were not, though, the only texts that represented (and sometimes tried to control) the ruptured, plural, terrifying, and marvellous temporalities experienced by sick bodies: different genres of medical writing also tried to order the body in time. We have already seen how medieval regimen inserted the body into a cyclical, ongoing routine of earthly maintenance. Astrological texts, on the other hand, depicted the patient's body as subject to the domination of particular planetary influences at particular times; those influences could be manipulated by medical practitioners for health or harm. Yet more temporal variety can be found in uroscopies: these not only required the practitioner to look forward to the future (in the act of prognosis) but also to deduce the past and present workings of the patient's body from their urine in order to issue a diagnosis. Accordingly, Henry Daniel, echoing the start of the Hippocratic *Prognostics* and Isidore of Seville's *Etymologiae*, claimed in his vernacular

---

[8] Alison Kafer, *Feminist, Queer, Crip* (Bloomington, IN, 2013), p. 28 also links different kinds of asynchronous time by stating that 'illness, disability and crip time are always already present in queer time'.
[9] Windeatt, ed., *The Book of Margery Kempe*, p. 272.
[10] Dinshaw, *How Soon Is Now?*, p. 114.

Liber Uricrisiarum that 'hit behovith him that shall be a leche for to knowyn thingis þat arn passid and wittin þingis þat nowe arn and for to sen beforn thingis þat arn for to comyn'.[11] This advice bestows the medical manipulation of time with an ethical dimension: prudence, classified by medieval thinkers as a cardinal virtue, was the ability to determine the most appropriate source of practical action through consideration of past events, present circumstances, and future consequences.[12]

As patchwork creations that often contain bits of astrological, uroscopic, and prognostic lore embedded within or attached to recipes, remedy books incorporate the temporal structures of all these medical genres; they are already, then, the perfect genre through which to explore temporal multiplicity. But remedies also contain their own distinctive—and plural—ways of structuring time. Some of these have already been studied: drawing on the work of Jack Goody, Lisa Cooper has explored how recipes and their literary rewritings could be simultaneously 'prescriptive and commemorative', recording past actions and mapping future ones.[13] In a similar way, Wendy Wall has highlighted the conceptual importance of 'preservation' for early modern culinary and medical recipes, exploring the various ways in which recipe writers and readers 'indulged in dreams of a world where humans might prevent or retard loss in a capacious sense'.[14]

In this chapter, I focus on two other temporal structures characterizing recipes and constructing bodies: firstly, some recipes prescribe incredibly long and convoluted processes of preparing medicines. At the same time, though, remedies often promise that the cure they describe will bring about the patient's recovery rapidly: drawn out labours can thus stand in stark contrast to miraculously quick results. Each of these temporal structures is also measured and marked in a multitude of ways: in hours or days, in the number of minutes it takes to speak the psalm *Miserere mei, Deus*, or in the

---

[11] HEHL, MS HM 505, f. 79v. See Lindsay, ed., *Isidori Hispalensis Episcopi*, Bk IV, p. 177, lines 1–2 and *Hippocrates: Volume II*, ed. by Jeffrey Henderson and trans. by W.H.S. Jones (Cambridge, MA, 1923), pp. 6–7. For further discussion, see Hannah Bower, '"Her ovn self seid me": The Function of Anecdote in Henry Daniel's Liber Uricrisiarum', in *Henry Daniel and the Rise of Middle English Medical Writing*, ed. by Sarah Star (Toronto, forthcoming), pp. 133–57.

[12] John A. Burrow, 'The Third Eye of Prudence', in *Medieval Futures: Attitudes to the Future in the Middle Ages*, ed. by J.A. Burrow and Ian P. Wei (Woodbridge, 2000), pp. 37–48; on further connections between prudence and medicine, see Kathryn Crowcroft, 'Reconsidering Sense: Towards a Theory of Medieval Preventative Medicine', *Postmedieval: A Journal of Medieval Cultural Studies*, 8 (2017), 162–9.

[13] Cooper, 'Recipes for the Realm', p. 197. See also Jack Goody, *The Domestication of the Savage Mind* (Cambridge, 1977), pp. 129–45.

[14] Wall, *Recipes for Thought*, pp. 167–8.

time it takes to walk a certain number of miles.[15] Time can also be marked by seasonal and astrological events, by prayer times, and, in later recipes, one also finds occasional references to clocks, a relatively new late medieval urban phenomenon: for instance, a remedy for the pestilence which was probably copied in the second half of the fifteenth century instructs the reader to gather herbs 'bytwyn viij and ix of þe clocke'.[16]

The most obvious conceptual lens through which to interpret this contrast between prolonged labour and rapid recovery is perhaps that of Christian salvation: through church iconography, sermons, and all kinds of written text, medieval people were surrounded by reminders of humanity's fallen, sinful, labouring state and, at the same time, its miraculous redemption through the healed, resurrected body of Christ. Some writers and readers do evoke this history in their interpretations of recipe temporalities. But it was not the only interpretative lens available: as we shall see, other possible contexts include secular debates about what counted as proper and productive labour and satirical critiques of temporal abuses. Each provides different ways of viewing recipe times, showing how both prolonged preparation and rapid recovery could be poised between the marvellous and the mundane, the wondrous and the ridiculous. What is more, in some texts, a potential conflict exists between the two temporalities: spending too long preparing a cure could *prevent* the possibility of any kind of recovery for a sick patient, rapid or otherwise.

It is worth remembering, of course, that to a greater extent than modern readers, medieval people were used to combining, representing, and coexisting in multiple temporalities. In his study of 'church time' and 'merchant time', Jacques Le Goff argued that the introduction of mechanical clocks allowed merchants to measure, buy, and sell their time accurately. This contrasted and sometimes conflicted with the church's view that man's time belonged to God and could not be sold for profit. Le Goff acknowledged, though, that for merchants, church time could function as a 'second horizon', framing their religious life.[17] Subsequent discussions of medieval time by Linne Mooney, Chris Humphrey, Paul Brand, Caroline Barron, and Paul

---

[15] Examples of recipes using this psalm to measure time occur in TCC, MS O.2.13, ff. 102v, 129r; it is not clear why this psalm specifically was chosen. Examples of time measured by walking distances occur in BodL, MS Douce 78, ff. 8r, 11r, 13v, 14r, 14v, 16r, 17r.

[16] BodL, MS Laud misc. 553, f. 66v. For time measured by prayer times, see TCC, R.14.39, f. 40r and, for a recipe structured around midsummer, see BodL, MS Ashmole 1438, Part I, p. 101.

[17] Jacques Le Goff, *Time, Work and Culture in the Middle Ages*, trans. by Arthur Goldhammer (Chicago, IL, 1980), pp. 29–42 (p. 37).

Strohm have developed this emphasis upon multiplicity beyond the purview of merchants, arguing that individuals of many different walks of life made use simultaneously of different ways of measuring time, not all of which were compatible.[18] Medieval writers sometimes reflected upon this incommensurability, particularly in the collision between human and eternal time: addressing God, St Augustine wrestled with the untranslatability of eternity into human terms: 'everything tomorrow and beyond, everything yesterday and before, all of it you will make, and you have made, your "today"'.[19] Augustine also presented time as something experienced, measured, and conceptualized subjectively in the mind (and specifically the memory), rather than as part of any objective reality: 'Within you, O my mind, I measure times'.[20] It is clear that, for Augustine and those influenced by him, individual minds were sites where multiple temporal frameworks were continuously competing, interacting, and pulling in different directions. Indeed, Augustine acknowledged that, as he tried (and failed) to understand the passing of time, he felt himself being painfully 'ripped apart by turbulent vicissitudes'.[21] Time and change are here linked to a pain that is simultaneously imaginative and bodily.

This chapter contends then that, because recipes are concerned with bodies in states of flux and change, and because remedy books are patchwork compilations absorbing influences from all kinds of medical and non-medical writings, they are—in spite of their ostensibly linear and sequential form—the perfect genre through which to explore medieval experiences of temporal plurality. In the subsequent pages, I explore how various meanings might be attached to recipes' temporal structures of prolonged preparation and rapid recovery by medieval readers. Some of these readers are medical thinkers; some are poets who repurpose recipes creatively. Other readers are

---

[18] Linne R. Mooney, 'The Cock and the Clock: Telling Time in Chaucer's Day', *Studies in the Age of Chaucer*, 15 (1993), 91–109; Chris Humphrey, 'Time and Urban Culture in Late Medieval England', in *Time in the Medieval World*, ed. by Chris Humphrey and W.M. Ormrod (Woodbridge, 2001), pp. 105–17; Paul Brand, 'Lawyers' Time in England in the Later Middle Ages', in *Time in the Medieval World*, ed. by Humphrey and Ormrod, pp. 73–104; Caroline Barron, 'Telling the Time in Chaucer's London', in *'A verray parfit praktisour': Essays Presented to Carole Rawcliffe*, ed. by Linda Clark and Elizabeth Danbury (Woodbridge, 2017), pp. 141–51; Paul Strohm, *Social Chaucer* (Cambridge, MA, 1989), pp. 110–43.

[19] Augustine, *Confessions: Books 1–8*, ed. and trans. by Carolyn J.B. Hammond (Cambridge, MA, 2014), p. 17.

[20] Augustine, *Confessions: Books 9–13*, pp. 248–9. He continues: 'What I measure is the actual present impressions produced in you by passing events; and which remains when those events have passed'. For further discussion, see Dinshaw, *How Soon Is Now?*, pp. 13–14.

[21] Augustine, *Confessions: Books 9–13*, pp. 254–5.

manuscript compilers who (intentionally or not) place recipe collections next to texts which function as commentaries on recipe time and open up even more multi-layered and intersecting temporal horizons. We return here to Arthur Bahr's notion of 'compilational reading', a subjective mode of reading in which readers interpret different textual fragments as belonging to 'an interpretably meaningful arrangement'.[22] As Bahr notes, compilations—produced and rearranged through time and reformulated in the event of each reading—are themselves products, and producers, of a 'nexus' of different temporalities.[23] In this chapter, we shall see that remedy compilations not only demand that readers move flexibly between temporal perspectives, envisaging their bodies in mundane *and* marvellous time, but that they also consistently redefine what counts as 'marvellous' and 'mundane'.

Laborious Preparations

Certain medieval medical treatments were renowned for their complex composition and time-consuming preparation. For instance, the most esteemed Montpellier variety of *theriac*, a late medieval panacea, allegedly contained eighty-three different substances.[24] Although many of the cures in remedy collections only contain a handful of ingredients and a few simple instructions, there are often remedies within larger collections that seem far more convoluted. Some of these recipes require even more ingredients than the Montpellier *theriac*. For example, this recipe for a medicinal concoction called 'water of antioche' is from a large late fifteenth-century collection copied by one hand after the herbal *Agnus castus*; it may have been used in a professional or domestic context. Rubrication is marked in bold:

> **For to make the water of antioche that is the most principalle water and the best that mai be founde For that shal hele al maner sores** Take . woderoue . bugle . pygle . sanycle . tormentille . scabiouse . ambrosye . betayne . mousere . mousepese . palma Christi of euerich **v . vncer** . irenharde wodebynde . redebrere . feldethorne herbe iohn herbe water . herbe robert wodesoure coluerfote tanasye of euerich **iij vnce** consolida maior . consolida minor brounewort osemound of euerich . **v . vnces** fumetorie

---

[22] Bahr, *Fragments*, p. 3.   [23] Ibid., p. 15.
[24] Paul Freedman, *Out of the East: Spices and the Medieval Imagination* (New Haven, CT, 2008), p. 68.

egremonie warmode . southernewode of euerich . **ij vnce** tauke auance mader **as moch wight as of all the other herbis before** hayryfe ʒarewe . ribbewort weibrode ysope watercresse . sauge . lauendre off euerich **an handfull** dytaundre **v . vnce** crowesope brome . verueyne . hemp rede dokke . rede netele . the rote of redes that groweth in water orpyne . rede cowele of euerich **ij . vnces and halfe** violett daundelion vrtica greca colombyne . herbe yue . solsequye . todewort persile . rewe of euerich **an vnce and a quarter** flos campi . **iij vnces** . croyser . morell . hillewort . puliol ryall . flexe hokkes . clytheren houndestong . baume . peritorie . radiche . horehounde of euerich **an vnce and half** astrologia rotunda . watercarse . weyhore eufragie toutsayen . merche moderwort moggewort wild tesyle bornet of euerich **an vncer and iij quarter .** Gracia dei . centorie radix gladioli pympernole . saxefragie . filipendula . calamynte of euerich . **iij handful** . origoun . streberi wyse . prymerose cowslippe . houndestonge . spygernole . endeyue . yuy of the oke . rede rose maidenhere . holihokke of euerych **v . vnces** cryspe malowe . vartelon rosemaryne maiorana . caraway . cerefoyl peruynk . leke sedewale affodylle of everich **ij . vnces and a quarter .** groundeswelie **ij vnces** smerewort lombestonge valeryane . lauriole leues . mercurie . borage . costemarye . wilde tansie . quyntefoyle of euerich **ij vnce and a quarte** filles dragaunce . softe . bursa pastoris rede mynte . haymayde of everich . **ij . vnces.**[25]

I have concluded that the recipe requires 125 herbs and substances.[26] Other recipes in the collection contain similarly large numbers of ingredients: for example, a remedy for gout requires thirty-eight herbs and a recipe for a salve requires sixty-one.[27] Intriguingly, the collection also contains another recipe for 'water of antioche' but it is much shorter, only requiring fourteen different herbs, honey, and white wine.[28] Perhaps this less time-consuming and expensive recipe was considered a more practical alternative to that above. Like the recipes examined in Chapter 3, which were distinguished by their use of the finest ingredients, the lengthy recipe may only have been included because it suggested wealth: the owner of the recipe book *could* purchase all of these ingredients *if* he or she chose to do so.

---

[25] HEHL, MS HM 58, f. 85r-v.
[26] I have counted 'flexe hokkes' as two plants (flax and *hok*, the latter relating to plants of the genera Malva and Althæa; see MED, *hok*, n. 1, entry 1(a)); however, it could have been a scribal mistake for *flex hoppes*, the seed pods of the flax.
[27] HEHL, MS HM 58, ff. 51v-52v, 66r-v, respectively.   [28] Ibid., f. 90r.

In other lengthy recipes, it is not the number of ingredients which makes them appear time-consuming, but the number of stages involved in their preparation and the way those stages are described. The remedy below is for a fistula. It comes from a large remedy collection in a mid-fifteenth-century manuscript copied predominantly in one hand which also contains Walter Hilton's devotional guide *On the Mixed Life* and an English translation of the encyclopaedic, pseudo-Aristotelian text, the *Secreta Secretorum*. The fact that Hilton's *On the Mixed Life* is addressed to a wealthy layman may suggest that the manuscript functioned in a lay household as a repository of bodily and spiritual advice. The recipe in question reads:

> A medecyn for the comyne festre / tak hardys / and hak theym and wet hem wel in lyes of ale / that ys ymad of whete and soth hem wel and bynd hyt so vppon the sore a hol ny3t / and a hol day /and thanne tak hyt away and wasch the sor wyth mannys pysse / and lok thou haue poudre alredy ymad in thys manere Tak the grete fetheres of the gos and do away the rowe and thanne bren hem and mak a poudre therof and do hyt in a molour and lay that poudre on the sore and vppon that lay lard of the bor or of a barw and sauge / and vppon al that a wortlef and after tak goud stal ale that ys mad of whete clene wythoute barly or any other corn and fyl therof a pot that be hol and newe and put therto salt / and pych and arnement of eche elyche moche / and of wex more thane of any othyr and seth al thys ry3t wel tylle at hyt be thykke and set yt thanne adoun and lat hyt kele and sattelyn and thanne make a plastere ther of and lay to þe festre / Fyrst laye the forsayd poudre and thanne the plastere and thanne the lard / and thanne þe lofd and chaunge at morwe / and at euen /and 3yf hym drynke eche morwe anence for that day þat he drynketh hyt he shal not greue[29]

> [*hardys* = the coarse part of flax; *lye3* = sediment; *molour* = handheld stone for grinding substances; *barw* = castrated boar; *sauge* = sage; *wortlef* = cabbage leaf; *arnement* = iron or copper sulphate; *lofd* = error for leaf?; *morwe anence* = towards morning]

The extended paratactic, polysyndetic structures ('and...and...and') and temporal conjunctions ('Fyrst...thanne...thanne') make explicit to the reader the number of stages involved in the remedy's preparation; twenty-six different imperatives communicate the labour's varied and protracted

---

[29] BodL, MS Laud misc. 685, ff. 83v–84r.

nature. Furthermore, extended sequences of pre- or postmodifiers such as 'goud stal ale that ys mad of whete clene wythoute barly' suggest that locating ingredients or apparatus that are just right might take the reader a significant amount of time.

The ingredients in the recipe also have to be left for a particular number of days if they are to prove efficacious: the mixture of flax and ale sediment must be left for 'a hol nyȝt / and a hol day'. In other collections, ingredients have to be left for much longer periods: for example, a fifteenth-century remedy for wounds instructs the reader to hang up a herbal mixture 'a fourtnyght befor myssomer and a fourtnyght after' and a fifteenth-century remedy for gout requires the reader to bury a pot of henbane leaves deep in the ground before taking it up 'and þat day a xij monthe þat þou didest hit in þe erþe'.[30] These recipes both have a ritualistic air about them: the symmetry of two weeks before and two weeks after midsummer and the pleasing circularity of one year suggest that these time spans may have been selected, in part, for their aesthetic appeal. In the above remedy for a fistula, the aesthetic dimension to this ritualistic experience is communicated—and heightened—by the fact that the period of time for which the ingredients must be left is communicated through a nicely balanced but circumlocutory structure: 'a hol nyȝt / and a hol day'. It would have been simpler to write 'a nyȝt and day'. The circumlocution in this phrase and the emphatic tone of 'hol' underscore that waiting for the ingredients to combine is, like the rest of the recipe, a process that will extend through, and take up, time.

This fistula remedy not only records a time-consuming and laborious process; it is also time-consuming to read. As well as stringing together imperatives, it moves back and forth in time in a way that is hard to follow. The recipe begins by telling the reader to make and apply a concoction to the patient's sore; it then instructs him or her to make a particular powder but it simultaneously shifts back in time because it tells the reader that he or she should already have made it: 'lok thou haue poudre alredy ymad in thys manere'. Afterwards, the reader is instructed to lay the powder to the sore, followed by the fat of a boar, sage, and a cabbage leaf. Next, instructions are given to make a plaster. Immediately after, however, another moment of temporal confusion occurs: the reader is again instructed to apply 'the forsayd poudre', the fat, and the leaf, only this time the application of the plaster is inserted between that of the powder and the boar's fat. Although this

---

[30] Respectively, BodL, MS Ashmole 1438, Part I, p. 101 and BodL, MS Laud misc. 553, f. 63r.

seems to be a repetition of, and addition to, the earlier application sequence, it is initially unclear whether it is a correction to it. Such temporal ambiguity gives the remedy a cyclical and confusing feel, encouraging a reader to reread it in an attempt at clarification. The remedy therefore not only depicts a time-consuming process, it also creates one, complicating most readers' instinctive assumption that recipes plot linear, sequential temporalities. The laboriousness of both these processes also contrasts with the rapidity with which the treatment is claimed to work once inside the body: 'that day þat he drynketh hyt he shal not greue'. The incredibly long preparation and rapid working of the remedy seem carefully juxtaposed: each works to make the temporal characteristics of the other more noticeable.

In this account of preparing a cure, then, there is no urgency. Only occasionally do medical recipes explicitly urge the reader to be hasty in their preparations.[31] One might contrast this lack of explicit haste with the sustained urgency of other types of writing concerned with the sick. For example, a widely copied devotional text, which scripts a speech of Christian reassurance to be delivered to the sick and dying alongside the last rites, survives in a fifteenth-century manuscript where several other late medieval hands have copied remedy collections.[32] This combination of religious and medical texts is not surprising: religion was thought to be an effective remedy for the soul *and* the body, because bodily afflictions were sometimes (though by no means always) considered the result of spiritual sickness.[33] Every person—ageing, mortal, and on the path to death—was in fact already in a state of physical infirmity because of original sin. Accordingly, the Fourth Lateran Council of 1215, which tried to implement a range of changes to confessional practice, decreed that, before offering medical treatment to a patient, it was the physician's responsibility to ensure that the

---

[31] Exceptions include recipes on TCC, MS R.14.39, f. 19r and TCC, MS 0.1.13, ff. 65r, 151r, which promise alleviation if the medicine is administered 'betymys' ('promptly') and an acephalous recipe on BodL, MS Ashmole 1477, Part I, f. 34r, which instructs the reader to strain a mixture 'as faste as thow may wythoute taryynge'. See also Chapter 2 for discussion of some verse remedies that—sometimes as filler lines to complete the rhyme—urge haste.

[32] BodL, MS Ashmole 750, ff. 11v–14r. Substantial recipe collections occur between ff. 142r–147v; 169v–179r; and 184r–194r. On this *ars moriendi* text, see Amy Appleford, *Learning to Die in London, 1380–1540* (Philadelphia, PA, 2015), pp. 18–54.

[33] Naoë Kukita Yoshikawa, 'Introduction', in *Medicine, Religion and Gender in Medieval Culture*, ed. by Naoë Kukita Yoshikawa (Cambridge, 2015), pp. 9–17. Scholars have shown, however, that spiritual sickness and disability were not always connected and the latter was not necessarily negative: see Metzler, *Disability in Medieval Europe*, pp. 38–64.

patient had already confessed his or her sins.[34] It is therefore no surprise that, like others of its kind, this *Ars moriendi* text urges haste: at various intervals, the script is punctuated by commands such as 'Of thu maist noȝt for haste of deth seie al this befor: begyn here.'[35] Whereas the temporal distortions in the recipe text threatened to prolong and confuse the process of medical treatment, the temporal leap in this *Ars moriendi* text encourages the reader to skip through the text in cases of severe sickness, hastening the provision of spiritual remedies.

One might explain these different levels of urgency in the remedy and religious text by arguing that, for medieval writers and readers, the stakes of saving the soul were (discursively at least) far higher than those of saving the body. But this fails to convince because, though urgency is often absent from the remedies' description of preparing cures, it is not absent from the remedies altogether: as we shall see later in this chapter, many recipes contain reassurances that, once the patient has used or ingested the remedy, he or she will be cured within a small number of days. This reassurance shows that the authors and copiers of the remedies *were* concerned with lessening bodily pain in this life. Perhaps, then, the lack of urgency in the cures is better understood as a pragmatic acknowledgement of the fact that some processes cannot be sped up: because of the seasons and astrological movements of the planets, herbs need to be collected at particular times and prepared in particular ways; substances need time to react with one another. Medieval readers clearly recognized and made provision for these delays: just as the remedy for a fistula assumes that the reader will have preprepared the required powder, others instruct the reader to place the remedy into boxes ready for future use: 'put hit yn a box of horne or of copre and whan þou wylt... put a lytylle yn þyn eyȝen'.[36] A minority of recipes also instruct the reader to purchase ingredients or preprepared mixtures from an apothecary.[37] Those purchases may have been more common in practice than the infrequency of these explicit instructions imply. All of these examples of foresight are ways for the practitioner to exercise prudence—to show his or her ability to use past and present experience of effective cures and

---

[34] Carole Rawcliffe, 'Curing Bodies and Healing Souls: Pilgrimage and the Sick in Medieval East Anglia', in *Pilgrimage: The English Experience from Becket to Bunyan*, ed. by Colin Morris and Peter Roberts (Cambridge, 2002), pp. 108–40 (p. 119).

[35] BodL, MS Ashmole 750, f. 13r. For similar exhortations to haste, see 'Lerne to Dye', in *Hoccleve's Works: The Minor Poems*, ed. by Frederick James Furnivall and Israel Gollancz, EETS es 61, 2nd edn (London, 1970), lines 365–6, 459, 772, and 904–10.

[36] BodL, MS Ashmole 1438, Part II, p. 3.   [37] E.g. TCC, MS O.1.65, ff. 253r, 254r.

commonplace ailments to calculate which remedies he or she might need at hand in the future.

The possibility that practitioners made some of these time-consuming cures in advance does not, however, change the fact that they invested significant time and effort in doing so. Even if the recipes were *never* put into practice, it is still interesting that scribes took the time to copy them alongside shorter, more convenient cures. Anthropologists such as Claude Lévi-Strauss and Pierre Bourdieu have shown that time is integral to understanding, or misunderstanding, cultural practices. They demonstrate this through gift exchanges: if a gift is reciprocated too soon, it suggests that the recipient felt under an obligation to return the gift; if the same gift that is given is returned immediately, the gift may have been rejected; if the return of the gift is decided upon when it is given, then some kind of loan is in place.[38] Bourdieu also argues that the strategic manipulation of time is at work even in cultural rituals which seem fixed and formulaic in nature—like recipes.[39] This idea of strategic manipulation can offer a useful way of interpreting lengthy cures: at what point do protracted labour and its written representation become spectacles, which are not merely responses to unalterable seasonal factors but are also intended, by means of their elongated nature, to impress an onlooker or reader? The above recipes—with their endless lists of herbs, pronounced temporal structures ('a hol day and a hol night'), and climactic juxtaposition of slow process and rapid result ('that day þat he drynketh hyt he shal not greue')—are certainly written in a way that shapes extended labour, or its written representation, into a spectacle to be marvelled at.

Of course, those spectacles might serve their own practical healing purpose, convincing patients of the practitioner's sophistication and prowess or the cure's ritualistic, occult potency. Furthermore, the recipes could have functioned as healing narratives. Narrative was well recognized in the Middle Ages as a healing tool, with medical practitioners such as John Arderne instructing practitioners to tell their patients comic, tragic, and biblical stories in order to distract, please, and uplift them. Read as narratives, each consecutive stage in these recipes could function as a new affirmation that the patient's affliction is being—or will be—methodically,

---

[38] Claude Lévi-Strauss, *The Elementary Structures of Kinship*, trans. by James Harle Bell and others (Boston, MA, 1969), pp. 52–3; Bourdieu, *Theory of Practice*, pp. 5–9.
[39] Bourdieu, *Theory of Practice*, p. 7.

meticulously, and diligently cured.[40] Such reassurances may have eased patients of their distress and, in doing so, actually improved their condition. But the protracted nature of the spectacle might also be interpreted negatively: at what point does the enacted or represented labour involved in the cure appear excessive and, therefore, absurd? At what point does the wondrous teeter into the ridiculous or inappropriate?

A literary text which recalls late medieval recipe discourse affirms this close relationship between time, wonder, and the ridiculous: John Gower's *Confessio Amantis* (c. 1390) is composed from a series of narratives, all of which are framed by the story of an ageing lover confessing his sins to the priest of Venus.[41] In Book V, the protagonist is told the story of Jason and Medea as a warning against the moral trials of love. Gower depicts Medea labouring extensively to produce a 'medicine' to restore Jason's ancient father, Eson, to his youth; time's onward, linear passage is here to be reversed.[42]

Gower's lengthy and detailed portrayal of this episode is closely based on Ovid's similarly lengthy representation in Book VII of *Metamorphoses*.[43] In the *Confessio*, Medea's labour is drawn out across 200 lines and divided into five stages: the gathering of ingredients (V. 3957–4022) is followed by a sacrifice to the Gods (V. 4023–58); next comes the performance of a ritual around Eson's body (V. 4059–114) and the preparation of the medicine (V. 4115–54), followed by the eventual administration of it (V. 4154–74). The labour required for each stage is described in great detail with consistent emphasis on its duration and difficulty: for instance, we are told that 'In daies and in nyhtes Nyne, | With gret travaile and with gret pyne, | [Medea] was pourveid of every piece' needed to concoct her remedy for old age. The superfluous prepositions in the temporal phrase 'in daies and in nyhtes Nyne' recall the circumlocutory phrase 'a hol ny3t / and a hol day' in the remedy for a fistula. Medea's remedy, however, goes well beyond even the most extravagant of medieval theriac recipes in the number of ingredients it

---

[40] E.g. *Treatises of Fistula in Ano, Hæmorrhoids, and Clysters*, ed. by D'Arcy Power, EETS os 22 (London, 1910), pp. 7–8. On the broader relationship between sickness and narrative, see Turner, 'Illness Narratives'.

[41] On other connections between Gower's poem and medical discourse, see Stadolnik, 'Gower's Bedside Manner'.

[42] *The English Works of John Gower*, ed. by G.C. Macaulay, EETS es 81-2, 2 vols (London, 1900–1), II, V. 4119, 4154. Future line references are within the text.

[43] Ovid, *Metamorphoses*, ed. and trans. by Frank Justus Miller, 2 vols (London, 1916), I, Bk VII, lines 179–293.

contains: it is allegedly composed from over 1,000 different substances (V. 4139).

Many of the ingredients used in the medicine and the rituals that accompany it are familiar from genuine remedies: like Ovid, Gower refers to 'warm melk' (V. 4048), 'hony' (V. 4049), and herbs such as 'fieldwode and verveyne' (V. 4039), all of which are common remedy ingredients.[44] Even ingredients such as the 'blod' from 'a wether which was blak' (V. 4045–6), which seem more mysteriously specific, have parallels: the blood of many different animals is used in medieval recipes and remedies often call specifically for parts of a black (rather than a white) sheep: for instance, a fifteenth-century remedy for aching joints calls for 'a pece of blake lambe skynne', adding that this is preferable to white skin but not explaining why.[45] In both the recipe and the *Confessio*, the blood of the black ram hovers precariously between possessing powers that are occult (or hidden) in the innocuous sense of natural magic and powers that seem more dangerously occult and liable to be connected with demonic magic.

It is notable, though, that many of Gower's lexical choices in the passage seem designed to soften (or at least nuance) Medea's associations in classical and medieval writing with witchcraft and sorcery: for instance, he twice describes Medea's concoction as a 'medicine' (V. 4119, 4154), using this to replace Ovid's term 'carmina' ('charms'), which has stronger associations with magic.[46] Moreover, when describing how Medea prepares the ram, Gower—unlike Ovid—writes, 'The blake wether tho sche tok, | And hiewh the fleissh, as doth a cok' (V. 4071–2).[47] This comparison not only evokes culinary recipes and domestic kitchen practices; it also evokes the culinary analogies frequently found in household remedies: 'for the goute take an owle and...opyn hym as þu woldyst ete hym'.[48] All of this suggests that Gower recognized the parallels between Ovid's depiction of Medea's protracted labour and that represented in contemporary recipes, approaching the former, in part, through the lens of the latter. It is impossible, however,

---

[44] See Ovid, *Metamorphoses*, I, Bk VII, lines 224–33, 247, and 244.
[45] BodL, MS Ashmole 1438, Part II, p. 24. For recipes requiring similar ingredients see BodL, MS Ashmole 750, f. 185r; TCC, MS O.1.13, f. 46r, and TCC, MS R.14.39, f. 8r.
[46] Ovid, *Metamorphoses*, I, Bk VII, lines 167, 253. On Medea's medieval reputation, see Ruth Morse, *The Medieval Medea* (Cambridge, 1996), pp. 185–236.
[47] Later in the poem, when Medea again proves her rejuvenation skills on an old ram at the house of Pelias, Ovid does describe Medea boiling a ram, but he never uses culinary processes as analogies for Medea's medical preparations. See Ovid, *Metamorphoses*, I, Bk VII, lines 312–17.
[48] BodL, MS Ashmole 1438, Part II, p. 112.

to construct any clear-cut or fixed opposition between the marvellous and the mundane: recipe books may have provided Gower with some of the softening, domestic language that he deploys, but they could also depict the same marvellous temporalities as Ovid. A remedy in Oxford, Bodleian Library, MS Ashmole 1443, the large, potentially quasi-professional medical collection examined in Chapter 3, also promises to make the patient 'ʒonglyche' ('youthful'), and the writer claims that the remedy was used by a man who lived to 150 years old.[49] Turning back and elongating time was not, then, just a preoccupation of poets, but also recipe writers and readers who found themselves drawn towards extraordinary temporalities.

Like the writer of the fistula remedy who carefully contrasts a lengthy preparation process with miraculously quick relief ('that day þat he drynketh hyt he shal not greue'), Gower artfully underlines the elongation of Medea's labour by contrasting it, at the beginning of the episode, with his own marvellous temporality, writing 'For tho [Medea] thoghte to beginne | Such thing as semeth impossible, | And made hirselven invisible' (V. 4024–8). The sequential language of beginnings in the opening line contrasts with the instantaneousness with which Medea—in the space of line 4028—achieves the apparently impossible and makes herself invisible. But, if Medea can perform *this* marvellous feat so rapidly, why does Eson's rejuvenation require so much time and labour? Is it because the turning back of time is such a momentous, near-impossible undertaking? This is one possible way of interpreting the clash of temporalities and it enhances the marvellousness of Medea's spectacle of labour, emphasizing the scale of her endeavour. But that hovering suggestion of difficulty and impossibility threatens consistently to undercut Medea's labour: is it all in vain? Gower certainly punctuates his description with passages that encourage readers to entertain the possibility that Medea's labour might be absurd, misguided, and futile. For example, he adds the following passage to Ovid's account:

> Sche made many a wonder soun,
> Somtime lich unto the cock,
> Somtime unto the Laverock,
> Somtime kacleth as a Hen

---

[49] BodL, MS Ashmole 1443, p. 270. See also William Rogers, 'Old Words Made New: Medea's Magic and Gower's Textual Healing', *South Atlantic Review*, 79 (2014), 105–17, which notes some general parallels between Gower's description and medieval medical and cosmetic treatises on retarding age.

> Somtime spekth as don the men:
> And riht so as hir jargoun strangeth,
> In sondri wise hir forme changeth
>
> (4098–104)

The varied and protracted nature of Medea's labour is again represented through a repetitive rhetorical structure that focuses the reader's attention onto the passing of time: 'Somtime... Somtime... Somtime...'. But here that labour is bathetically undermined because Medea's 'wonder soun'—her own kind of specialist discourse—is reduced to the sub-linguistic noises of various birds. In the Middle Ages, bird noise was often mockingly associated with nonsense speak: although the modern meaning of *jargon* as 'technical terminology' was not established until the late fifteenth century, the Middle English word *jargoun* could apply both to the chatter of birds and the meaningless chatter of humans.[50] Julie Orlemanski has shown how other parodies of medical recipes push medical terminology towards the semantic debasement of noise.[51] By drawing on these associations of bird noise with nonsense, Gower also edges his representation towards parody, teasing readers with the possibility that Medea's impressive and protracted performance might not have any healing effects at all: it might turn out to be mere noise or empty spectacle—excessive, unprofitable, and ridiculous.

This subversive suggestion of futile labour fits with Medea's medieval reputation as a pagan sorceress descended from pagan gods: in Christianity's salvation narrative, labour was part of the punishment for original sin and thus an emblem of mortality, but it was also embedded in a teleological narrative of redemption and, for commentators like St Augustine, it could be penitentially productive, drawing the labourer closer to God who would bring about that labourer's ultimate bodily rejuvenation.[52] As a pagan, Medea was, of course, exempt from that teleological narrative of productiveness and redemption, and this awareness may inform the sharp irony of Gower's description: Medea ends up—through her exaggerated and protracted bodily labours—reminding readers of the bodily degradations and limitations she is seeking to transcend; trying to stop the disintegration of one pagan body requires so much labour that it threatens the disintegration

---

[50] See *MED*, *jargoun*, n., and Orlemanski, 'Jargon and the Matter of Medicine', pp. 395–6.
[51] Orlemanski, 'Jargon'.
[52] For an overview, see Jeremy Kidwell, 'Labour in St. Augustine', in *The Oxford Guide to the Historical Reception of Augustine*, ed. by Karla Pollmann (Oxford, 2013), pp. 779–84.

of another, even when that other pagan body is (like Medea) of divine descent.

This concern with profitable uses of time and body infused late medieval secular and religious writings. Analysing the works of Ricardian poets, Gregory Sadlek recently claimed that, in the later Middle Ages, 'more and more emphasis was given to the value of productivity over and above the need just to keep busy'. He adds, 'writers not only expressed the urgent nature of time's passing... but also underscored the need to produce something of value for the common good'.[53] Kellie Robertson has also emphasized the role of fourteenth-century labour laws in shaping definitions of industry and productivity: although the laws were mainly intended to regulate the labour of agrarian workers, Robertson claims the laws 'had a powerful effect on "immaterial" labourers: preachers, pilgrims, and poets all found themselves forced to articulate not only the social benefits that accrued from their labours, but also to define their work in increasingly material ways'.[54] This is also true of medical writers: one example of such a definition occurs in John Arderne's fourteenth-century surgical treatise, *Fistula in ano*. Here, in a miniature redemption narrative, Arderne claims that the cure for anal fistulae was revealed to him by God as a reward for his protracted search for it. A fifteenth-century English translation, closely following Arderne's Latin original, renders this as follows:

> In hard thingis it spedith to studiers for to perseuere and abide, and for to turne subtily thair wittes. ffor it is opned not to þam that ar passand but to tham þat ar perseuerand. Therfore to the honour of god almyȝti that hath opned witte to me that I shuld fynde tresour hidde in the felde of studiers that long tyme and [with] pantyng breest I haue swette and trauailed ful bisily and pertinacely in diuanudiis.[55]

Despite the manual nature of his surgical work, Arderne and his translator follow many earlier surgical writers in depicting surgery as a rational and *intellectual* pursuit ('felde of studiers' or 'agro studencium' in the Latin).[56]

---

[53] Gregory M. Sadlek, 'Otium, Negotium, and the Fear of Acedia in the Writings of England's Late Medieval Ricardian Poets', in *Idleness, Indolence and Leisure in Literature*, ed. by Monika Fludernik and Miriam Nandi (London, 2014), pp. 17–39 (p. 24).

[54] Robertson, *The Labourer's Two Bodies*, p. 4.

[55] Power, ed., *Treatises of Fistula in Ano*, p. 3, lines 6–13. For a copy of Arderne's Latin text, see BodL, MS Ashmole 1434, f. 1v.

[56] BodL, MS Ashmole 1434, f. 1v. On the tradition of depicting surgery as a science see Michael McVaugh, *The Rational Surgery of the Middle Ages* (Tavarnuzze, 2006).

Ironically, though, he simultaneously frames his prolonged intellectual labour as highly physical work by describing it as a 'felde' to be traversed and by depicting himself panting and sweating during his labour. This may have been done to make his academic toil seem more tangible, arduous, and dramatic. That labour, after all, participates in a cyclical, symbiotic relationship with the reward of medical discovery: protracted labour makes the reward seem more precious and desirable, whilst referring to the reward as a 'tresour' makes the labour seem worthwhile in the first place. This dynamic could also be at work in the recipes examined earlier: the promise of marvellous results makes the labour worth undertaking, but the wondrously protracted labour also makes it seem more likely that a remedy of healing value will be produced.

Arderne's treatise has been read by some scholars as a text where the surgeon successfully juxtaposes his intact, mannered, knightly body against the fragmented, ailing bodies of patients; other scholars have argued that Arderne foregrounds his body's weaknesses in order to communicate his own socially precarious position as a surgeon.[57] Whichever way one reads the treatise, it is clear that Arderne's over-defined body risks introducing an element of bathos into his self-presentation, reducing him to a grotesque corporeality. The same is true of Medea. During her lengthy preparations, Medea is said to 'gaspe and gone' (V. 4064), which means to gasp for air and to gape or yawn.[58] She is also said to 'gaspeth with a drecchinge onde' upon the water three times (V. 3975). These actions can be understood as part of Medea's ritual (as they are in Ovid's version), but they are also signs of bodily exhaustion. In these moments of heightened corporeality, Medea and Arderne resemble Chaucer's sweating Canon's Yeoman who risks becoming grotesquely comic by his extended alchemical toil, part of which is also aimed—through the philosophers' stone—at reversing and arresting bodily time: beginning to embody the alchemical labour that he conducts, the Canon's Yeoman sweats 'as a stillatorie'.[59] All of these authors suggest, then, that extended medical labour can demean as well as dignify. This is true whether the labourer is a pagan sorceress, an alchemist prying sinfully into God's secrets, a surgeon studying with divine approval, or the enactor of a humble household medical recipe: in all of these texts, any human attempt

---

[57] See Jeremy J. Citrome, *The Surgeon in Medieval English Literature* (New York, 2006), pp. 113–38 and Turner, 'Illness Narratives', pp. 76–7.
[58] See *OED*, *gasp*, v., entry 1 and *MED*, *gaspen*, v.; see *MED*, *gonen*, v., entries 1(a), 1(b).
[59] Chaucer, *The Canon's Yeoman's Tale*, in *Riverside*, ed. by Benson, line 580.

to escape the body's mortal, temporal limits ultimately returns you to that body, to its extensive, drawn-out, corporeal labours in *this* life.

This episode from the *Confessio* enables us to see, then, to return to Bourdieu's argument, how integral the timing and duration of an action is to our interpretation of it. In the medical context, drawn-out labour—or its written representation in recipes—could have impressed or amazed and the sheer length or complexity of that labour might have reassured a patient that specialist expertise informed the action. But such labour could also have felt excessive, futile, impractical, and ridiculous; it might have reminded the reader of the impossibility of ever fully escaping the body's mortal constraints. Protracted labour could also raise questions about the medic's motivations: medieval writers such as John of Mirfield criticized professional physicians for protracting their healing labours in the interests of financial gain.[60] One might hear echoes of such criticism in Chaucer's claim that his gold-loving physician 'kepte his pacient a ful greet deel | In houres by his magyk natureel'.[61] Long recipes, unapologetically leisurely in their requests for hundreds of herbs, might seem detached from such polemic. But, because they are often surrounded by much shorter cures, they stand out in collections and encourage a reader to think about *why* they have been included. Just like the instances of extreme accumulation examined in Chapter 3, these long texts—connected to multiple interpretative contexts and poised between the pragmatic, the marvellous, and the ridiculous—elude predictable reader responses and reductive narratives of practical motivations.

Rapid Recoveries

In contrast, and sometimes in tension, with these protracted preparations, one finds promises that patients will be cured of their illness within a fixed, and often impressively small, number of days. Whilst lengthy preparation processes are only a feature of some recipes within remedy collections, these forecasts of rapid cures appear in the vast majority of recipes, both in Latin and English collections. They are usually structured by time or by

---

[60] Aldridge and Hartley, ed. and trans, *Johannes de Mirfield*, pp. 48–9.
[61] Geoffrey Chaucer, *General Prologue*, in *Riverside*, ed. by Benson, lines 415–16. The MED translates the phrase to 'kepen in houres' as 'to keep (a patient) under favourable planetary influence' (*MED*, *houre*, n., entry 2(c)), but it could have had a double meaning for readers.

repetition: for instance, whilst one recipe concludes, 'drynke þerof þre dayes... and he schal be sauf',[62] another predicts that the patient 'schal be hole within iij tymys drynkyng'.[63] Similarly, a Latin recipe guarantees that a perfect cure ('cura perfecta') will be completed 'in 3º vel 4º die' ('in the third or fourth day').[64] Although one does sometimes find longer cure times of seven, nine, and twelve (or more) days, there is a marked preference in the remedy collections for alleging that a cure will prove effective within three days or three repetitions of its application. Three may have been popular because of its aesthetic and mnemonic appeal in rhetoric, poetry, and art or because of its related prevalence in folklore and scripture: most notably of all, Christ—who was frequently referred to as *Christus medicus* and presented as a kind of physician in religious writings—was resurrected on 'the third day'.[65] The sparse temporal narratives of the recipes are again symbolically enriched through a possible connection with Christian salvation narrative.

This is not, however, the only interpretative lens available: multiple allusions and motivations cluster around the recipes' temporalities, layering or weaving together the spiritual, aesthetic, and physiological. For instance, the number three might have become popular in remedies for different ailments because it was already central to medical discourses about fevers: three-day cycles were considered integral to the way particular types of fever came and went.[66] Medieval understandings of critical days—the astrologically important days in which the appearance of particular symptoms could be used to foretell the outcome of a fever or disease—may also have informed writers' choices: 'good' critical days, such as the fifth, seventh, ninth, or eleventh days after the onset of the illness, were often (though not always) odd; on these days, certain prognostic tokens could be interpreted more positively than if they appeared on 'bad' days, perhaps explaining guarantees in recipes of seven- or nine-day cures.[67]

Whatever the reason, or combination of reasons, for these different temporal guarantees, John of Mirfield's late medieval medical treatise, the *Breviarium Bartholomei*, suggests that a cure time of three days became so popular in medical discourse that patients began to structure their

---

[62] BodL, MS Douce 84, f. 3r.   [63] BodL, MS Ashmole 1389, p. 20.
[64] BodL, MS Ashmole 1413, p. 86.
[65] On the history of the concept of *Christus medicus*, see R. Arbesmann, 'The Concept of "Christus Medicus" in St. Augustine', *Traditio*, 10 (1954), 1–20.
[66] I am indebted to Daniel McCann for this suggestion.
[67] On critical days, see Daniel, *Liber Uricrisiarum*, pp. 85–6, lines 184–213.

expectations through it, expecting to feel some kind of upturn in their health in three days or less:

> Multi infirmi modernis temporibus valde impacientes sunt. Nolunt enim sicut antiquitus facere solebant expectare vsque ad quartum vel quintum diem vel amplius si necesse fuerit, quousque materia peccans fuerit digesta et vtiliter euacuata. Verum nisi statim in prima die sentiant alleuiamen de medico diffidunt euisque medicinas respuunt et contempnunt.
>
> Many patients in these modern days are particularly impatient, and are unwilling to wait until the fourth or fifth day or more for the morbid matter in the body to be digested and usefully evacuated, as was the custom in the olden days: for in truth, unless such people feel relief immediately on the first day, they distrust their physician and despise and reject his prescriptions.[68]

It seems that patients were willing to tolerate a long preparatory process but, after the medicine had been administered into the body, they expected it to bring about relief rapidly and within a designated period. This might explain why some imprecise forecasts in medical recipes are disguised as precise ones: 'vse a quantite of this water … 12 . or. 14 . dayes'.[69]

These examples show that recipes usually dealt with what scholars in disability studies have referred to as 'curative time': prologues to remedy collections often reassured readers that whoever followed the remedy book's advice 'may be sekir to be hole of his euille'.[70] Recipe books therefore invited readers to reimagine their disabilities or illnesses—however long-lasting, chronic, or recurring they were—as short-term disruptions, capable of being remedied quickly once medicines were applied or ingested. Irina Metzler observes that this attitude was embedded in the intellectual traditions informing medieval medicine: 'The medical model, since the Hippocratic school, thought in terms of processes: people fall sick and then either die or get better, but a lingering chronic condition was not something a medieval physician or surgeon wrote about much.'[71] This linear model may well have left some medieval readers, whose experiences of chronic

---

[68] Aldridge and Hartley, ed. and trans, *Johannes de Mirfield*, pp. 50–1.
[69] HEHL, MS HM 64, f. 170v.   [70] BL, MS Sloane 213, f. 138r.
[71] Irina Metzler, 'Disability in the Middle Ages: Impairment at the Intersection of Historical Inquiry and Disability Studies', *History Compass*, 9 (2011), 45–60 (p. 48).

pain did not align with, or respond to, those forecasts of rapid cure, troubled and confused.

Such privileging of curative time also shows the problem with unthinkingly describing household remedy collections as mundane, everyday texts. Exploring the slipperiness and exploitability of the concept of 'the everyday', Rita Felski observes that we often think of everyday life as 'the essential, taken-for-granted continuum of mundane activities that frames our forays into more esoteric or exotic worlds'. This continuum is structured by repetition and habit and the body forms an integral part of its conception: 'everyone, from the most famous to the most humble, eats, sleeps, yawns, defecates'.[72] It is true that many of the ailments dealt with in remedy books, particularly of the domestic kind, are for common ailments, such as headaches, colds, and nosebleeds, which recur regularly in most human lives. But those ailments are represented through a recipe discourse which (unlike *regimen*) does not approach the body through daily cycles of repetition but, instead, represents the afflictions troubling that body as exceptional, extraordinary, and abnormal, as disturbances to be remedied and returned *to* normal. This troubles any rigid or fixed association between medical recipes and 'the everyday'.

The cure that makes that experience of illness short, unusual, and extraordinary (by ending it) is also a potential object of wonder, or at least a signifier for the idea of the marvellous. For example, in a compendium of Middle English translations of John Arderne's surgical writings, a patient with a swollen leg is cured within three days: 'And within þre daies without any oþer medicyne he was perfitely cured, whar-of many men wondred'.[73] This emphasizing of perceived marvellousness patterns for readers the response that the three-day cure should induce within them. A similar pattern is suggested by an episode in *The Boke of John Mandeville*, a widely circulating travel account of pilgrimage routes that was created out of numerous earlier writings and is well known amongst modern scholars for its descriptions of exotic Eastern marvels. In chapter 19, Mandeville describes a well which 'men seyn...cometh out of paradys'; it is alleged that 'whoso drynketh .iij. tymes fasting of water of þat welle he is hool of alle

---

[72] Rita Felski, 'The Invention of Everyday Life', in Rita Felski, *Doing Time: Feminist Theory and Postmodern Culture* (New York, 2000) pp. 77–98 (pp. 77, 79).

[73] Power, ed., *Treatises of Fistula in Ano*, p. 52, lines 21–3. This edition is based on BL, MS Sloane 6, ff. 141r–174v.

maner sykeness that he hath'.[74] Coming from terrestrial Paradise but perhaps evoking—through the mention of three—Christ's miraculous resurrection, the cures worked by this fountain are, like the forecasts in the remedy books, sites of multiple, intersecting temporalities. In contrast to the cures in remedy books, the water in this well, associated with the labour-less realm of Paradise, does not require protracted bodily labour to turn it into a cure. Nevertheless, the similarity between the temporal instructions in Mandeville's text and the recipes suggests that the earthly marvels of medicine were discursively programmed to evoke awe in the same way as the unearthly miracles of the divine.

The final way that wonder may be cultivated by these rapid recipe forecasts also creates a discursive connection between the natural and the supernatural. In recipe collections, rapid cures are sometimes juxtaposed with a long period of former suffering. For example, a remedy for hoarseness concludes 'þis medicun was previd on a man in . 2 . days þat was 30 . wynter hors'.[75] Elsewhere, a reader is assured that 'þou ne schalt neuer haue [epilepsy] after þey þou haddist had hit xxx^ti^ winter afore'.[76] Wonder is generated here when the seemingly impossible suddenly becomes possible. Such claims recall, and were perhaps intended to evoke, the supernatural healing miracles attributed to saints: when Cardinal Peter of Luxembourg was nominated for canonization in 1390, he was said to have healed a widow's arm which had been swollen for three months and to have cured a man of permanent blindness.[77] In these examples, then, the temporal perspective of the recipes shifts slightly to accommodate something more akin to chronic illness, to illness as everyday experience. Nevertheless, it is implied that chronic illness was simply the result of misguided medical treatment in the past; it can now, the recipes suggest, be subjected to a marvellous curative resolution.

Not all readers probably responded to these texts' invitations to wonder. Readers like Robert Henryson and Francesco Petrarch, who, as we saw in Chapters 1 and 3, were liable to read recipes' extravagant claims with a sceptical eye, probably doubted whether such formulaic rhetoric would ever come true. Other readers may have converted the promises' conventional

---

[74] *Mandeville's Travels*, ed. by Paul Hamelius, EETS os 153–4, 2 vols (London, 1919–23), I, p. 113, lines 13–14, 5–7. On the use of marvellous waters and springs in medieval healing, see Lorraine Daston and Katharine Park, *Wonders and the Order of Nature, 1150–1750* (New York, 1998), pp. 137–8.

[75] BodL, MS Rawlinson C. 506, f. 93r.   [76] BodL, MS Laud misc. 553, f. 46v.

[77] Robert Bartlett, *The Natural and the Supernatural in the Middle Ages* (Cambridge, 2008), pp. 10–11.

hyperbole back into more realistic terms, believing that recipes might offer them a cure but inferring that it would not be *as* quick as promised. Reducing the promises to these three categories—marvellous, false, and hyperbolic—is, however, to overlook some subtleties in the way that they represent healing time. For instance, it is significant that the recipes very rarely guarantee to cure the patient in less than a day. The small number of examples I have found of a cure being forecast in hours are usually only for analgesics: a remedy for aches copied in the second half of the fifteenth century guarantees to 'mitigate the payne withinne an eure or ij'[78] and another recipe from the first half of the fifteenth century promises to stop a wound aching 'withyn half an oure'.[79] Similarly, the long remedy for a fistula examined earlier only declares that the patient shall not 'greue' ('suffer') the same day that he uses the treatment; it does not promise to cure the fistula that day. These examples suggest that remedy writers could be more hesitant, discriminating, and (perhaps) realistic in the way that they deployed time than the prevalence of formulaic, three-day guarantees implies. They also suggest that copiers or compilers of remedy collections moved flexibly between credible and incredible timescales and expected their readers to do so too.

An example of a medical writer who clearly expected such flexibility is John Arderne. As we have seen, Arderne did claim to have performed wondrously rapid cures. However, he also offers some very different cure narratives. In the same compendium of Middle English translations of Arderne's surgical writings that the three-day cure appears, his treatment of a swollen arm is described at great length:

Þe arme of a certane manne biganne sodenly for to ake & prik in the buȝt of þe arme and afterward gretly to bolne fro þe shulder to þe fyngers... At þe last he soȝt & asked my help... ffirst I made hym ane emplastre of tartare of ale... I put þe emplastre on his arme, and alsone he feled alegeance of akyng. Þe 3 day, forsoþ, remeuyng þe emplastre, þe bolnyng in party was slaked. Bot in þe buȝt of þe arme al þe colleccion of gedryng abode stille, schewyng as it schuld gadre to ane heued. Þe which y-sene, I putte to ane emplastre maturatyue of maluez y-soþen and y-brissed, with grese 3 daies or 4, and neþerles I perceyued neuer þe soner for to be matured, bot þe bolnyng abode mych stil.[80]

---

[78] BodL, MS Ashmole 1432, p. 20.   [79] TCC, MS R.14.32, f. 132r.
[80] Power, ed., *Treatises of Fistula in Ano*, p. 49, lines 15–34. For a copy of the Latin version of this passage, see BL, MS Sloane 347, f. 64r.

[*bu3t of þe arme* = angle of the elbow; *bolne* = swell; *alegeance* = relief; *colleccion of gedryng* = accrual of pus and suppurative matter; *maturatyue* = medicine promoting suppuration; *malue3* = mallow; *y-sopen and y-brissed* = boiled and crushed]

The account, which closely follows its Latin source, continues in this way for approximately 400 words before the arm is cured. Within this episode, Arderne and his translator do evoke the motif of the three-day cure but they simultaneously undercut it: after the plaster is removed on the third day, the swelling ('bolnyng') is only 'in party...slaked'. Preparation and cure times consequently blur as Arderne is compelled to prepare and administer new treatments multiple times in response to a body that cannot be confined by neat three-day cures, stretching the second set of three days into four and ultimately elongating the treatment well beyond anything that might be considered rapid. Of course, this account does not necessarily represent 'real time', if such a thing can even be captured in language: Arderne's surgical writings are often flagrant acts of self-publicity and, like some of the spectacles of extended labour examined earlier, this passage is designed to showcase his marvellous perseverance, ingenuity, and skill in the face of prolonged difficulty.

Nevertheless, given that much medieval medicine did probably progress by extended trial and error, Arderne's account is likely to be closer to reality than the conventional three-day guarantees, even if it is partly patterned by them. Like the recipes—with their extraordinary three-day cures and more pragmatic hour-long analgesics, and their long preparations suspended between the pragmatic and the spectacularly impossible—Arderne's writings demonstrate that medical writers expected and encouraged their readers to move flexibly between multiple temporalities, imagining their bodies both in realistic and marvellous time.

Recipe Time in Romances

More consistently imaginative genres, such as romance, require a similar flexibility: romances frequently demand that a reader suspend his or her normal sense of time by depicting an extraordinarily rapid or amazingly protracted battle or an unrealistically quick descent into lovesickness. Although a few scholars have explored the shared manuscript space and imaginative exchanges connecting romances and medical writings, the temporal dimension to these exchanges has not been investigated.[81] In the final sections of this chapter, I will argue that romance writers actually used recipe discourse within their writings to signify or draw attention to polytemporality and to stimulate imaginative flexibility amongst readers; they considered recipes a means—and an easily importable and reinscribable one—for playing with bodies in, and out of, time.[82]

My first example of possible borrowing or overlap occurs in the Auchinleck copy of the anonymous romance *Bevis of Hampton* (c. 1300). In the surviving copies of this poem, the lines quoted below only appear in this manuscript, copied in the 1330s. In this passage, Josian (the Armenian wife of the English hero Bevis) attempts to protect herself from a forced marriage to one of Bevis's enemies by making herself appear as a leper or *mesel*. She does so through the power of an unnamed herb:

> While ȝhe was in Ermonie,
> Boþe fysik and sirgirie
> She hadde lerned of meisters grete
> Of Boloyne þe gras and of Tulete,
> Þat ȝhe knew erbes mani & fale,
> To make boþe boute & bale.
> On ȝhe tok vp of þe grounde,
> Þat was an erbe of meche mounde,
> To make a man in semlaunt þere,
> A foule mesel alse ȝif a were.
> Whan ȝhe hadde ete þat erbe, anon
> To þe Sarasines ȝhe gan gon,
> ...
> Þai nadde ride in here way
> Boute fif mile of þat contray,
> Ȝhe was in semlaunt & in ble
> A foule mesel on to se.[83]

---

[81] Corinne Saunders, 'Bodily Narratives: Illness, Medicine and Healing in Middle English Romance', in *Boundaries in Medieval Romance*, ed. by Neil Cartlidge (Woodbridge, 2008), pp. 175–90; Orlemanski, 'Thornton's Remedies', pp. 246–50.

[82] Recipes' capacity to be reinscribed resembles that which Emily Steiner has associated with late medieval legal documents: she claims that legal documents were 'citable' because of their 'conciseness' and 'portability' and that 'the document, because it was citable as a text, became a means of thinking through intergeneric problems about the status of textuality in late medieval England' (Steiner, *Documentary Culture*, pp. 3–4).

[83] *The Romance of Sir Beues of Hamtoun*, ed. by Eugen Kölbing, EETS es 46, 48, 65 (London, 1885–94), lines 3671–88. Future references are within the text. In other manuscripts either

168 MIDDLE ENGLISH MEDICAL RECIPES AND LITERARY PLAY

The episode is structured like an inverted remedy, depicting the transformation into, rather than out of, leprosy. The power of the herb Josian uses is also expressed in the same infinitive and third-person format that many recipe titles take: 'To make a man...'. Intriguingly, there is a close parallel for this episode in a large fifteenth-century remedy collection which contains a recipe for making a person *seem* like a leper, perhaps in the interests of securing more charitable donations when begging:[84]

> For to make won to seme A M3SELLE
>
> Take C3R6SE and doo hit in his potages whiles hit is hoote and eete hit and he schalle seme m3sel and if thou wilte delyver hit awaye take the iuce of fynelle or fyngkille and leete hym dryngke hit 3 dayes and also anoynte his face therewithe and vyneger togeres[85]
>
> [*ceruse* = white lead; *potages* = soup or stew; *fynelle or fyngkille* = both names for fennel]

Just as the herb Josian uses is identified only as an 'erbe of meche mou*n*de', the name of the crucial ingredient in this recipe—*ceruse*, white lead—is partially obscured through the use of a simple code. In both instances, the ingredient seems to have been obscured in order to create a sense of mystery. The century and a half separating these texts and a lack of other witnesses make it impossible to establish any specific connection between the pieces.[86] We can be sure, though, that both texts, the instructional *and* the literary, have a similar imaginative interest in disguise and intrigue.

Saber or Josian apply the ointment and the episode is described without any mention of leprosy or time passing: for example, 'Iosyan haþ maad an oynement; | Here skyn, þat was boþe bry3t & schene, | þere wiþ sche made 3elew and grene' (see Kölbing, ed., *Beues*, pp. 181–2 for variant versions). I have not cited the latest edition, *Sir Bevis of Hampton*, ed. by Jennifer Fellows, EETS os 349–50, 2 vols (Oxford, 2017), because Fellows uses CUL, MS Ff.2.38 and Naples, Biblioteca Nazionale, MS XIII.B.29, not Auchinleck.

[84] For a possible motivation as to why the owner of this recipe would wish to know how to make someone appear as a leper, see the entry for the plant *tapsia* in the copy of the herbal known as *Circa instans* in BodL, MS Ashmole 1443, f. 174: 'with þis erbe sum fayturs makiþ hem as mesel to bygyle þe pepil in beggyng'. In that text, vinegar is also used to remove the disguise.

[85] HEHL, MS HM 64, f. 102v. On leprosy's many divergent associations, see Carole Rawcliffe, *Leprosy in Medieval England* (Woodbridge, 2006).

[86] The Auchinleck *Bevis* was composed several decades before the explosion of vernacular medical writing in the late fourteenth century; this explosion, however, did not come from nowhere and English medical recipes were in existence (though in far smaller numbers) at the beginning of the fourteenth century. Alternatively, the author could have read Latin medical recipes.

The temporal dynamics of the Auchinleck episode also evoke recipe discourse. The author of the lines includes a precise temporal description of Josian's rapid transformation, alleging that 'Þai nadde ride in here way | Boute fif mile of þat contray...'. In contrast, the Anglo-Norman source text of the romance is far less specific in its medical and temporal allusions, simply claiming 'Un herbe achata, unkes meylur ne vist, | Tut en tent son cors e son vis',[87] translated by Judith Weiss as 'she bought a herb—you never saw a better—and with it she dyed all her body and her face'.[88] Amy Burge has noted that *Bevis* often displays a much greater sensitivity to the passing of time than the Anglo-Norman *Boeve* and that time is frequently measured through space in the romance.[89] She does not, however, note that, in this instance, the temporal allusions may have strengthened the connection to recipe discourse in the minds of writers and readers. Recipes often represent time through space: for instance, in a fifteenth-century collection, ingredients are to be boiled 'þe space of a qwarter of a myle way'.[90] Very occasionally the time taken for a cure to work is also expressed in this way: in a remedy for worms in a man's ear, it is claimed that 'within a myle weye [the sap of the herb lovage] schal sle þe vermyn'.[91]

This echo of recipe discourse in *Bevis* forges a possible connection between the marvellous, imaginary world of the romance and the concrete, practical world—and everyday means of measuring time—of the reader. The familiarity of these rapid recovery formulae does not, however, seem to have decreased their potential to arouse wonder in the eyes of the author: the negative construction prefacing the description of the miles walked, 'Þai nadde...', simultaneously assumes and instils readerly awe. But there is one divergence from recipe formulae: whilst the recipes normally predict recoveries in days (carefully reserving promises in hours for analgesics), Josian's inverted cure takes place in the short time it takes to ride five miles. According to Chaucer's *Treatise on the Astrolabe*, walking five miles takes one hour and forty minutes, so riding would be even quicker.[92] It seems that,

---

[87] *Beuve de Hamptone: Chanson de Geste Anglo-Normande de la Fin du xIIe Siècle: Édition Bilingue*, ed. by Jean-Pierre Martin (Paris, 2014), lines 2779–80.

[88] *Boeve de Haumtoun and Gui de Warewic: Two Anglo-Norman Romances*, trans. by Judith Weiss, (Tempe, AZ, 2008), p. 77.

[89] Amy Burge, 'Desiring the East: A Comparative Study of Middle English Romance and Modern Popular Sheikh Romance' (unpublished doctoral thesis, University of York, 2012), pp. 76–7.

[90] BodL, MS Douce 78, f. 8r.   [91] TCC, MS R.14.39, f. 2v.

[92] Chaucer, *A Treatise on the Astrolabe*, in *Riverside*, ed. by Benson, Part I, 16.15–16: '3 mile-wei maken an houre'.

though the recipes' temporal formulae could have functioned within different text-types as a cultural shorthand for wonder, those formulae needed exaggerating if they were to impress in the already wondrous world of romance.

Crucially, though, Josian's transformation never becomes instant: despite inhabiting a fictional landscape where marvellous transformations and temporalities *could* occur (if the author desired it), her body does not escape time and is still tied to mundane means of measuring time. This returns us to recipes' capacity to function as sites of plural, non-linear time for medieval writers and readers: despite their ostensibly linear and sequential form, they seem to have been thought of as nexuses where different temporal structures could criss-cross in explicit and pronounced ways and as textual arenas where the body could cheat or evade time whilst, simultaneously, remaining subject to its constraints and degradations.

This becomes even more apparent through the creative reinscription of recipes in Thomas Malory's Arthurian prose epic, *Le Morte d'Arthur* (*c.* 1469–70). The temporal coordinates of this romance narrative are often vague and dreamlike: it is composed out of endless chivalric quests and battles joined together by paratactic structures such as 'and...and...' or 'and then...and then...'.[93] Aside from feast days, the time taken for the body to heal after it has been wounded is one of the few ways in which the linear onward motion of time is marked precisely. But amazingly quick cures occur very sparingly in the narrative; recovery times normally stretch to weeks or months. For example, Malory writes, 'Sir Trystrams was so wounded that unnethe he myght recover, and lay at a nunrye half a yere' (p. 143, lines 21–2) and 'Sir Gawayne lay syke and unsounde thre wykes in hys tentis with all maner of lechecrauffte that myght be had' (p. 912, lines 21–3). Given the licence for magic afforded by the genre, a reader might expect cures in romances to be rapid or instantaneous and certainly not described in weeks or months. But, ironically, the forecasts in recipes seem more marvellous than the recoveries narrated in this romance.

In the light of these protracted recoveries, it is revealing that one of the few wondrously quick cures that *does* occur in Malory's narrative is phrased in language closely resembling that of a medical recipe. When Gawain and Sir Pryamas injure one another in combat in Book V, Sir Pryamas takes it upon himself to heal them both:

---

[93] E.g. Thomas Malory, *Le Morte D'Arthur*, ed. by P.J.C. Field, 2 vols (Cambridge, 2013), I, 191, lines 5–16. Future references are included within the text.

'Now fecche me,' seyde Sir Pryamus, 'my vyall that hangys by the gurdyll of my haynxman, for hit is full of the floure of the foure good watyrs that passis from Paradyse, that mykyll fruyte in fallys that at one day fede shall us all. Putt that watir in oure fleysh where the syde is tamed, and we shall be hole within foure houres.'

Than they lette clense theire woundys with colde whyght wyne, and than they lete anoynte them with bawme over and over, and holer men than they were within an houres space was never lyvyng syn God the worlde made. (p. 180, lines 14–22)

The imperatives 'fecche' and 'putt' recall recipes, as do the 'colde whyght wyne' and unspecified 'bawme' or balsam, both common ingredients in cures. The clearest echo of recipes, however, is Pryamus's confident assertion 'we shall be hole within foure houres'. A few lines later this wondrously quick recovery time is further reduced to less than 'an houres space'. As in the Auchinleck episode, the day-long promises of real recipes are exaggerated to suit the already marvellous world of romance.

In spite of the supernatural assistance of 'the foure good watyrs…from Paradyse', the knights' cure is, however, still not instant; it fills 'an houres space'. What is more, just as the cure does not become instant, the treatment does not become labourless: the paradisal waters must be accompanied by white wine and balm which should be applied 'over and over', evoking Medea's seemingly endless labour. These ingredients in turn generate additional temporalities. Balsam, considered to be hot and moist, was often associated with rejuvenation: it was believed to replace the heat and moisture intrinsic to the sustenance of human life and depleted during old age. Precisely because of these associations with rejuvenation, however, balsam was often used—alongside white wine—to embalm the corpses of the rich and powerful.[94] Both ingredients are simultaneously associated with life and death, corruption and rejuvenation.

Once again, then, despite recipes' immediate formal associations with linearity and sequentiality, the recipe form functions counterintuitively as a vehicle for signalling plurality and atemporality, overlaying the labourless time of Paradise and instantaneous resurrections of salvation with the spectre of bodily corruption, laborious earthly endeavours, and recoveries constrained to take place *in* time. In other words, while the earlier

---

[94] On these associations of balsam, see Elly Rachel Truitt, *Medieval Robots: Mechanism, Magic, Nature, and Art* (Philadelphia, PA, 2015), pp. 103–11.

descriptions of Tristram and Gawain's bodies follow a sequential, linear trajectory of illness and recovery, this interpolated recipe discourse enables Malory to imagine multiple temporalities at work on the knights' bodies simultaneously and even to imagine those time-travelling bodies *out*side of time: we are told that 'holer men than they were...was never lyvyng syn God the worlde made'. The knights' bodies are at once embedded in Christian temporalities and transported outside of them to an unimaginable time before all creation.

Of course, the hyperbole in this assertion that the knights' health has no comparison in the entire history of salvation heightens the potential for bathos hovering beneath the rest of the description. Along with the staged reduction of the cure time to one hour, and the simultaneous reminder that the body cannot ever really escape time, this assertion encourages readers to view the passage as a gentle parody of recipe discourse and its inflated promises. The forecasts, belonging half to the unearthly world of romance and devotional discourse and half to the world of the everyday, therefore come to signify both the wondrous *and* the far-fetched in Malory's text. Returning to the recipes themselves, and viewing them in part through the lens of these literary writings, one can see how the recipes' promises of recovery might have encouraged a similar variety of emotional and affective responses: although they may have appeared extravagant, ridiculous, and conventional to some, others might at least have entertained their credibility or considered them an emblem of hope. John of Mirfield's account certainly suggests that some patients continued to believe in rapid cures, becoming impatient if the remedy took more than a day to bring relief. A modern-day parallel might be the many miracle creams lining the shelves of pharmacies: like the remedies, these creams guarantee wrinkle-, blemish-, or spot-free skin in a specific number of days or weeks. Though the results are never as promised—and we often anticipate that they will not be when we buy them—many of us still purchase the creams in the *hope* that this time they might work.

Of course, hope could also have been supplemented by faith for medieval readers: God might not have granted a rapid cure this time, but he might on the next attempt. When it comes to sickness, hope and faith can be powerful affective tools, encouraging individuals to suppress their doubts. They can also make a patient feel physically and emotionally better. The recipes' promises of rapid recovery may, then, have invited a response similar to the wilful and continual resuppression of rational objection which Steven Justice argues structured medieval belief in miracle stories and saints' lives—texts that are often far more conventional and seemingly far-fetched than medical recipes.[95]

Reading Practices

As the preceding analysis has shown, medieval readers were used to imagining their bodies from different temporal perspectives at one time or in quick succession. This habit was also engrained through means of producing manuscripts: the very process of compiling a collection of texts in a manuscript—a process undertaken by increasingly more amateur lay readers in the later Middle Ages—frequently demanded that successions of writers and readers constantly adjust their temporal outlook.[96] For example, in one composite manuscript containing medical and other kinds of household texts, a late fifteenth- or early sixteenth-century hand has composed a list of the number of miles that separate different ports.[97] Earlier in this manuscript, however, a different fifteenth-century hand has composed a list of the distances between different planets and between the heavenly spheres: a round-trip between earth and the sphere that Christ resides in would take 7,700 years to walk.[98] Like many recipes, both lists appear—in their layout and structure—mundane and unimaginative. Nevertheless, they ask the reader to imagine him or herself in very different scenarios: one is realizable within the constraints of earthly time but the other requires a creative expansion of that familiar temporality.

The same flexibility is required by a late fifteenth-century manuscript containing medical recipes and devotional poems.[99] This manuscript demonstrates how recipe timescales can interact with those of different genres (whether or not that interaction was intended by the manuscript's compiler). Here, twenty-eight medical recipes have been copied between two devotional poems.[100] The recipe collection stands out because of its explicit concern with time. Firstly, it gives much more precise timings for preparing medicines than many other recipes do and it often measures the time of

---

[95] Steven Justice, 'Did the Middle Ages Believe in Their Miracles?', *Representations*, 103 (2008), 1–29.
[96] Meale, 'Amateur Book Production'.   [97] CUL, MS E.e.15, f. 129r.
[98] Ibid., f. 73r.
[99] BodL, MS Douce 78. The manuscript—continuing the medical theme—also contains a copy of *Titus and Vespasian*, a romance in which one of the protagonists suffers from leprosy.
[100] The recipes occur in BodL, MS Douce 78, ff. 7v–17v.

these actions in hours: 'lay hit in warme watur þe space of. 1 . oure'; 'ete non mete no drynke aftur þe space of an houre or more'; 'sethe ham in faire watur þe space of an houre or more'.[101] Secondly, it uses the word 'time' a lot. Consider this extract:

> ... þen drynke þerof vere warme xx sponefulle *at a tyme* And loke at *euery tyme* þat þou layste þe sayd medycyn to þe saide steche; also *oftyn tymys* schalte þou drynke xx sponefulle of þe saide mylke. Vse þese medycynes if hit be nede as *often tymes* as þou wylte.[102]
>
> [*steche* = sudden pain or stitch]

The last line also points towards another way in which the temporal vision of the recipes differs from many other collections discussed in this chapter: although it does contain a few examples of recoveries being guaranteed within a small number of days, the recipes more frequently instruct the reader/patient to use the medicine for as long as he or she needs to: for example, 'drynke þerof warme euery day furste and laste XV days togedur and more if hit be nede'.[103] These instructions—which add another layer to recipes' polytemporal texture—depict the reader engaged in a process of self-healing that can extend through time in a leisurely fashion.

In the manuscript that survives today, the text of the recipes seems incomplete, the final recipe breaking off without the usual application instructions and efficacy guarantees; pages also appear to be missing between the recipes and the devotional poem that follows them (which also survives incomplete), though both the recipes and the poems are copied by the same hand and with the same decoration style.[104] It is possible, then, that at one point in time there was more text in between the two. However, the off-print onto the recipes of the poem's rubricated capital 'O' suggests that—at least at the point of rubrication—the poem followed the recipes (see Figures 4.1 and 4.2). Readers would, then, have been able to draw connections and contrasts between the two. The most obvious contrast between

---

[101] BodL, MS Douce 78, ff. 8r, 15r. Other examples occur on ff. 13v, 12r. The collection also often gives precise durations using spatial measurements such as miles and furlongs: e.g. ff. 8r, 11r, 13v, 14r, 14v, 16r, and 17v.
[102] Ibid., f. 8v, italics mine.
[103] Ibid., f. 14r. The only examples of these rapid recoveries occur on ff. 8v, 12r, 16v, and 17v. For more instructions commanding the reader to use the medicine for as long as required, see ff. 8v, 9v, 10v, 11r–11v, 12v, 13v, 14r, 15v, 16v, and 17r.
[104] Versions of this poem also survive in at least two other manuscripts: for full details, see *DIMEV* 4079, 3870, and 6019.

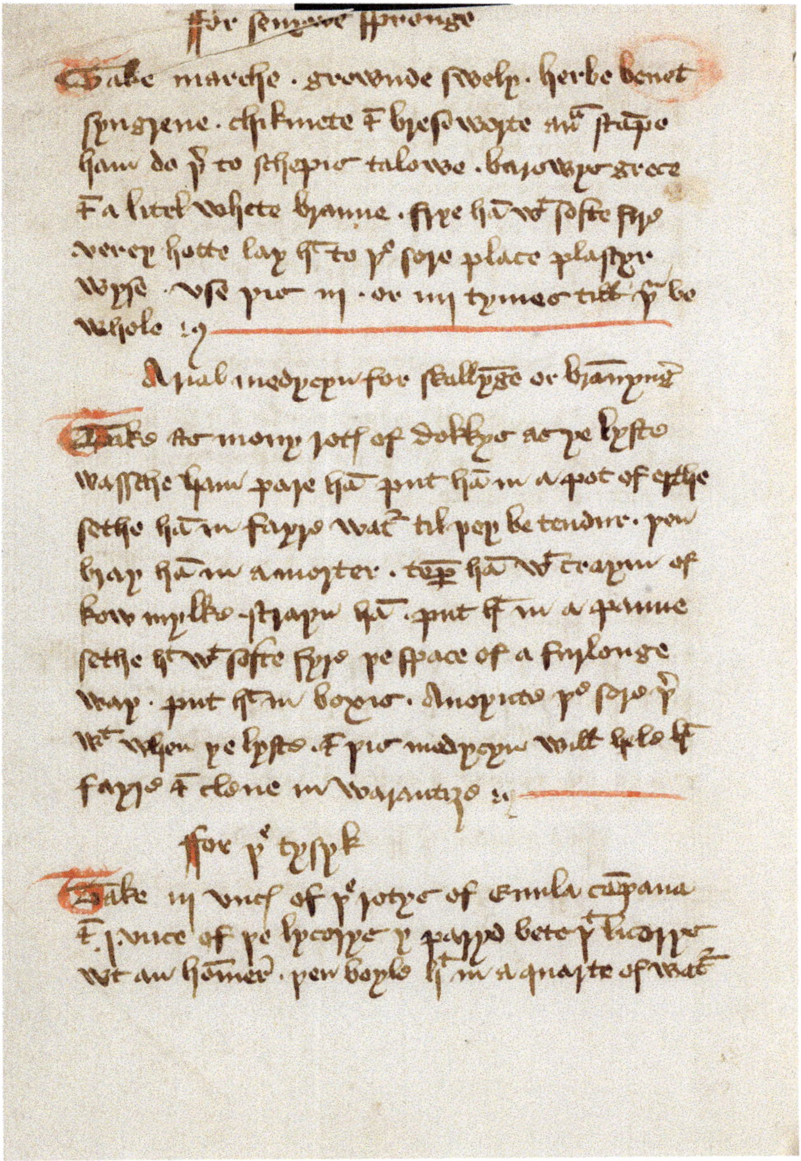

Figure 4.1 Recipes surviving alongside a devotional poem. The Bodleian Libraries, University of Oxford, MS Douce 78, f. 17v. Reproduced with kind permission from the Bodleian Libraries, University of Oxford through the Creative Commons licence CC-BY-NC 4.

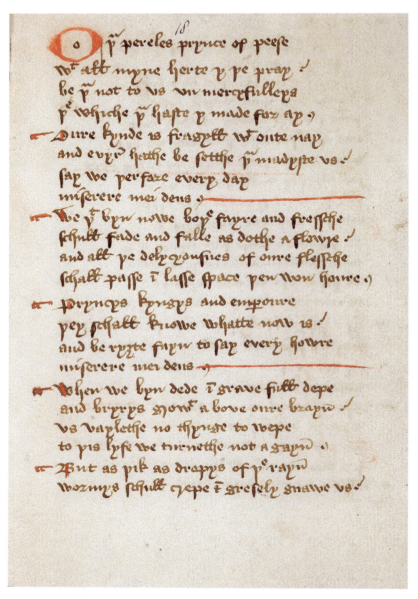

Figure 4.2 A devotional poem copied next to recipes. The Bodleian Libraries, University of Oxford, MS Douce 78, f. 18r. Reproduced with kind permission from the Bodleian Libraries, University of Oxford through the Creative Commons licence CC-BY-NC 4.

the texts concerns time. Below are the first four stanzas of the poem; they encapsulate that work's temporal perspective:

> O þou pereles prynce of peese
> with alle myne herte y þe pray.'
> be þou not to vs vnmercyfulleys
> þe whiche þou haste ymade for ay.
>
> Oure kynde is fragylle withoute nay
> and evyre hathe be setthe þou madyste vs.'
> say we þerfore every day
> miserere mei deus.
>
> We þat byn nowe boþe fayre and fressche
> schulle fade and falle as dothe a flowre.'
> and alle þe delycyousnes of oure flessche
> schalle passe in lasse space þen won houre.
>
> Pryncys kyngys and emperoure
> þey schalle knowe whatte now is.'
> and be ryȝte fayn to say every howre
> miserere mei deus.[105]

The poem encapsulates a dizzying array of temporal perspectives, encouraging the reader to inhabit another version of Dinshaw's polytemporal, non-linear, embodied time; when the body becomes the subject of conscious attention and reflection, it seems inevitable that temporalities will multiply. Firstly, the hypothetical, sickening individual body of the remedies is here made general and ubiquitous, as man's frail and ailing mortal state is emphasized ('Oure kynde is fragylle withoute nay | and euyre hathe be setthe þou madyste vs'). The poem thereby inverts the recipes' presentation of illness as an extraordinary, sporadic, temporally finite experience, turning it into a chronic condition for all of fallen humanity and underlining the provisional, shifting nature of all temporal perspectives: individuals are both whole and sick simultaneously.

Furthermore, while the remedies show humanity engaged in a protracted and leisurely process of repairing this sick body, the poem predicts—either in the rapid and ageing trajectory of life or at the point of death—a swift process of decay for humankind, which inverts the hour-long recovery

[105] BodL, MS Douce 78, f. 18r.

depicted in Malory's reinscription of recipe discourse in *Le Morte d'Arthur*: in an echo of Isiaiah 40.6–8, it is proclaimed 'alle þe delycyousnes of oure flessche | schalle passe in lasse space þen won houre'. As life (or death) is telescoped into less than an hour, we are shown to have very little time to heal and repair our bodies or souls. In fact, human temporal measurements are shown to be entirely inadequate for understanding the time we have as that hour is reduced into the ever elusive and indefinable present moment: 'Pryncys kyngys and emperoure... schall knowe whatte now is'. In the next few lines, temporal perspectives are then multiplied and compacted with increased fervour as those same princes are, in a sudden dilation of time, encouraged to say their psalms 'every howre' so they might eventually be made by God to last for 'ay'. Divine rejuvenation and preservation replace and efface all human attempts.

Wendy Wall has observed that, in early modern household books, medical and culinary recipes are often copied in close proximity to family records of births and deaths, encouraging subsequent readers to reflect on the simultaneous desirability and impossibility of everlasting earthly preservation.[106] In this medieval compilation, the links between the recipes and the devotional poem are even more pronounced: the temporal precision and concern for 'hours' in the recipes and the appearance of the same phrasing ('þe space of an houre') in both recipes and poem directly encourage a reader to contrast the temporal perspectives offered by the texts: one depicting earthly recovery *in* time and *through* prolonged human labour, the other depicting instantaneous destruction and resurrection at the hands of the divine. The poem could be interpreted as a corrective rebuke to the recipes that reminds readers of the vanity of tending extensively and leisurely to their body's earthly needs: 'Hyt helpythe fulle lytylle aȝenste dethe to rage | for sone sche wylle overcome alle vs'.[107] However, the decision of the scribe or the compiler to copy the poem *and* the recipes suggests that both visions of time offered him or her something valuable: recognition of the body's corruptibility on earth did not stop individuals, plagued by pain and discomfort, spending time tending to it. Faith and healing action each offered their own temporal vision and the collision and multiplication of those temporalities seem sometimes to have been a comfort for readers rather than the painful 'ripping apart' which Augustine experienced.

---

[106] Wall, *Recipes for Thought*, pp. 198–208.   [107] BodL, MS Douce 78, f. 18v.

The proximity of these texts thus demonstrates, once again, medieval readers' ability to hold different temporal perspectives in their minds simultaneously without those perspectives necessarily being in tension. It seems that such flexibility was a more common part of reading experiences than we might assume, operating within compilations of all kinds, including remedy collections and practical manuscripts. Not only do recipes and recipe collections require just as much flexible, polytemporal thinking as romances and devotional writings, but they—frequently dismissed by modern scholars as mundane, everyday, earthly texts—are used within those *un*earthly, fantastical genres as a creative means of manipulating time. Imaginative writings in themselves, they also functioned for poets as imaginative tools and stimulants, consistently destabilizing within their superficially linear, formulaic structures any consistent relationship between the marvellous and the mundane. To reduce the recipes to practical, instructional writings translated straight into action is, then, to overlook the creative reading they invite and the creative thinking they stimulated in other medieval writers concerned with the protraction, contraction, and evasion of time.

5
Experiencing Boundaries

The coexisting, intersecting, and conflicting temporal structures examined in Chapter 4 are just one of many ways in which recipe compilations invite readers to cross—and recross—boundaries: medieval medical writing consistently confuses the categories of human and object, the marvellous and banal, and the permitted and prohibited in ways that could have discomforted, amazed, and intrigued contemporary readers. For example, in remedy collections, marvellous transformations of human bodies were imagined not only through the assistance of exotic and extraordinary substances, but also through strange applications of otherwise mundane objects. Similarly, charms and amulets using familiar and orthodox scriptural language were condemned by some pastoral writers as demonic and otherworldly. Finally, commonplace herbs were claimed in empirical *experimenta* to affect the body in ways that could not be explained or rationalized by prevailing academic theories.[1] Because of this blurring of categories, it can be very difficult to establish where the different boundaries were drawn by medieval thinkers between the marvellous and the mundane, the natural and the supernatural, the licit and the illicit.

A few canonical texts offered guidelines which were recopied throughout the Middle Ages. St Augustine condemned charms, divination, and astrology, as well as all healing uses of herbs, stones, and animal parts that exploited those substances' occult powers rather than their known, natural ones; he argued that such practices brought individuals into dangerous contracts with demons.[2] Also influential was Gratian's *Decretum*, a twelfth-century legal textbook which drew heavily on Augustine's writings and included divination, charms, amulets, and unorthodox uses of religious

---

[1] On attitudes to charms and amulets, see Skemer, *Binding Words*, pp. 21–73; Catherine Rider, *Magic and Religion in Medieval England* (London, 2012), pp. 55–61; Eamon Duffy, *The Stripping of the Altars: Traditional Religion in England c.1400–c.1580* (New Haven, CT, 1992), pp. 266–98.

[2] Augustine, *De doctrina christiana*, ed. and trans. by R.P.H. Green (Oxford, 1995), pp. 91–101.

rituals amongst its examples of *sortilegium* ('sorcery').³ In the later Middle Ages, however, these views were challenged by large-scale changes, such as the thirteenth-century establishment of natural magic as an acceptable alternative to demonic magic.⁴ In addition to these broad shifts, individual scholars, churchmen, and lawyers found their own ways of defining the marvellous, supernatural, and forbidden. The negotiations the learned members of these intellectual circles made in relation to charms, natural magic, and ritual magic (all of which could be used to heal) have been the subject of many recent studies.⁵

Less attention has been paid to the way that such categories were negotiated in anonymous, untheoretical remedy books with uncertain or looser connections to academic environments and stronger connections with informal or amateur medical practice.⁶ Although general studies of magic and medicine have considered the attitudes and actions of the laity as well as those of religious and scholarly communities, they do not pay close or sustained attention to such remedy books.⁷ Perhaps this is because these collections, conglomerations of multiple fragmentary sources, do not usually contain a sustained commentating voice marking particular practices as marvellous, distasteful, or taboo in the way that scholastic and theological writings do. Consequently, it is easy to assume that every recipe or type of practice represented in a collection was embraced and trusted by its owner in the same way. The fact that we have little biographical information about the scribes and owners of such manuscripts also makes it difficult to speculate about their views. We do know that the dangers of potentially demonic practices—such as charms, divination, and judicial astrology—were

---

³ Rider, *Magic and Religion*, p. 14.
⁴ See Page, *Magic in Medieval Manuscripts*, pp. 18–28 and Chapter 1 for further discussion of natural magic.
⁵ E.g. Lea T. Olsan, 'Charms and Prayers in Medieval Medical Theory and Practice', *Social History of Medicine*, 16 (2003), 344–66; Rider, *Magic and Religion*, pp. 25–69; Catherine Rider, *Magic and Impotence in the Middle Ages* (Oxford, 2006), pp. 53–207; Sophie Page, *Magic in the Cloister: Pious Motives, Illicit Interests and Occult Approaches to the Medieval Universe* (Philadelphia, PA, 2013); Frank Klaassen, *The Transformations of Magic: Illicit Learned Magic in the Later Middle Ages and Renaissance* (Philadelphia, PA, 2013); Richard Kieckhefer, *Forbidden Rites: A Necromancer's Manual of the Fifteenth Century* (Cambridge, 1989).
⁶ An exception is the PhD thesis of Laura Mitchell which explores the ways boundaries are negotiated and used to construct identities in four personal or household manuscripts containing various kinds of magical texts, some of which could serve healing purposes. See Laura T. Mitchell, 'Cultural Uses of Magic in Fifteenth-Century England' (unpublished doctoral thesis, University of Toronto, 2011), pp. 96–242.
⁷ E.g. Kieckhefer, *Magic*, pp. 56–94; Richard Firth Green, *Elf Queens and Holy Friars: Fairy Beliefs and the Medieval Church* (Philadelphia, PA, 2016); Michael D. Bailey, *Fearful Spirits, Reasoned Follies: The Boundaries of Superstition in Late Medieval Europe* (Ithaca, NY, 2013).

communicated to the laity through sermons and vernacular writings such as the fifteenth-century dialogic text *Dives and Pauper*.[8] But, like the denunciations in patristic, legal, and academic writings, the strict prescriptions of these vernacular texts do not reflect the wide range of intertwined practices that existed and the variety of attitudes these could attract.

In many instances, a recipe's inclusion in a collection probably *did* signal some form of acceptance by a scribe or compiler. However, there are different kinds of acceptance. Copying a cure might mean that the scribe was seriously considering translating it into practice. But his engagement with the recipe could also be more tentative, hypothetical, and imaginary, motivated by curiosity or intellectual interest. Some scribes might have copied morally or intellectually ambivalent recipes because they offered them the idea (but not necessarily the reality) of solving their problems. As Laura Mitchell has demonstrated, magic texts, charms, and recipes in personal and household collections were often aimed at redressing the kind of social, sexual, and economic problems that people experienced on a day-to-day basis.[9] Other scribes may have copied particular remedies because they were intrigued by, and simultaneously disapproving of, their transgressive potential. Such a response could lie behind one late fifteenth-century scribe's annotation of healing charms: he writes that practice of the charms, which he himself has copied, is prohibited by the Catholic church.[10] There is clearly an awareness here that a social and cultural boundary is being, or is about to be, crossed.

Written evidence like this, which testifies unequivocally to scribes' and readers' sense of liminality and transgression, is rare in recipe collections but not as rare as the lack of critical attention suggests. Close reading the remedies reveals that some scribes and readers were sensitive to, and sometimes troubled or excited by, those texts' potential to stray into marvellous, strange, disgusting, and illicit territories. This reminds us of the importance of perspective in constructing the wonderful, strange, revolting, or taboo: how these deviations from the familiar and accepted are understood depends upon the norms of cultures and individual readers. The perspectives of most individual medieval readers are now impossible to recover, but this chapter speculates about the range of connotations that ingredients and

---

[8] On sermons and the handbooks informing them, see Bailey, *Fearful Spirits*, p. 33. See *Dives and Pauper*, ed. by Priscilla Heath Barnum, EETS os 275, 323 280, 3 vols (London, 1976–2004), I, Part I, pp. 119–59.
[9] Mitchell, 'Cultural Uses of Magic', pp. 202–3.
[10] HEHL, MS HM 58, ff. 69r, 75v, 84r.

practices *could* have had for readers, arguing that this semantic plurality may have lent recipe collections, and their construction of specific boundaries, a shifting, metamorphic quality in readers' eyes. This is similar to the flexible dynamic characterizing the recipes' temporal structures. Here, however, the stakes are sometimes higher, as it is not merely the boundary between the magical and the mundane which is crossed and recrossed, but also the threshold demarcating sin.

Often this metamorphic quality seems unintentional: it occurs because the objects, actions, and ingredients in the recipes participate in a large number of discursive networks at once. This instability is exacerbated by the compilatory form of recipe collections which means that texts drawn from different sources—each with their own ideas about the permitted and the possible—are copied in close proximity. In some instances, though, it seems possible that this metamorphic effect was more deliberate and that compilers playfully exploited the mechanics of perspective when they arranged their collections. So, whilst extant scholarship has concentrated upon where the boundaries are drawn in medical texts in order to speculate about *extra-textual* medical practices, I shall end this chapter by redirecting attention back onto the texts themselves as affective arrangements. I speculate that boundaries, though they may be shifting and unpredictable, were central to experiences of writing, reading, and interpreting recipe books.

Explicit Boundaries

Occasionally, the scribes of recipe collections left explicit clues that they anticipated the crossing of a boundary. In Chapter 1 we saw how similes could be used to help readers negotiate unfamiliar medical processes or ailments. Comparing the preparation of animal carcasses to the preparation of meats more commonly used in cooking is one recurring type of simile: for instance, in a recipe for removing earwigs from an ear, the reader is instructed to take a cat and 'bowelle yt as ye doo a rabett' and then 'roste yt as ye doo a rabett'.[11] Similarly, in a remedy for a swollen throat, the reader is instructed to 'farse þe cate with-in als þou farses a gose'.[12] One might be surprised that these analogies were needed given that cats appear frequently in remedy collections and are used to treat a range of ailments including

---

[11] CUL, MS Ee.1.15, f. 132r.
[12] Ogden, ed., *The 'Liber de diversis medicinis'*, p. 36, lines 32–8.

menstrual pain and backache.[13] The fact that an ingredient appears often in cures might lead one to suppose that medieval readers considered it a familiar healing substance. But how frequently an ingredient appears is just one way of measuring its familiarity, and it can be misleading. After all, the authors and scribes of the above recipes clearly assumed that their readers would be unsure how to prepare cats; otherwise there would be no need to borrow analogies from the related genre of the culinary recipe.[14]

One might counter this point by arguing that analogies with other types of meat were merely part of the cures' formulaic language and were copied from manuscript to manuscript unthinkingly; they do not necessarily testify to an *individual's* experience of crossing a boundary.[15] In support of this counter-argument is the fact that the same analogies appear in other kinds of recipes in other languages: for instance, an unusual recipe for roasting and eating a cat in a fifteenth-century copy of a Catalan cookbook also instructs the reader to cut up the cat like one would a rabbit.[16] The rabbit comparison seems, then, to have become commonplace in instructional writing. And yet, the fact that scribes continued to invest the effort of copying it might suggest that medieval readers were not *using* the recipes they copied as often as we assume: in other words, they did not become desensitized to the strangeness of disembowelling a cat.

Similar traces of writers and readers crossing into unfamiliar territory occur in relation to unpleasant ingredients.[17] Medieval recipes contain animal products, such as faeces, fat, bones, or genitals, that modern readers might balk at ingesting or rubbing into their skin. Such recipes, however, are usually copied without comment, making it easy for modern scholars to assume that medieval readers were entirely comfortable using such products.[18] But this is not necessarily the case: a handful of recipes that I have

---

[13] For a remedy for menstrual pains that involves a cat see Dawson, ed., *A Leechbook*, p. 89 (no. 238). For remedies for back and sciatic pain involving the fat of a cat see BodL, MS Rawlinson C.506, ff. 65v, 68v.

[14] The similes draw additional attention to the proximity of cooking and medicine: both were prepared in the kitchen, medicines were administered with meals, and foodstuffs with particular humoral properties could function as medicines.

[15] Barbara Rosenwein, *Emotional Communities in the Early Middle Ages* (Ithaca, NY, 2006), p. 27 acknowledges the difficulties that all generic conventions pose to understanding medieval emotional responses.

[16] See *Libre del Coch*, ed. by Veronika Leimgruber (Barcelona, 1977), p. 77, no. 122.

[17] On the belief of Nicholas of Poland, an educated thirteenth-century practitioner, that God had instilled the most disgusting substances with the greatest healing powers, see William Eamon, *Science and the Secrets of Nature: Books of Secrets in Medieval and Early Modern Culture* (Princeton, NJ, 1994), p. 77.

[18] E.g. Rawcliffe, 'Curing Bodies and Healing Souls', p. 122.

examined contain instructions to conceal the distasteful ingredient from the patient, perhaps for fear that he or she will refuse the medicine. For instance, the following powder is suggested for those who become drunk too easily or are already drunk:

> Medicine for man or woman þat wil be liȝtly dronke or is dronke. Take swalewes and brene hem and make pouder þer of... and after þat time schal he neuer be dronke more but late not þat man be ware what he drinkeþ[19]

Here, it could be the swallows that are concealed from the recipient *or* it could be the (potentially unpopular) fact that the concoction will inhibit future intoxication.[20] Elsewhere remedy ingredients are more obviously problematic: in a remedy for epilepsy, the sting of a bee is to be concealed in ale so that the patient 'wete it not',[21] and in a remedy for jaundice earthworms should be crushed 'so small that þe syke may nat se ne witt what it is for lothynge (nausea)'.[22] A final example of anticipated distaste occurs in a remedy for a tooth cavity:

> Tak a rauenes turde and put hit in þe holewe toght bot furst colore hit with <peletur> þe ius of peletur of spayne þat þe seke knowe noht what hit be[23]

[*rauenes turde* = raven's dung; *holewe toght* = hollow tooth; *ius of peletur of spayne* = sap of pellitory of Spain]

Animal excrement is one of the most common ingredients in medieval remedies but, in this recipe, it is concealed from the patient through dye made from plant sap.[24] All of these recipes demonstrate that the ubiquity of an ingredient within recipe collections did not necessarily mean that it was

---

[19] BL, MS Additional 34210, f. 22r.

[20] On the use of swallows in early modern medicine (but with applicability to the medieval period), see Michelle DiMeo and Rebecca Laroche, 'On Elizabeth Isham's "Oil of Swallows": Animal Slaughter and Early Modern Women's Recipes', in *Eco-Feminist Approaches to Early Modernity*, ed. by Jennifer Munroe and Rebecca Laroche (New York, 2011), pp. 87–104.

[21] BL, MS Harley 2378, f. 142v.

[22] Dawson, ed., *A Leechbook*, p. 154 (no. 465). See Norri, *Dictionary*, s.v., *loathing*. In the same recipe in another collection, the word 'wlatyng' is given for nausea: see BL, MS Sloane 3666, ff. 44v–45r.

[23] TCC, MS O.2.13, f. 113v.

[24] Ironically, the plant pellitory of Spain which is here used as a disguise has long been considered to have healing properties in Ayurvedic medicine. In medieval healing, unpleasant-*tasting* medical ingredients were also regularly concealed in sweeter substances: see Mount, *Dragon's Blood*, pp. 115–16, 134.

considered mundane or unremarkable by readers: the disguises reflect—and promote—a reader response which considers certain ingredients to be affronts to the normal relationship between human and animal bodies.

In *We Have Never Been Modern*, Bruno Latour claims that, since the seventeenth century, modern society has sharply segregated humans and things, subjects and objects, nature and culture, and that this segregation has paradoxically arisen because modern society produces more hybrid forms than any preceding culture. It avoids acknowledging this by rigidly delimiting these categories.[25] This anxiety about hybridity may be one reason why modern popular culture has often portrayed medieval medical practice as grotesquely at ease in its mixing of bodies, things, animals, and plants. Latour, however, suggests that premodern cultures actually thought carefully and constantly about hybrids, dwelling 'endlessly and obsessively on those connections between nature and culture'.[26] The above analogies and instructions are also evidence that medieval writers and readers worried about the appropriate relationship between their bodies and those of the creatures around them and that they could be disgusted by certain conjunctions of human and animal. Perspective is, however, integral to the construction of these boundaries: an unexperienced amateur medical practitioner may find it strange to chop up cats, but an experienced one might be very familiar with the process. This may seem like an obvious point, but it is easy to forget and assume that, because recipes are often formulaic texts, they always invited formulaic responses.

Shifting Boundaries

This kind of written recognition of boundaries is rare in remedy collections. But what is clear is that the substances and practices represented in the collections belonged to a multitude of distinct but overlapping discursive networks, which could each imbue those substances and practices with a specific set of associations. By examining these different discursive networks, we can begin to reconstruct the variety of perspectives available to readers of vernacular remedy books and the multitude of ways they may have constructed the strange, familiar, permitted, and forbidden. Scholars such as Lea Olsan and Catherine Rider have already reconstructed the range

---

[25] Bruno Latour, *We Have Never Been Modern*, trans. by Catherine Porter (Cambridge, MA, 1993), p. 41.
[26] Latour, *We Have Never Been Modern*, p. 41.

of attitudes certain practices attracted in pastoral, legal, and academic medical writings: these include charms, lists of lucky or unlucky days, and texts using divination to predict the fate of the sick.[27] Each of these could appear marvellous or mundane, permitted or prohibited to different readers. Less studied, however, is the *stuff* cluttering the recipes: the objects, animal parts, and herbs which also drew multiple discourses and categories into conversation.

One possible way of defining what a mundane recipe would have looked like to a medieval reader is by the things within it. Rita Felski argues that 'the characteristic mode of experiencing the everyday is that of habit', and so a mundane recipe might contain ingredients that were habitually visible and proximate.[28] This could include herbs such as sage, betony, and rue, which were all native to England. It might also include objects present in households of most means. For instance, a remedy for staunching blood requires 'þe felte of an olde hatte'[29] and a cure for epilepsy involves urinating in a shoe and giving the sick that urine to drink.[30] In another remedy for the scab, the writer or scribe explicitly evokes a mundane domestic space by instructing the reader to collect 'þe soot of the howse'.[31] Part of an unremarkable, everyday environment, these things are quite literally *mundanus*, which in medieval Latin meant 'of this world'.[32]

But even these mundane ingredients could become marvellous. For example, tutty, made from zinc oxide, is a fairly common ingredient in medical recipes.[33] Because *tutie* could be made from the char inside chimneys, it closely resembles the 'soot of the howse'. However, unlike that soot, tutty was considered a spice by medieval writers: the Florentine merchant Francesco Pegolotti claimed that tutty came from Alexandria, Egypt.[34] This shows how two very similar substances could evoke completely different connotations: while one was part of the everyday domestic environment, the other was a product of the exotic Eastern spice trade, which, as Paul Freedman has claimed, had uncertain geographical coordinates for many people in the West.[35] Freedman argues that the perceived mysteriousness of the East must have imbued these spices with a marvellous, otherworldly quality.[36]

[27] Lea T. Olsan, 'Charms and Prayers' and Rider, *Magic and Religion*, pp. 55–61.
[28] Felski, 'The Invention of Everyday Life', p. 81.
[29] TCC, MS R.14.51, f. 25r. See also TCC, MS O.1.65, f. 249r.
[30] CUL, MS Dd.10.44, f. 131v.
[31] BodL, MS Ashmole 1477, Part I, ff. 35v–36r. See also NLW, MS 572, f. 11v.
[32] See *DMLBS*, *mundanus*, adj., entry 2. [33] See *MED*, *tutie*, n., entry 1(a), (b).
[34] Freedman, *Out of the East*, p. 13.
[35] Ibid., pp. 95–103. [36] Ibid., pp. 2, 5, 104.

This process, however, also works in reverse: the marvellous can rapidly become mundane. Medieval thinkers were very sensitive to the importance of distance and rarity in the cultivation of wonder: St Augustine's claim that the reaction of lime to fire would appear marvellous to readers if it occurred in India and was heard of rarely was often repeated.[37] This illuminates conceptions of spices: though the spice trade spanned continents, the apothecaries, spicers, and grocers who sold the spices to medical practitioners and amateur healers were an established part of many urban scenes.[38] As Christopher Bonfield argues, there was a 'proliferation of apothecaries' stalls and shops in the later Middle Ages', offering substances such as sweet-flag root, pulp of cassia, and fistula fruit, which came from the same distant shores as the spices.[39] So, although many spices were still relatively expensive and therefore luxurious, their marvellous and exotic qualities may have been circumscribed by their proximity.[40] This is the implication in Chaucer's *Pardoner's Tale* when one of the three revellers attempts to buy poison from an apothecary. While no mention is made of the exotic origins of the apothecary's wares, Chaucer's account emphasizes the reveller's quick and easy transition from village to town, thereby suggesting the closeness and convenience of the apothecary shop:

> And forth he gooth, no lenger wolde he tarie,
> *Into the toun*, unto a pothecarie[41]

Integrated into the everyday world of commerce, the seller of spices and his wares here becomes part of the mundane urban environment.

Other substances could also metamorphosize between categories: Jerry Stannard used the term 'magiferous' to describe herbs such as vervain and St John's wort which change their properties under particular forces or

---

[37] Caroline Walker Bynum, *Metamorphosis and Identity* (New York, 2001), p. 48.
[38] On apothecaries, their guild structure, and their role in the community, see Getz, ed., *Healing and Society*, pp. xxix–xxx.
[39] Christopher Bonfield, 'The First Instrument of Medicine: Diet and Regimens of Health in Late Medieval England', in *'A verray parfit praktisour'*, ed. by Clark and Danbury, pp. 99–119 (p. 112).
[40] Freedman, *Out of the East*, pp. 126–9. Bonfield, 'The First Instrument', p. 112 also makes this point.
[41] *The Pardoner's Tale*, in *Riverside*, ed. by Benson, lines 851–2, italics mine. See also *The Nun's Priest's Tale*, in *Riverside*, ed. by Benson, line 2948: 'Though in this toun is noon apothecarie...'.

conditions.[42] Vervain, hot and dry according to medieval humoral theory, is often used in unremarkable herbal concoctions.[43] And yet, since classical times, the plant has also been connected to magicians and necromancers. According to Pliny the Elder, vervain was used by past civilizations to cleanse and purify houses; he claimed that Zoroastrian Persian Priests asserted that those who are rubbed with vervain obtain their wishes, win friends, eradicate fevers, and cure all diseases.[44] This reputation endured into the later Middle Ages and beyond. In a short fifteenth- or sixteenth-century series of recipes added to spare leaves at the end of a manuscript containing a wealth of learned medical and scientific texts, a reader is instructed to use vervain tempered with wine or water and crushed with various other herbs to heal bites from venomous beasts, fevers of various types, and gall or kidney stones.[45] The herb still seems to be working here through its natural humoral qualities. However, immediately after these remedies, it is written, 'Also whoso berithe verven vppon them shulle haue gret loue of euerybody so haue his askyng yf it be resonabulle'.[46] In another medical and miscellaneous collection, it is claimed that if someone drinks the juice of vervain, he or she will be invisible until they drink holy water; a thief will expose himself if touched with vervain, and a man who wears the herb upon him shall not be injured by his enemies.[47] It is not made clear whether seasonal changes or changes in planetary influences could be partially responsible for these various powers.

In these examples, multiple boundaries are crossed: the visible becomes invisible, active agents become passive targets, and victims become vanquishers. In the process, a commonplace, easily attainable herb capable of healing everyday afflictions through its natural qualities is also shown to have extraordinary powers, working in ways that may be considered magical: these workings could have been interpreted as a kind of natural magic, but the fact that the invisible drinker of vervain will become visible

---

[42] Jerry Stannard, 'Magiferous Plants and Magic in Medieval Medical Botany', in *Herbs and Herbalism in the Middle Ages and Renaissance*, ed. by Katherine E. Stannard and Richard Kay (Aldershot, 1999), pp. 33–46.

[43] See BL, MS Harley 2390, f. 119v for a list of the humoral qualities of different herbs.

[44] Pliny, *Natural History*, trans. by H. Rackham, W.H.S. Jones, and D.E. Eichholz, 10 vols (London, 1938–63), VII, Bk XXV, ch. LIX. Cited in Stannard, 'Magiferous Plants', p. 38.

[45] TCC, MS R.14.52, f. 270r. On this (predominantly vernacular) manuscript and its possible connection to the Hammond scribe, see *Sex, Ageing, and Death in a Medieval Medical Compendium: Trinity College Cambridge MS R.14.52—Its Texts, Language, and Scribe*, ed. by M. Teresa Tavormina (Tempe, AZ, 2006), pp. 1–17.

[46] TCC, MS R.14.52, f. 270r.   [47] BL, MS Additional 12195, f. 149r–v.

after drinking holy water suggests that that recipe could also have been perceived to have shadier, demonic workings.

These herbs and spices demonstrate, then, the metamorphic quality of recipes: the penumbra of connotations surrounding individual ingredients means that they can appear marvellous or mundane, licit or illicit, depending upon the perspective from which they are viewed and the prior experience or knowledge of the reader. Focusing upon the beaver hat that belongs to Chaucer's Merchant, Kellie Robertson has recently argued that this semantic instability means that 'premodern subjects are often shown to be at the mercy of "their" things'.[48] Robertson claims that, whilst human beings select which objects in their surroundings to focus upon, wear, and adorn their houses and texts with, those objects carry with them a penumbra of connotations that cannot be deployed selectively or dispelled at will by their human owners.[49] This effect seems even more intense in recipe collections, where texts using ingredients in different ways are copied in close proximity to one another. Because there is no continual authoritative voice circumscribing this play of connotations, it is left up to later readers to decide how, or whether, a boundary is constructed between such recipes.

Dead Men's Heads

This lack of explicit boundaries could have dangerous moral consequences. The author of one of the above texts on vervain recognized this: although he does not explain how vervain ensures that all the requests of a man or woman will have favourable outcomes, he acknowledges that such a power could be misused, circumscribing it by stipulating that whoever uses the herb in this way will only 'haue his askyng yf it be resonabulle', a word which could mean 'rational', 'appropriate', 'sensible', or 'natural'.

In most collections, though, there is no authorial or scribal voice to resolve the moral dilemmas created by the ingredients and practices represented in recipes, not all of which were unequivocally licit. Human remains are one such problematic substance. In the collections that I have consulted, at least five recipes require body parts of dead human beings. A remedy for epilepsy in a fifteenth-century collection requires the sick to drink powder

---

[48] Kellie Robertson, 'Medieval Things: Materiality, Historicism, and the Premodern Object', *Literature Compass*, 5 (2008), 1060–80 (p. 1063).
[49] Robertson, 'Medieval Things', p. 1070.

made from a 'ded mannes hed', and another remedy in a different late medieval manuscript for the same affliction instructs the reader to make the bone of a dead man into a powder and drink it.[50] Elsewhere, two similar remedies for sore penises call for the powdered 'bone of a dede man'.[51] Finally, a fifteenth-century remedy for warts requires 'þe erþe within a dede manys schulle (skull)'.[52] Three of these remedies occur in intellectually accessible recipe collections written partly or predominantly in the vernacular, which may have been copied by individuals for private use.[53] The fourth occurs in a similarly accessible collection copied by multiple hands, perhaps in a collaborative enterprise.[54] The fifth—the wart remedy—occurs in MS Ashmole 1443, the manuscript examined in Chapter 3 because it contains accessible, vernacular texts but also sometimes displays a more learned theoretical and Latinate style.[55] It is likely, then, that remedies involving human remains occurred in collections read by people with different levels of knowledge and experience.

The remedies for a sore penis are the only ones listed for that affliction on the manuscript page on which they appear. In contrast, the other three remedies for epilepsy and warts are surrounded by alternative cures for the same ailments. Although the humoral workings of these alternative cures are not made explicit, many deploy innocuous herbs and animal substances, such as sheep's fat, tormentil, and animal excrement, which appear frequently in the theoretically grounded remedies and empirical *experimenta* gathered in scholastic collections. Two of the manuscripts, however, also contain a large number of cures which appear to work through different, potentially less acceptable means.[56] In these collections, there are a large number of charms and amulets, some of which are made from herbs and some of which are made from less easily attainable ingredients such as wolf's skin.[57] It is never explicit whether these amulets are working purely through natural occult properties, divine power, or demonic mediation. Furthermore, though many of the charms or ritual behaviours to be performed involve Christian language, others use unfamiliar names; this second kind had long been considered problematic by pastoral writers because

---

[50] Respectively, BodL, MS Laud misc. 553, f. 46r and BodL, MS Rawlinson C.506, f. 104v.
[51] BodL, MS Ashmole 1438, Part II, p. 23 and TCC, MS R.14.39, f. 63v.
[52] BodL, MS Ashmole 1443, p. 328.
[53] BodL, MS Ashmole 1438, Part II, p. 23; BodL, MS Rawlinson C.506, f. 104v; TCC, MS R.14.39, f. 63v.
[54] BodL, MS Laud misc. 553, f. 46r.   [55] BodL, MS Ashmole 1443, p. 328.
[56] BodL, MS Rawlinson C.506, f. 104v and BodL MS Laud misc. 553, f. 46r.
[57] BodL, MS Laud misc. 553, f. 46r.

it could lead to individuals unwittingly evoking the assistance of demons.[58] In these manuscripts, then, the remedies involving human remains are surrounded by texts belonging to many different areas of medical practice, some of which are ambiguously poised between the licit and the illicit. Because of such instability, this framework of surrounding texts offers us limited help in interpreting the five recipes.

The use of skeletons and corpses for healing purposes is itself a practice embedded in several discursive networks, some of which are also morally problematic. It is therefore surprising that this body of ingredients has received little attention in studies of magic and medicine.[59] One lens through which to interpret the remedies is provided by the Arabic and Greek sources from which they might have derived: the Persian medical authority, Avicenna, recommended using human skulls to treat epilepsy.[60] Another Arabic-speaking thinker, Ibn al-Baytār, attributed to Galen the claim that human bones can be used to dry surplus humours in the body.[61] It is not clear whether Galen ever did directly advocate this practice; as Caroline Petit notes, it seems unlikely that he would recommend it explicitly, given that he described Xenocrates's therapeutic uses of human bones as 'forbidden by law'.[62] Interestingly, though, he also writes that such practices are 'not perverted' ('aselgē'), suggesting that he did not find them naturally or morally wayward.[63]

The cures in the above remedy books could also have been viewed by late medieval readers as examples of natural magic, as the head of a corpse was sometimes claimed to possess an inherent vivifying power: in an Arabic work by Ibn Al Jazzar (d. 974), known in its Latin translation as *De proprietatibus*, it is written that when the skull of an old man is placed in a dove or pigeon cote, the birds will increase in number greatly.[64] As already noted,

---

[58] Rider, *Magic and Religion*, p. 56.
[59] An exception is Richard Sugg, *Mummies, Cannibals, and Vampires: The History of Corpse Medicine from the Renaissance to the Victorians* (London, 2011), but this discusses little medieval material.
[60] Housni Alkhateeb Shehada, *Mamluks and Animals: Veterinary Medicine in Medieval Islam* (Leiden, 2013), p. 356, note 105.
[61] Shehada, *Mamluks and Animals*, p. 356, note 105.
[62] Caroline Petit, 'Galen, Pharmacology and the Boundaries of Medicine: A Reassessment', in *Collecting Recipes: Byzantine and Jewish Pharmacology in Dialogue*, ed. by Lennart Lehmhaus and Matteo Martelli (Berlin, 2017), pp. 51–79 (pp. 56, 57, and 61 for Greek and English versions).
[63] Petit, 'Galen', pp. 56, 57, and 61.
[64] See Oxford, Corpus Christi College, MS 125, f. 124v and Sophie Page, *Magic in the Cloister*, pp. 71, 186. On the text's connection to natural magic, see Maaike Van der Lugt,

natural magic became more acceptable from the thirteenth century onwards and these associations with intellectually acceptable medical theories probably explain why cures involving human remains come to be copied alongside more innocuous herbal preparations in late medieval remedy books.

These traditions, however, are not referenced in the remedy books and it is unlikely that all readers would have had prior knowledge of them. Other cultural discourses might have offered models for this therapeutic practice that were more accessible to the varied readership of vernacular remedy collections. One such discourse is hagiography, which was communicated to the laity through texts, paintings, church architecture, and feast days.[65] Aptly, a particularly close parallel appears in the story of the patron saints of physic and surgery, Cosmas and Damian.[66] These third-century physicians, piously devoted to the early Christian cause, were credited with the miraculous cure of a churchman from Rome whose leg was consumed by infection. After praying to Cosmas and Damian, the churchman dreamt that the brothers amputated his leg and replaced it with the leg of a black Ethiopian man buried in a local churchyard on the same day. When he woke, he found that the transplant had really occurred and his leg had been cured.[67] This narrative has particularly close parallels with one of the above remedies for a sore penis because that remedy specifically instructs the reader to 'take a boon of a dede man *in þe chyrche ȝerde*'.[68] Physically, it would have been easy for a medieval reader to attain the required bones: medieval churchyards were very full and graves were normally unmarked and shallow, meaning that, as the ground was being prepared for a burial, remains of older corpses were disturbed.[69] The story of the two saints seems to affirm

---

'"Abominable Mixtures": The *Liber Vaccae* in the Medieval West, or the Dangers and Attractions of Natural Magic', *Traditio*, 64 (2009), 229–77.

[65] See Elizabeth King, 'Clockwork Prayer: A Sixteenth Century Mechanical Monk', in *Blackbird: An Online Journal of Literature and the Arts*, 1 (2002), n.p. for an anecdote surrounding a sixteenth-century healing use of a dead saint's head.

[66] See K.J.P. Lowe, *Nuns' Chronicles and Convent Culture in Renaissance and Counter-Reformation Italy* (Cambridge, 2003), pp. 369–70; *One Leg in the Grave Revisited: The Miracle of the Transplantation of the Black Leg by the Saints Cosmas and Damian* ed. by Kees Zimmerman (Groningen, 2013); and Toni Mount, *A Year in the Life of Medieval England* (Stroud, 2016), p. 238 for information about these saints and the iconographical traditions surrounding them.

[67] Jack Hartnell, *Medieval Bodies: Life, Death, and Art in the Middle Ages* (London, 2018), pp. 92–4.

[68] TCC, MS R.14.39, f. 63v, italics mine. There is also a possible pun here as *yerd* could mean penis: see *MED*, yerd, n. 2, entry 5(a).

[69] N.J.G. Pounds, *A History of the English Parish: The Culture of Religion from Augustine to Victoria* (Cambridge, 2000), pp. 420–5.

that such action is morally and spiritually permissible if performed by one pious person for another with good will and healing intent.

This does not, however, seem to have been a common view in the everyday social, legal, and religious practices of late medieval life. As Caroline Walker Bynum notes, by the twelfth century, there was a widespread insistence that Christian remains needed to be buried in consecrated ground, be this a churchyard, ossuary, or reliquary in a religious house; burial in non-consecrated ground marked one as a sinner.[70] Punishments issued to those who disturbed graves—sometimes in the interests of anatomic dissection—show that the removal of Christian remains from sacred sites, even in the interests of medical progress, was strongly prohibited in medieval Europe.[71] Viewed from this perspective, then, the remedies ask a reader to perform an action that was widely considered sinful.

Human remains also had a troubling association with more illicit forms of magic. In his Latin medical handbook, *Rosa medicinae*, John of Gaddesden cites the claims of earlier medical writers Constantine the African (d. before 1099) and Urso of Salerno (d. 1225) that placing a needle with which a dead man has been sewn up in one's bed or clothes causes impotence, preventing the erection of the penis.[72] Impotence is here presented as a product of harmful symbolic magic: the needle resembles and brings about the affliction of the man's genitals. This connection between impotence and magic involving dead bodies perhaps explains why the bone of a dead man is used in the above remedies to treat a sore penis: magic—be it natural or demonic—may have been thought more likely to cure magic.[73]

Human bones and skulls were associated with necromancy as well: this was a more explicit type of black magic, unequivocally condemned by ecclesiastical and civic authorities because it involved invoking demons and spirits of the dead to see the future or achieve one's ends. For example, John Metham's fifteenth-century romance *Amoryus and Cleopes*, set in the pagan past, depicts a necromancer using human remains to collaborate with evil

---

[70] Caroline Walker Bynum, *The Resurrection of the Body in Western Christianity, 200–1336* (New York, 1995), p. 204.

[71] Danielle Jacquart, 'Medical Scholasticism', in *Western Medical Thought from Antiquity to the Middle Ages*, ed. by Mirko D. Grmek and others (Cambridge, MA, 1998), pp. 197–240 (p. 224); Katherine Park, 'The Criminal and the Saintly Body: Autopsy and Dissection in Renaissance Italy', *Renaissance Quarterly*, 47 (1994), 1–33 (p. 7).

[72] Rider, *Magic and Impotence*, p. 163.

[73] Epilepsy was also often associated with magical causes. See Catherine Rider, 'Demons and Mental Disorder in Late Medieval Medicine', in *Mental (Dis)order in Later Medieval Europe*, ed. by Sara Katajala-Peltomaa and Susanna Niiranen (Leiden, 2014), pp. 47–69 (pp. 49–55, 64, and 67).

spirits in the construction of a magical sphere: he 'gadyrryd a multytyde of mennys bonys... For as clerkys wryte, the damnyd spyrytys have delectacion | Amonge tresur and ded mennys bonys to make ther mancion'.[74] This connection between skulls and necromancy is also affirmed by a legal case heard by the King's Bench in 1371: a man named John Crok was ordered before the King's justices because his bag allegedly contained a dead man's head. When he was questioned, Crok claimed that the head was the head of a Saracen ('capud... Sarisini') that he had purchased in Spain.[75] He argued that he needed the head to act as a container to house a magical spirit; the spirit could then speak through the head's mouth and listen through its ears. The bag and all of its contents were subsequently burnt and Crok was ordered to swear upon the Gospels that he would not henceforth use such things in a way that contravened the faith of the Holy Church.

Although none of the five remedies described above involve using human remains in necromantic rituals, the scribe who copies the epilepsy remedy that instructs the reader to drink the powder of 'a ded mans bon' also copies several Latin and English texts that involve conjuring spirits for purposes such as knowing whether a man shall live or die.[76] The epilepsy remedy occurs over sixty folios after these necromantic texts (with many natural herbal remedies in between), so it is not certain that the scribe connected the two. Nevertheless, the necromantic texts reveal that the scribe was interested in exploring such illicit practices and render it possible that he was aware of the shadier associations of possessing human skeletons.

Viewed through the lens of these associated discourses, then, the use of human remains to heal the sick seems poised between the permissible and the prohibited. There is one thing, though, which may have made many of these associated contexts more socially acceptable: the corpses of social or religious outsiders are used. Crok's punishment, after all, seems fairly lenient and, although the court record justifies this by claiming that he had not yet done any harm with the head, it also probably had something to do with the fact that the head belonged to a 'Saracen', a wide-ranging term applicable to

---

[74] John Metham, *Amoryus and Cleopes*, ed. by Stephen F. Page (Kalamazoo, MI, 1999), lines 489–91.
[75] See *Select Cases in the Court of King's Bench Under Edward III: Volume VI*, ed. by G.O. Sayles, Selden Society 82 (London, 1965), p. 163 for the original Latin and an English translation. This anecdote is also described in Getz, *Medicine in the English Middle Ages*, p. 79.
[76] BodL, MS Rawlinson C.506, ff. 39r–41r. The manuscript is discussed in Mooney, 'Manuscript Evidence', pp. 196–9, where Mooney notes that it was associated with a 'Humphridus Harrison, capellanus' (chaplain) in the late fifteenth century. For further discussion in this book of the manuscript, see Chapter 3.

a Turk, Muslim, or Arab person but usually shorthand in medieval texts for a non-Christian religious enemy.[77] 'Saracen' heads were frequently mocked, abused, and mistreated in medieval culture: for example, the romance *Richard Coeur de Lion* depicts the English King Richard I eating the head of a Saracen.[78] In her analysis of this romance, Nicola McDonald demonstrates that late medieval culinary recipes existed instructing readers how to bake pies in the shape of Saracen heads; she also shows that the cannibalism in the romance is described in language borrowed from culinary recipes. Through this discourse, the author of the romance 'renders what is otherwise alien and forbidden a familiar, and thus edible, food; it effectively diffuses the taboo that makes man-eating, if not unthinkable, unpalatable'.[79]

In the other associative contexts outlined above, the unthinkable is made similarly thinkable for medieval readers through the use of outsider bodies: in the hagiography of Cosmas and Damian the churchman's new leg is taken from a Christian buried in consecrated ground, but the Christian is explicitly identified as Ethiopian. In many medieval western European narratives, religious otherness is marked by dark skin.[80] In this hagiography, skin colour is not indicative of religion but, as a racial marker, it could still function as a sign of otherness; there was, after all, believed to be a large population of Christian Ethiopians living in India, a realm considered distant and mysterious by many western writers and readers.[81] In another surviving European narrative, the remains of an unbaptised baby were allegedly prepared for healing purposes at a crossroads where criminals were hanged.[82] The unbaptised baby is an outsider to the Christian religion; the liminal space of the crossroads was also associated with outsiders as it was where criminals were hanged so that their spirits could not torment the living.[83] The use of outsider bodies therefore functions as an ambiguous sign in these accounts: on the one hand, it exacerbates the demonic element of

---

[77] Sayles, ed., *Select Cases in the Court of King's Bench*, p. 163. See *MED*, *Sarasin*, n. 1, entries 1(a), (b), (c) and *DMLBS*, *Saracenus*, n., entries 1, 2.

[78] See *Der Mittelenglische Versroman über Richard Löwenherz*, ed. by Karl Brunner (Vienna, 1913), lines 3194–3226.

[79] Nicola McDonald, 'Eating People and the Alimentary Logic of *Richard Coeur de Lion*', in *Pulp Fictions of Medieval England: Essays in Popular Romance*, ed. by Nicola McDonald (Manchester, 2004), pp. 124–50 (p. 134). See Brunner, ed., *Der Mittelenglische Versroman*, lines 3088–93.

[80] For example, *King of Tars*, where the sultan's skin turns from black to white when he is converted.

[81] Freedman, *Out of the East*, pp. 95–103.   [82] Kieckhefer, *Magic*, p. 59.

[83] Derek A. Rivard, *Blessing the World: Ritual and Lay Piety in Medieval Religion* (Washington, DC, 2009), p. 75, note 97.

the magic rituals, signalling that the enactor is crossing a boundary between the licit and the illicit and transitioning from a social insider to an outsider. On the other hand, it simultaneously renders those rituals less shocking: using the bodies of those outside central social and religious institutions would have seemed far less of an affront—and threat—to those within.

In the light of this, it is surprising that the recipes in the Middle English collections described above do *not* specify that the skeletons must come from perceived outsiders. Instead, as we have seen, one explicitly instructs the reader to take the bone from *inside* a churchyard. Furthermore, four of the recipes are clear that the bones themselves are to be used in the cures. This contrasts with recipes in both academic and informal collections where the body is not treated by the remains themselves but by things that have fleetingly come into contact with them: for instance, a remedy for a *mormal* (a scabbed ulcer) involves washing it with 'þe water þat a ded mon was ywasche wyþ'.[84] Dead bodies are there skirted around and circumvented.

Why are the authors, compilers, and scribes of recipe collections not equally cautious? Laura Mitchell has recently examined other informal, miscellaneous recipe collections requiring ingredients that, like human skulls, were used in necromantic rituals (for instance, the hoopoe).[85] The texts often claim to fulfil everyday social, sexual, and economic desires such as helping a man attract women or protecting him in the marketplace. Consequently, Mitchell argues that the recipes, regardless of whether they were actually attempted, offer relief from—and gratification of—these everyday needs through the imagined idea of fulfilment. This could also be true of the epilepsy and impotence remedies: they offer the prospect of an empowering cure, even if the scribe was not truly willing to translate them into action.

Another reading, however, is also possible: given that some of the remedies are surrounded by alternative cures for epilepsy and impotence which use less problematic ingredients, it could be that satisfaction was derived less from an imagined endpoint and more from an imagined *means*: the cures satisfied readers' desires to envisage transgressive actions, such as stealing a body, without actually demanding that they perform any wrongdoing. This appeal to dark impulses is heightened in the remedy which

---

[84] BL, MS Additional 33996, f. 134r. This ingredient also recalls *mummia*, a secretion from embalmed bodies which was frequently listed in medical remedies, including those originating from learned authorities. See *MED*, mummie, n.

[85] Mitchell, 'Cultural Uses', pp. 199–200. The remedy for epilepsy using human remains on BodL, MS Rawlinson 506, f. 104v is also followed by a remedy for epilepsy involving a hoopoe.

explicitly instructs the reader to locate the body in 'þe chyrche ȝerde'. Such specificity—which seems gratuitous in a practical sense given that everybody knows where to find a dead body—recalls the less controversial descriptions of plant habitats that one sometimes finds in herbals and remedies: 'take...an handfull of pelatory that growyth ouer schurche wallis or castell wallys'.[86] Just like the use of recipe language in *Richard Coeur de Lion* to describe the eating of a human head, this familiar discourse both normalizes and renders strange the transgressive act: for a moment, it makes the action seem tantalizingly possible, mundane, and culturally acceptable, but, as soon as one fully comprehends the nature of the act, one feels doubly alienated from it through this contrast with the familiar. The instruction seems designed to put in motion a peculiar dynamic of temptation and restraint. A similar effect is cultivated in one of the remedies for epilepsy: the scribe explicitly states that it is 'þe best' of the medicines listed, which can be read as a playful challenge to the reader to translate it into action.[87]

The responses such recipes may have evoked can be productively considered alongside those *deliberately* cultivated in late medieval fabliaux, literary narratives powered by witty deceptions and inappropriate desires which invite readers to imagine crossing all kinds of socially enforced boundaries. The plots of these narratives often involve dead bodies in taboo practices: corpses are buried, exhumed, disguised, imitated, and debased; they are given the exact opposite of the properly observed burial rites so highly esteemed in medieval culture. For example, *Dane Hew, Munk of Leicestre* is a comic narrative which only survives in sixteenth-century print but which, on the basis of linguistic evidence, probably circulated in the fifteenth century or before.[88] In this tale, the eponymous monk is killed by a tailor after attempting sexual relations with his wife. After he has been killed, however, he is hanged once and slain another four times when his corpse—made to look alive for the purposes of trickery—is used to deceive a string of unwitting individuals. Only at the end of the tale is Dane Hew finally buried. Analysing a French analogue for this narrative, Howard Bloch suggests that circulating corpses in fabliaux act as an analogy for the unstable relationship between signifier and signified which these tales—with their puns, linguistic deceptions, and misunderstandings—draw out:

---

[86] BodL, MS Ashmole 1389, p. 203.   [87] BodL, MS Rawlinson C.506, f. 104v.
[88] *Ten Fifteenth-Century Comic Poems*, ed. by Melissa M. Furrow (New York, 1985), p. 161.

The body is a shifter. As it circulates it derives its significance from the subject with which it comes into contact, the subject who is obliged to invest it with meaning. Where the process becomes complicated, however, is in its very multiplicity.[89]

Bloch argues that, because the body, passed from person to person, can mean anything to anyone, it—like language—risks meaning nothing at all. There are clear parallels here with the way fragmented human corpses work in the recipes: participating in multiple cultural discourses and surrounded by other ambiguous remedies, they too can function as empty and ambiguous signifiers which can mean very different things to different people.

In fabliaux, though, readers know what to expect: we find ourselves in a fictional world where there are different, and often fewer, rules about what it is acceptable to desire and do, but we are not usually invited to apply them to the real world. The recipes are less clear in this respect: although they may not actually have been translated into practice, the imperatives they contain invite readers to imagine translating them into action more emphatically than fabliaux. One might wonder what the relationship was for readers between these transgressive recipes and the more orthodox ones surrounding them. Do the orthodox texts make the remedies' illicit elements stand out more, or are the subversive recipes contained, and rendered safe, by those reminders of more acceptable practice? These questions echo those raised by Bakhtin's theory of the carnivalesque and its many critical permutations: it has long been debated whether the violation of convention that carnivalesque rituals involve actually ends up reaffirming order, rather than subverting and challenging it as Bakhtin claims.[90] Allon White and Peter Stallybrass have warned against trying to essentialize carnival by proclaiming it 'intrinsically conservative or radical'.[91] This warning seems apt in relation to remedy collections: because there is no guiding narrative voice, there is no way of knowing how the scribes of these collections understood the relationship between orthodox and transgressive remedies. Inscription marks and annotations by later readers in many manuscripts show that these collections often passed through multiple hands and multiple

---

[89] Howard Bloch, *The Scandal of the Fabliaux* (Chicago, IL, 1986), pp. 67–8.
[90] A summary of the arguments questioning this aspect of Bakhtin's theory appears in Peter Stallybrass and Allon White, *The Politics and Poetics of Transgression* (London, 1986), pp. 13–14.
[91] Stallybrass and White, *Politics and Poetics*, p. 15.

generations: these later readers would have been free, within some of the cultural parameters outlined above, to construct such relationships as they liked.[92]

Playing with Boundaries

In the above examples, the metamorphic dynamic of the remedy books seems largely to be the result of the formal conventions of the genre and its typical manuscript layout: whether the remedy books are scruffy personal notebooks or neatly executed productions, they all list recipe after recipe, bringing countless ingredients, processes, and discourses into unpredictable conversations. Form produces effect. Sometimes, though, it seems possible that this process was reversed and that compilers consciously arranged their collections around a simple kind of perspectival play. This seems most likely in recipe collections which contain a mix of medical cures, miscellaneous household recipes, and practical jokes.[93] One scruffy, early Tudor collection of recipes, Oxford, Bodleian Library, MS Ashmole 1389, contains an extensive collection of medical recipes but, copied in the middle of this medical collection and only separated from it by two blank leaves, are a large number of instructions, some in Latin, some in English, to make men and women take off their clothes; to make men dance; to make quicksilver into a contraceptive; to prepare an anaesthetic for animals that will make them seem dead; to make a man seem headless; to make all men in a house have two heads; to make eggs leap out of a pan; to make vinegar from wine; to ensure that a man shall never be drunk; to make oneself invisible; to make a dead capon cry out when roasted upon the spit; to make a solution from birdlime and oil; to make a copper penny appear silver; and to make glue that will not come loose in fire or water. Then there are a few more fishing, agricultural, and household recipes for things such as making boras (a mineral used in medical preparations but also to solder metals) and removing

---

[92] Although we often have little biographical information for owners of medieval recipe collections, it seems likely that some were handed down through families in the same way that Elaine Leong has demonstrated several early modern recipe collections were: Elaine Leong, 'Collecting Knowledge for the Family'. However, the role of women in recording this knowledge was less frequently documented in the fifteenth century than in the sixteenth and seventeenth centuries. On female ownership of medieval medical writings, see Green, 'The Possibilities of Literacy'.

[93] On the mode of knowing advocated by these miscellaneous and jokey recipes, see Jahner, 'Literary Therapeutics'.

stains from clothing. Amongst these there is also a mysterious recipe, simply entitled 'a marwylle' ('marvel'), which involves casting the blood of a duck into an oil lamp.[94] The recipes, then, work through a mix of mechanical illusion and ambiguously occult processes; texts promising seemingly mundane results are mixed in amongst those promising more spectacular outcomes.

In MS Ashmole 1389, the miscellaneous recipes are separated from the bulk of the medical remedies by two blank leaves, but in other manuscripts they are intermingled with them.[95] Consider the late fifteenth- or early sixteenth-century codex now often known as the *Tollemache Book of Secrets*: alongside marvellous recipes for feats such as carrying fire with bare hands, growing parsley in two hours, and becoming invisible, the collection also contains medical recipes to stop bleeding, remove warts, stay free from cuts, know if a woman is pregnant with a boy or a girl, and make hair grow.[96] So, these 'books of secrets' (collections of tricks, illusions, and empirical 'experimenta') were never fully separate from medical recipes.[97]

Like the text on the miscellaneous virtues of vervain, these trick texts cross boundaries of all kinds: headless men seem to cross and recross the borderline between life and death; recipes to make copper seem silver change the appearance of one substance into that of another; instructions for making eggs leap out of a pan render the inanimate animate. The recipes also map a back-and-forth movement across the boundary between change and inertia: they promise to make a transformation and yet they acknowledge that the change will only be an illusion. Consider the following recipes from MS Ashmole 1389:

For to make men to davnce

Take a pype of ellertre and pyke awaye the pythe and put ther in a <here> here of a ded body and stoppe þe iude with virgyn wax and ley it owur þe dore ther as þou wyllt men to davnce

...

For to seme þat a manes hed ys of

---

[94] The miscellaneous recipes occur in BodL, MS Ashmole 1389, pp. 39–47. Blank leaves occur on pp. 38, 48.
[95] E.g. BodL, MS Ashmole 1438, Part I, p. 23 and BL, MS Sloane 1315, ff. 88r–149r.
[96] *The Tollemache Book of Secrets*, ed. by Jeremy Griffiths and A.S.G. Edwards (London, 2001), pp. 46–52.
[97] On the tradition behind books of secrets see Eamon, *Science and the Secrets of Nature*, pp. 15–90.

Take brymstone and put it in a lampe with fyre and let it hang were as men cum in and they shalle seme þat ther heddes be of þat be within

For to make alle men in a howse to havee too heddes

Take a quantyte of azure and as moche of quickesiluer and as moche of sulphur ^brymston^ and put these iij together in a brynnyng lampe and euery man shall seme þat he hathe too heddes[98]

[*ellertre* = elder tree; *pyke awaye* = pick away; *pythe* = column of tissue in the centre of a tree[99]]

While the first recipe promises to bring about real change through ambiguous occult means, the last two recipes openly acknowledge that they are delusions: it will only 'seme' as though the transformation has occurred. This crucial verb compels readers to qualify the idea of recipe collections as purely practical compositions because it makes clear that the recipes do not actually 'get anything done'; they entertain and amuse by virtue of the fact that they only appear to have done so. Recipes such as these are therefore another potential source of carnivalesque energy within mixed medical collections, not only complicating the practical bent of a collection but also making light of taboos and socially censured practices such as nudity.

This capacity to turn accepted codes of behaviour topsy-turvy is heightened by the fact that the actions the recipes map out are all imagined in tightly bounded, interior spaces: the tricks are played upon those who are 'within', are inside 'a howse', or have passed through a 'dore'. Such explicit demarcation of domestic space does not usually occur in the titles of medical recipes, despite the fact that these are usually considered 'household texts'; the demarcation recalls the unusual example of the skeleton in the 'þe chyrche ʒerde'. It also recalls the domestic setting of many fabliaux: Chaucer's *Miller's Tale* and *Reeve's Tale* take place in houses and bedrooms, and crucial events, such as Absolon's misdirected kiss at Alison's window, occur at domestic thresholds.[100] A similar use of space characterizes *Jack and His Stepdame*, a fifteenth-century tale in which the eponymous Jack is given a magical pipe that will make everybody dance. The climax of this tale, which seems to have been part of the same imaginative network as the above

---

[98] BodL, MS Ashmole 1389, pp. 39–40. Individually and in other combinations, these recipes occur in other manuscripts too. E.g. see BL, MS Sloane 1315, f. 115r; BodL, MS Radcliffe Trust e.10, f. 61v; and BodL, MS e.Museo 52, f. 61v.
[99] *MED*, *pith*, n., entry 1(a).
[100] Geoffrey Chaucer, *The Miller's Tale*, in *Riverside*, ed. by Benson, line 3727.

recipe for making everybody dance, is marked by the movement of the pipe and the mischief it unleashes towards the hall, or 'howse', of Jack's father and the bounded space of the local court.[101] These circumscribed, ordered, and hierarchal domestic settings make the overturning of order more palpable. In both the recipes and the fabliaux, then, the violation of social, sexual, and conceptual thresholds is mapped onto the imagined violation of physical ones.

In her study of several similar miscellaneous collections, Laura Mitchell claims that 'there is no discernible pattern to the order in which things appear', adding that this 'unorganised order...makes [the scribe's] alternative interests available to the reader almost simultaneously'.[102] While it is certainly true that many miscellaneous recipes may have been copied together because the owner of the manuscript wished to have all of his or her recipes in one conveniently accessible book, there does sometimes seem to be more thought behind the arrangement. In collections such as MS Ashmole 1389 and *The Tollemache Book of Secrets*, overtly marvellous or playful recipes—such as making men seem headless or making men breathe fire—are copied amongst medical and household recipes that, if copied individually, would appear mundane, unexciting, and utilitarian: these include removing a stain from clothing, catching fish, staunching blood, and making hair grow.[103] The last two recipes often appear in unremarkable head-to-toe medical compendia.[104] When these mundane recipes are copied alongside the other marvels, however, their marvellous, transformative qualities are also drawn out: just as herbs such as vervain could shift unpredictably from recipe to recipe between signifying the marvellous and the mundane, these texts metamorphosize in relation to one another, shifting between the wondrous and the quotidian. The capacity to make hair grow, warts disappear, and blood stop flowing suddenly seems more wondrous when equated with making parsley grow in two hours. Just like the tricks and illusions surrounding them, these medical recipes bring about a physically demonstrable result, which can be performed before and used to impress spectators in a way that the curing of a headache and other internal ailments cannot. It seems possible then that, at least at one stage in their

---

[101] *Jack and His Stepdame*, in *Ten Fifteenth-Century Comic Poems*, ed. by Furrow, pp. 124–31, lines 319–84.
[102] Mitchell, 'Cultural Uses of Magic', pp. 162–3.
[103] On BodL, MS Ashmole 1393, ff. 1v–2v, similar recipes for making hair fall away and for catching rabbits are copied amongst obvious marvels. The same kinds of texts appear, then, to have been incorporated into these marvel networks, perhaps suggesting that certain combinations became conventional.
[104] E.g. YM, MS XVI.E.32, ff. 17r–v, 58r–59r.

transmission, a scribe chose to place these miscellaneous and medical texts alongside one another because he recognized this similarity and potential for semantic interplay.

Recipes also move each other across the boundary between the licit and the illicit and the serious and the funny. This occurs in a passage on the virtues of lily in the Middle English verse herbal discussed in Chapter 2. The author of these lines claims that if a lily-based mixture is placed in a dunghill, it will produce worms. The following uses can be made of those worms once powdered:

> And cast it on clothys þat folk han on
> ȝey schull noȝt slepyn be dayes iij
> Whil þe clothis on hem be
> ...
> ȝif þou take netys mylk also
> And þis powdir þou medyl þerto
> And who þer of etyn schall
> In to a feuer schal he falle[105]

The itching powder initially seems like a playful practical joke. But because the recipe immediately after it is for inducing a fever, it retrospectively appears more sinister. Once again, the transgressive aspects of one recipe draw out those in another. There are several other recipes in the herbal which could also be used to torture or control others: these include bringing about discord between a husband and wife, depriving someone of sleep until the herb dragonwort is removed from under his or her head, and making everyone appear like devils.[106] In the longest surviving versions of the herbal, though, there is a pronounced sense of balance: although instructions are given for bringing about injury and harm, there are also remedies for these afflictions. There are numerous remedies for fevers, instructions for protecting oneself against the devil, and a recipe for bringing about unity between a husband and wife.[107] This suggests another kind of thoughtful arrangement: the author may have enshrined within the poem a reassuring sense of equilibrium. But it is significant that, for a reader progressing

---

[105] Stephens, ed., *Extracts in Prose and Verse*, lines 994–1002.
[106] Ibid., lines 810–14, 1136–8, and 943–4.
[107] Ibid., lines 472, 594, 694–6, 716, 721, 729, 758–9, 803–4, 871–6, 1062, 1100, 1238, 1261, and 1412–15.

linearly through the herbal, this equilibrium is experienced as a playful dynamic between transgression and atonement: balance may ultimately be restored but the push and pull—the crossing and recrossing of boundaries—has to take place first.

These dynamic patterns in the verse herbals and miscellaneous recipe collections may indicate that some compilers built into their collections a simple but effective kind of perspectival play. In his seminal study of play, *Homo Ludens*, Johan Huizinga claims that play has an 'aesthetic' quality and is described by 'terms with which we try to describe the effects of beauty: tension, poise, balance, contrast, variation, solution, resolution etc'.[108] The contrasts, tensions, and resolutions in the recipe collections and herbals may be simple and the combinations of recipes—copied from manuscript to manuscript—may have become formulaic, but they still have the potential to produce satisfying aesthetic effects.

Huizinga claims, though, that play is formed through rules, boundaries, and the demarcation of a finite 'playground'.[109] In a few recipe collections, such boundaries are made explicit: for instance, in MS Ashmole 1389, the separation of the marvellous recipes from the surrounding medical ones by two blank leaves implies that the compiler wished to demarcate his 'playground', separating the comic from the serious.[110] Often, though, such boundaries are hard to discern: was it as acceptable to some readers to steal human remains from a churchyard as it was to gather betony and sage or make someone appear headless? Usually, we are forced to speculate about the answers to such questions from omissions or silences. It is this very silence, however, which means that the things and actions recorded in recipes *can* produce multiple associations and responses. So, although we cannot be sure how individual readers responded to the collections, we can remain sensitive to the great range of reactions and interpretations available to them.

Furthermore, it seems highly likely that the recipes did not evoke stable, singular responses at all, but shifting, metamorphic ones which changed when the contents of the recipes were viewed from the alternative vantage points constructed by other remedies within the collection. Unlike rigid clerical denunciations of particular healing actions, the collections may, then, offer a more accurate reflection of the constant negotiations and

---

[108] Johan Huizinga, *Homo Ludens: A Study of the Play Element in Culture*, trans. by R.F.C. Hull (London, 1949), p. 10.
[109] Ibid.   [110] BodL, MS Ashmole 1389, pp. 38, 48.

renegotiations medieval people made in the face of ambiguous boundaries and ambivalent attitudes to practices associated with magic. Indeed, the compilatory form *encourages* such negotiations, stimulating the interpretative and imaginative faculties and underlining how a seemingly practical and convenient form could produce unexpected, unpredictable, and varied responses.

Conclusion

Lechecraft is man to hele . of all maner sekenesse
And to kepe hym hool þat is hol . as fer as craft may[1]

To be healthy in Middle English is to be 'hol', whole, uninjured, and intact; it is to be balanced, in proportion, and moderate. This study has shown, however, that the means of achieving that wholeness could be fragmentary, piecemeal, and inconclusive: in the pursuit of health, one had to engage with parts and fragments of texts and with cumulative assemblages that were elastic, extendable, and, perhaps, frighteningly incompletable. Books and bodies may well have been in tandem here: Julie Orlemanski's work has already shown how important bricolage and pastiche were to medieval conceptions of the embodied self, showing that bodies—at once universal types and stubbornly particular masses of flesh—were interpreted through a shifting matrix of medical, astrological, religious, and poetic models. What is more, individual strands of medical practice required healers to reach diagnostic, prognostic, and ethical judgements by patching together the evidence of different body parts: the translator of a Middle English physiognomic tract underlined this when he warned readers against hinging their ethical assessments on the appearance of just a nose, hand, or eye: 'Forsothe thow shalt not fasten thy jugementis vpon one of these signes neither sentence, but gadre the witnesse of all.'[2] 'Gadering' fragments was, then, integral to the act of appraising bodies *and* to acts of creating, compiling, reading, and interpreting medical texts—and particularly recipe collections.[3]

That fragmentariness could take many forms: this study has shown that, when opening their remedy collections, medieval people were frequently confronted with bits and pieces of knowledge that had been excised from any available theoretical underpinnings and from the diagnostic and

---

[1] BL, MS Sloane 340, f. 65v. The prologue—though prose—is lineated like verse (as discussed in Chapter 2).
[2] *Secretum Secretorum: Nine English Versions*, ed. by M.A. Manzalaoui, EETS 276 (Oxford, 1977), p. 113.
[3] For further discussion of acts of 'gadyring', see Chapter 3.

prognostic intelligence informing that knowledge's practical enaction in many medical encounters. Furthermore, although individual recipes within a collection often seem stylistically and visually formulaic, set out upon the page in the same way and employing the same syntactic structures and conventional phrases, they are simultaneously quirky, idiosyncratic, and inconsistent: syntactic patterns, playful puns, and sporadically careful rubrication all point to the many sources those recipes may have been extracted from, the changing hands involved in their copying, and the changing impulses or priorities of the persons responsible for their written form.

This fragmentariness is not, though, totally at odds with wholeness: the scribes, compilers, and readers who collected large numbers of medical recipes and those patients and practitioners who examined their bodies through different interpretative lenses may well have felt, through acts of accumulation and integration, that they were moving towards a state of fullness and completion, a state of impressive and all-encompassing encyclopaedic know-how. It is also possible that, though medical language could be seen to disturb, fragment, and adulterate literary discourses, it was simultaneously felt to be allusive and connected, and was understood to be embedded within larger intertextual webs: we have seen that recipes shared images, registers, and ideas not only with other practical, medical, and scientific writings but also with romances, fabliaux, devotional writings, and Chaucerian poetry. What is more, recipes could be excised from medical contexts and embedded wholesale within literary works, particularly romances. In that genre, they function both to punctuate texts with a different temporality and to enhance the marvellous temporalities already within the romance; they can be both complementary and 'other', circumscribing within the text a moment for a different kind of imaginative and temporal transportation.

So, because recipes were so reinscribable, and because recipe collections were patchwork creations produced through a variety of sources and hands, we need to practise a different mode of reading when attending to their quirks, ambiguities, and sporadic artfulness. On the one hand, this mode is more fragmentary: we need a way of reading which does not try to construct a single narrative of practicality or impracticality but is open to a shifting and unpredictable relationship between these things and the individuals involved in the texts' production and reception: after all, a collection's relationship with practicality can seem to shift from recipe to recipe or even from line to line.

At the same time, though, our way of reading needs to be more holistic and integrative, not only thinking about recipes and the manuscripts that contain them alongside literary texts and manuscripts, but also applying and testing the same analytical techniques. We can use this exercise to nuance, redefine, and expand familiar categories, such as the 'aesthetic', 'crafted', and 'careful'. For example, in Chapter 3, we saw how a recipe's insistence on the whitest and fairest of ingredients connected that text to culturally constructed ideas of beauty and aesthetic decorum. Another area that might benefit from such an integrative approach is the visual appearance of recipe collections in manuscripts. There was not space in this study to explore in much depth the ways in which the visual layout and ornamentation of a recipe collection could complicate our criteria for determining what is 'useful' or 'frivolous', 'careful' or 'scruffy', 'thoughtful' or 'thoughtless', but it was a question that repeatedly struck me as I consulted the manuscripts.[4] For instance, in one manuscript, a scribe has copied a set of Latin and English medical texts, including recipes, in a mid- or late-fifteenth-century neat secretary hand, with the heading for each recipe copied in a larger, bolder, slightly more calligraphic display script; thoughtfully, plenty of space for annotation has been left around the recipes.[5] There is no colour or fancy decoration but care has clearly been taken over the appearance and design of the collection (see Figure C.1). Similarly, in another codex, medical texts and recipe collections have been copied predominantly by a fifteenth-century smart bastard anglicana hand.[6] The *textura* influence upon this script suggests that the manuscript was carefully and slowly copied. The manuscript also contains the red and blue rubrication typical of many fifteenth-century manuscripts and used to separate the recipes from one another. And yet there is nothing impressively lavish or ornate about the manuscript; its small dimensions also suggest that it was intended for itinerant use (see Figure C.2). Are these manuscripts aptly described as 'plain' or 'embellished', 'carefully shaped' or 'pragmatically executed'? Questions such

---

[4] Remedy collections are frequently represented as belonging to two extremes: For instance, Mooney, 'Manuscript Evidence', pp. 187, 199 draws a sharp contrast between 'ornate collections for the aristocracy's leisured reading' which—judging from 'the expense of production' and the 'present condition of the manuscript[s]'—were 'not intended for daily use', and medical or scientific manuscripts intended for use which 'are usually made of paper, [and] often written by a single hand without rubric or embellishment of any kind'. See also Voigts, 'Scientific and Medical Books', p. 379.
[5] BL, MS Additional 19674, ff. 2r–50v. [6] CUL, MS Kk.6.33, ff. 11r–113r.

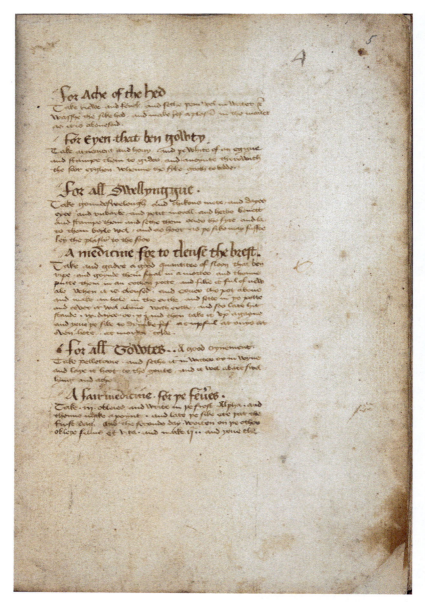

Figure C.1 Recipe collection with titles in a more elaborate display script. © The British Library Board, BL MS Additional 19674, f. 5r.

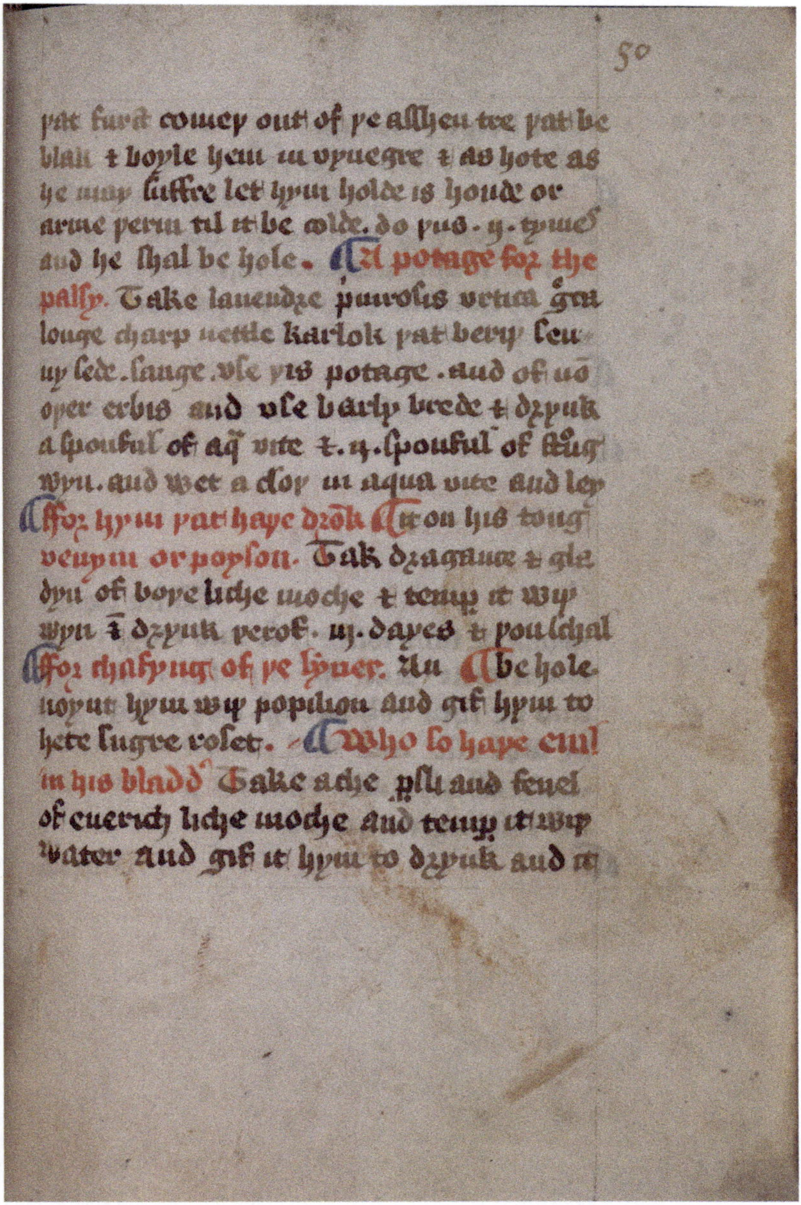

þat fond comey out of þe asshen tre þat be
blak t boyle hem in vynegre t as hote as
ye may suffre let hym holde is honde or
arme þerin til it be colde. do þus . v . tymes
and he shal be hole. ¶ A potage for the
palsy. Take lauendre piuroles vetica grā
longe charp nettle karlok þat bery seu-
uy sede . sauge . vse þis potage . and of no
oþer erbis and vse barly brede t drynk
a spouful of aq̄ vite t . ij . spouful of stūg
wyn. and wet a cloþ in aqua vite and ley
¶ For hym þat haþe droh ¶ It on his tong
venym or poyson. Tak dragance t gla-
dyn of boþe liche moche t temp it wiþ
wyn t drynk þerof. iij. dayes t þou shal
¶ For chafyng of þe lyuer. An ¶ Be hole
noynt hym wiþ popilion and gif hym to
ete sugre roset. ¶ Who so haþe euil
in his bladd' Take ache psli and fenel
of euerich liche moche and temp it wiþ
water and gif it hym to drynk and it

Figure C.2 Recipe collection using red and blue rubrication. Cambridge University Library, MS Kk.6.33, f. 30r. Reproduced by kind permission of the Syndics of Cambridge University Library.

as these, and about the range of scribal choices made when presenting and copying recipe collections, invite further, integrative exploration.[7]

There is, then, much more of the recipes' story to write. It is also true that the stories of the collections examined in this book do not end in 1500. This is nicely exemplified by a poem copied by a seventeenth-century hand on a blank leaf shortly after several late medieval remedy collections examined in previous chapters.[8] The poem reads:

> A Censure of Some Writers
>
> Many haue their time and paines
> In writing cures imployd;
> But he that by experience gaines
> And writes what he hath tryed
> I hould him wiser then that sort
> Whoe for the thirst of fame
> With toyle doe labour to report
> What but retornes theyr shame.
> They hould their Readers with delight
> And hope of finding cure,
> When proofe concludes no point is right
> That did your health assure.[9]

As Paul Slack has shown, remedy collections were one of the most popular genres of vernacular medical writing produced by sixteenth-century English printers.[10] This poem, which draws attention multiple times to the act of 'writing cures', reflects the textual self-consciousness and heightened

---

[7] In relation to manuscripts containing devotional verse, Sawyer, *Reading English Verse*, p. 100 makes the thought-provoking observation from such codicological evidence that many 'smaller books which were manual and suitable for handling, were not purely utilitarian productions straining to make the most efficient possible use of space. Rather, those making small books observed aesthetic conventions and responded to literary form'.

[8] The poem appears after a series of remedy collections in different late medieval and early modern hands (see BodL, MS Ashmole 1438, Part I, pp. 6–31, 39–52) and before the 'Nicholas Neesbett' collection discussed in the Introduction and Chapter 3 (BodL, MS Ashmole 1438, Part I, pp. 57–71).

[9] BodL, MS Ashmole 1438, Part I, p. 55.

[10] Although Paul Slack counts only eighteen new remedy collections printed between 1486 and 1604, he notes at least ninety-seven editions of these: see Paul Slack, 'Mirrors of Health and Treasures of Poor Men: The Uses of the Vernacular Medical Literature of Tudor England', in *Health, Medicine and Mortality in the Sixteenth Century*, ed. by Charles Webster (Cambridge, 1979), pp. 237–73 (p. 243).

cultural commentary which surrounded those early modern acts of recipe-writing, both in manuscript and print: lengthy introductions, prologues, and dedicatory epistles became a hallmark of the latter format. As we have seen, medieval vernacular remedy collections are encircled by far less explicit commentary but they too could be shaped by 'delight' and 'hope', by long-term affective structures and more short-term emotions and impulses, by whimsy and play. The fragmentariness of those medieval collections takes on a new dimension when we consider that many of them were later punctuated by, bound with, and read alongside early modern recipe-writing. Inevitably, this shaped—in a very material way—how those medieval texts were handled, read, interpreted, and judged by early modern readers and, indeed, by ourselves. In the rich field of early modern recipe studies, there is still more to be done on the interpretative lenses these later material contexts created for viewing medieval texts.[11]

Opening up such questions is one of the central aims of this study. Within it, I have sought to demonstrate just how many stories there are still to tell about medieval recipes: recipes may be formulaic and repetitive, but they are also quirky, diverse, and eternally adaptable. Both their repetitiveness *and* their adaptability can be signs of—and stimuli for—care, creativity, and playfulness. The archives are full of more collections demanding close reading and attention: nuancing, enriching, and rewriting recipes' reputation in this way enables us not only to understand *them* better, but also the manifold textual, material, and literary networks they were creating and participating in.

---

[11] For an overview of scholarship on early modern recipe-writing, thought, and practice, see the Introduction.

APPENDIX 1

Vernacular Medical Collections Used in Sample

Manuscript	No. of Collections	Folios/Pages
BodL, MS Rawlinson C.506	4	15r–79v; 82r–109r; 115r–117v and 146r–166v and 171r–174v (collection is split); 130r–145r
BodL, MS Ashmole 1389	1	2–256
BL, MS Sloane 468	1	7v–80v
BL, MS Lansdowne 680	1	22r–73r
YM, MS XVI E 32	4	15r–19v; 82r–109r; 115r–117v and 146r–166v and 171r–174v (collection split during binding); 130r–145v
WT, MS London Medical Society 136	1	1r–95v
BodL, MS Laud misc. 553	1	34v–74v
HEHL, MS HM 1336	2	2v–18v and 29r–34v (collection split during binding); 19r–28v
HEHL, MS HM 64	4	104r–113r; 113v–120r; 143v–153r; 156v–176r
WT, MS Wellcome 542	1	1r–20v
WT, MS Wellcome 5262	1	3r–61v
BodL, MS Ashmole 1443	2	193–350; 401–60
BodL, MS Ashmole 1438	5	Part I: 8–25; 96–126; Part II: 1–57; 83–106; 120–61
BodL, MS Douce 84	1	1v–24v
TCC, MS R.14.32	1	116r–127v
BL, MS Additional 19674	1	2r–34v
BL, MS Sloane 1315	1	119r–149r
BL, MS Additional 33996	1	80v–148v

Manuscript	No. of Collections	Folios/Pages
BL, MS Sloane 3866	3	14r–52v; 62r–80r; 80r–89v
BL, MS Harley 2378	2	17r–61v; 121r–154v
BL, MS Additional 34210	2	5r–22r; 25r–48r
BL, MS Harley 1602	1	13v–23v
BodL, MS Hatton 29	1	89–95
BodL, MS Ashmole 750	1	184–94
BodL, MS Selden Supra 70	3	37r–64v; 65r–75r; 123r–129v

Bibliography

Manuscripts Consulted

(Manuscripts marked by * and accompanied by folio numbers contain a version of the verse herbal *DIMEV* 4171, discussed in Chapter 2)

Aberystwyth, National Library of Wales, MS 572
Aberystwyth, National Library of Wales, MS Brogyntyn II.1
Aberystwyth, National Library of Wales, MS Peniarth 369
Aberystwyth, National Library of Wales, MS Peniarth 388
Aberystwyth, National Library of Wales, MS Peniarth 403
*Cambridge, Gonville and Caius, MS 345/620 (ff. 33v–34v)
Cambridge, Cambridge University Library, MS Dd.6.29
Cambridge, Cambridge University Library, MS Dd.10.44
Cambridge, Cambridge University Library, MS Dd.11.45
Cambridge, Cambridge University Library, MS Ee.1.13
Cambridge, Cambridge University Library, MS Ee.1.15
Cambridge, Cambridge University Library, MS Kk.6.33
*Cambridge, Magdalene College, Pepys Library, MS 1661 (pp. 288–309)
*Cambridge, Trinity College, MS R.14.32 (ff. 134v–139v)
Cambridge, Trinity College, MS R.14.39
*Cambridge, Trinity College, MS R.14.51 (ff. 34v–47r)
Cambridge, Trinity College, MS R.14.52
Cambridge, Trinity College, MS O.1.13
Cambridge, Trinity College, MS O.1.65
*Cambridge, Trinity College, MS O.2.13 (ff. 179r–181r)
London, British Library, MS Additional 10440
London, British Library, MS Additional 12056
London, British Library, MS Additional 12195
*London, British Library, MS Additional 17866 (ff. 5r–16r)
London, British Library, MS Additional 19674
London, British Library, MS Additional 33996
London, British Library, MS Additional 34111
London, British Library, MS Additional 34210
*London, British Library, MS Additional 60577 (f. 119r–v)
London, British Library, MS Harley 1602
London, British Library, MS Harley 2375
London, British Library, MS Harley 2378
London, British Library, MS Harley 2390
London, British Library, MS Lansdowne 680
London, British Library, MS Sloane 4

London, British Library, MS Sloane 56
*London, British Library, MS Sloane 140 (ff. 52r–56v)
*London, British Library, MS Sloane 147 (ff. 94r–112r)
London, British Library, MS Sloane 213
London, British Library, MS Sloane 340
London, British Library, MS Sloane 468
London, British Library, MS Sloane 1315
*London, British Library, MS Sloane 1571 (ff. 14v–36v)
*London, British Library, MS Sloane 2457/2458 (ff. 2r–7r)
*London, British Library, MS Sloane 2460 (f. 34v)
London, British Library, MS Sloane 3160
London, British Library, MS Sloane 3466
London, British Library, MS Sloane 3866
London, Wellcome Trust, MS London Medical Society 136
London, Wellcome Trust, MS Wellcome 405
London, Wellcome Trust, MS Wellcome 542
London, Wellcome Trust, MS Wellcome 5262
*New Haven, Beinecke Rare Book and Manuscript Library, MS Takamiya 46 (ff. 3r–14v), accessed online at https://collections.library.yale.edu/catalog/16156709 [accessed 17/02/2021]
Oxford, Bodleian Library, MS Ashmole 750
Oxford, Bodleian Library, MS Ashmole 1389
Oxford, Bodleian Library, MS Ashmole 1393
*Oxford, Bodleian Library, MS Ashmole 1397 (ff. 117v–118v)
Oxford, Bodleian Library, MS Ashmole 1413
Oxford, Bodleian Library, MS Ashmole 1432
Oxford, Bodleian Library, MS Ashmole 1434
Oxford, Bodleian Library, MS Ashmole 1438
Oxford, Bodleian Library, MS Ashmole 1443
Oxford, Bodleian Library, MS Ashmole 1444
Oxford, Bodleian Library, MS Ashmole 1447
*Oxford, Bodleian Library, MS Ashmole 1477 (Part III, f. 3r–v)
Oxford, Bodleian Library, MS Ashmole 1505
Oxford, Bodleian Library, MS Bodley 686
Oxford, Bodleian Library, MS Digby 75
Oxford, Bodleian Library, MS Douce 78
Oxford, Bodleian Library, MS Douce 84
Oxford, Bodleian Library, MS e. Museo 52
Oxford, Bodleian Library, MS Eng Poet e.1
Oxford, Bodleian Library, MS Hatton 29
Oxford, Bodleian Library, MS Laud lat. 106
Oxford, Bodleian Library, MS Laud misc. 553
Oxford, Bodleian Library, MS Laud misc. 685
Oxford, Bodleian Library, MS Radcliffe Trust e. 10
Oxford, Bodleian Library, MS Rawlinson C. 506
Oxford, Bodleian Library, MS Selden Supra 73

Oxford, Corpus Christi College, MS 125
*Oxford, Corpus Christi College, MS 265 (ff. 55r–56v, only f. 55r–55v are in verse; the herbal entries on ff. 55v–56v seem to be prose summaries of the verse herbal's contents)
San Marino, Huntington Library, MS HM 58
San Marino, Huntington Library, MS HM 64
San Marino, Huntington Library, MS HM 505
San Marino, Huntington Library, MS HM 1336
San Marino, Huntington Library, MS HM 19079
*San Marino, Huntington Library, MS HU 1051 (f. 85r)
*Stockholm, Kungliga Biblioteket, MS X 90 (pp. 49–78)
*York, YM, XVI.E.32 (ff. 120r–121r)

Early Printed Books

Anglicus, Bartholomaeus, *Tractatus de proprietatibus rerum* (Nuremberg, 1483)
Anglicus, Gilbertus, *Compendium medicine* (Lyon, 1510)
De Gordonio, Bernardus, *Lilium medicinae* (Lyon, 1559)
Elyot, Thomas, *The Castell of Helth* (London, 1541)
Lloyd, Humphrey, *The Treasuri of Helth* (London, 1558)
Moulton, Thomas, *The Myrrour or Glasse of Helth* (London, 1580)
Turner, William, *A New Herball* (London, 1551)

Modern Editions of Primary Texts

Aldridge, Harold Richard and Percival Horton-Smith Hartley, eds and trans, *Johannes de Mirfield of St Bartholomew's, Smithfield: His Life and Works* (Cambridge: Cambridge University Press, 1936)
Aristotle, *The Physics*, trans. by Philip Wicksteed and Francis Cornford, 2 vols (London: Heinemann, 1929)
Aristotle, *On Sophistical Refutations; On Coming to Be; On Passing Away; On the Cosmos*, trans. by E.S. Forster and D.J. Furley (London: Heinemann, 1955)
Augustine, St, *De doctrina christiana*, ed. and trans. by R.P.H. Green (Oxford: Clarendon Press, 1995)
Augustine, St, *Confessions: Books 1–8*, ed. and trans. by Carolyn J.B. Hammond (Cambridge, MA: Harvard University Press, 2014)
Augustine, St, *Confessions: Books 9–13*, ed. and trans. by Carolyn J.B. Hammond (Cambridge, MA: Harvard University Press, 2016)
Austin, Thomas, ed., *Two Fifteenth-Century Cookery-Books*, EETS os 91 (London: Trübner & Co., 1888)
Bacon, Roger, *The Opus Majus of Roger Bacon*, ed. and trans. by Robert Belle Burke, 2 vols (Philadelphia, PA: University of Philadelphia Press, 1928)
Benson, Larry D., ed., *The Riverside Chaucer*, 3rd edn (Oxford: Oxford University Press, 1987; repr. 2008)

Boethius, *Anicii Manlii Severini Boethi Philosophiae Consolatio*, ed. by Ludwig Bieler (Turnhout: Typographi Brepols, 1957)

Brodin, Gösta, ed., *Agnus Castus: A Middle English Herbal Reconstructed from Various Manuscripts* (Cambridge, MA: Harvard University Press, 1950)

Brunner, Karl, ed., *Der Mittelenglische Versroman über Richard Löwenherz* (Vienna: Braumüller, 1913)

Butler, Sharon and Constance B. Hieatt, eds, *Curye on Inglysch: English Culinary Manuscripts of the Fourteenth Century (Including the Forme of Cury)*, EETS ss 8 (London: Oxford University Press, 1985)

Carr, David R., ed., *The First General Entry Book of the City of Salisbury 1387–1452* (Trowbridge: Wiltshire Record Society, 2001)

Choulant, Ludwig, ed., *Macer Floridus de viribus herbarum*, (Leipzig: Leopoldi Vossii, 1832)

Clarke, Mark, ed., *The Crafte of Lymmyng and the Maner of Steynyng: Middle English Recipes for Painters, Stainers, Scribes, and Illuminators*, EETS os 347 (Oxford: Oxford University Press, 2016)

Colton, James B., trans., *John of Mirfield: Surgery: A Translation of His Breviarium Bartholomei, pt. IX* (New York: Hafner Publishing Company, 1969)

Copeland, Rita and Ineke Sluiter, eds and trans., *Medieval Grammar and Rhetoric: Language Arts and Literary Theory AD 300–1475* (Oxford: Oxford University Press, 2015)

Corbeil, Gilles de, *Carmina Medica*, ed. by Ludwig Choulant (Leipzig: Leopoldi Vossii, 1826)

Dahiyat, Ismail M., ed. and trans., *Avicenna's Commentary on the Poetics of Aristotle: A Critical Study with an Annotated Translation of the Text* (Leiden: Brill, 1974)

Daly, Walter J. and Robert D. Yee, 'The Eye Book of Master Peter of Spain: A Glimpse of Diagnosis and Treatment of Eye Disease in the Middle Ages', *Documenta Ophthalmologica*, 103 (2001), 119–53

Daniel, Henry, *Liber Uricrisiarum: A Reading Edition*, ed. by Ruth E. Harvey, M. Teresa Tavormina, and Sarah Star (Toronto: University of Toronto Press, 2020)

Davis, Norman, ed., *Paston Letters and Papers of the Fifteenth Century*, 2 vols (Oxford: Clarendon Press, 1971–6)

Davis, R.T., ed., *Medieval English Lyrics: A Critical Anthology* (London: Faber and Faber, 1963)

Edwards, A.S.G. and Jeremy Griffiths, eds, *The Tollemache Book of Secrets* (London: Roxburghe Club, 2001)

Eldredge, L.M., ed., *The Wonderful Art of the Eye: A Critical Edition of the Middle English Translation of De probatissima arte oculorum* (East Lansing, MI: Michigan State University Press, 1996)

Faral, Edmond, ed., *Les arts poétiques du XIIe et du Xiii[e] siècle: Recherches et documents sur la technique littéraire du moyen âge* (Paris: É Champion, 1924)

Fenlon, Iain and Edward Wilson, *The Winchester Anthology: A Facsimile of British Library Additional Manuscript 60577* (Cambridge: Brewer, 1981)

Fox, Denton, ed., *The Poems of Robert Henryson* (Oxford: Oxford University Press, 1981)

Frisk, Gösta, ed., *A Middle English Translation of Macer Floridus de viribus herbarum* (Uppsala: Lundequistska Bokhandeln, 1949)
Furnivall, Frederick James and Israel Gollancz, eds, *Hoccleve's Works: The Minor Poems*, EETS es 61, 2nd edn (London: Oxford University Press, 1970)
Furrow, Melissa M., ed., *Ten Fifteenth-Century Comic Poems* (New York: Garland, 1985)
Getz, Faye, ed., *Healing and Society in Medieval England: A Middle English Translation of the Pharmaceutical Writings of Gilbertus Anglicus* (Madison, WI: University of Wisconsin Press, 1991)
Greco, Gina L. and Christine M. Rose, eds and trans., *The Good Wife's Guide: Le Ménagier de Paris: A Medieval Household Book* (Ithaca, NY: Cornell University Press, 2012)
Grymonprez, Pol, ed., *'Here men may se the vertues off herbes': A Middle English Herbal (MS Bodley 483, ff. 57r–67v)* (Brussels: Omirel, 1981)
Hamelius, Paul, ed., *Mandeville's Travels*, EETS os 153–4, 2 vols (London: Kegan Paul, Trench, Trübner, 1919–23)
Heath Barnum, Priscilla, ed., *Dives and Pauper*, EETS os 275, 323 280, 3 vols (London: Oxford University Press, 1976–2004)
Heinrich, Fritz, ed., *Ein Mittelenglisches Medizinbuch* (Halle: Niemayer, 1896)
Henderson, Jeffrey, ed., *Hippocrates: Volume II*, trans. by W.H.S. Jones (Cambridge, MA: Harvard University Press, 1923)
Hope Robbins, Rossell, ed., *Secular Lyrics of the XIVth and XVth Centuries*, 2nd edn (Oxford: Clarendon Press, 1964)
Horace, *Satires, Epistles and Ars Poetica*, trans. by H.R. Fairclough (Cambridge, MA: Harvard University Press, 1952)
Kölbing, Eugen, ed., *The Romance of Sir Beues of Hamtoun*, EETS es 46, 48, 65 (London: Kegan Paul, Trench, Trübner and Co., 1885–94)
Kooper, Erik, ed., *Sentimental and Humorous Romances: 'Floris and Blancheflour', 'Sir Degrevant', 'The Squire of Low Degree', 'The Tournement of Tottenham', and 'The Feast of Tottenham'* (Kalamazoo, MI: Medieval Institute Publications, 2006)
Leimgruber, Veronika, ed., *Libre del Coch* (Barcelona: Curial Edicions Catalanes, 1977)
Lindsay, W.M., ed., *Isidori Hispalensis Episcopi: Etymologiarvm sive originvm: Vol. 1: Libros I–X* (Oxford: Oxford University Press, 1911)
Macaulay, G.C., ed., *The English Works of John Gower*, EETS es 81–2, 2 vols (London: Oxford University Press, 1900–1)
MacCracken, Henry Noble, ed., *The Minor Poems of John Lydgate: Part II*, EETS os 192 (London: Oxford University Press, 1934)
Malory, Thomas, *Le Morte DArthur*, ed. by P.J.C. Field, 2 vols (Cambridge: Brewer, 2013)
Meier, Rudolf, ed. and trans., *Das Innsbrucker Osterspiel; Das Osterspiel von Muri: Mittlehochdeutsch und Neuhochdeutsch* (Stuttgart: Reclam, 1962)
Metham, John, *Amoryus and Cleopes*, ed. by Stephen F. Page (Kalamazoo, MI: Medieval Institute Publications, 1999)
Ogden, Margaret Sinclair, ed., *The 'Liber de Diversis Medicinis' in the Thornton Manuscript*, EETS os 207 (London: Oxford University Press, 1938)

Ogden, Margaret Sinclair, ed., *The Cyrurgie of Guy de Chauliac*, EETS os 265 (London: Oxford University Press, 1971)
Ogilvie-Thomson, S.J., ed., *Richard Rolle: Prose and Verse*, EETS os 293 (Oxford: Oxford University Press, 1988)
Ovid, *Metamorphoses*, ed. and trans. by Frank Justus Miller, 2 vols (London: Heinemann, 1916)
Parkinson, David. J., ed., *Robert Henryson: The Complete Works* (Kalamazoo, MI: Medieval Institute Publications, 2010)
Petrarch, Francesco, *Letters of Old Age: Rerum senilium libri*, ed. and trans. by Aldo S. Bernardo, Saul Levin, and Reta A. Bernardo, 2 vols (Baltimore, MD: Johns Hopkins University Press, 1992)
Petrarch, Francesco, *Invectives*, ed. and trans. by David Marsh (Cambridge, MA: Harvard University Press, 2003)
Petrarch, Francesco, *Res seniles: Libri IX–XII*, ed. by Monica Berté and Silvia Rizzo (Firenze: Casa Editrice Le Lettere, 2014)
Pliny, *Natural History*, trans. by D.E. Eichholz, H. Rackham, and W.H.S. Jones, 10 vols (London: Heinemann, 1938–63)
Power, D'Arcy, ed., *Treatises of Fistula in Ano, Hæmorrhoids, and Clysters*, EETS os 22 (London: Oxford University Press, 1910)
Sayles, G.O., ed. and trans., *Select Cases in the Court of King's Bench Under Edward III: Volume VI*, Selden Society 82 (London: Quaritch, 1965)
Seville, Isidore of, *The Etymologies of Isidore of Seville*, ed. and trans. by Stephen A. Barney and others (Cambridge: Cambridge University Press, 2006)
Somer, John, *The Kalendarium of John Somer*, ed. by Linne R. Mooney (Athens, GA: University of Georgia Press, 1998)
Stephens, George, ed., *Extracts in Prose and Verse from an Old English Medical Manuscript, Preserved in the Royal Library at Stockholm* (London: Society of Antiquaries, 1844)
Trevisa, John, *On the Properties of Things: John Trevisa's Translation of Bartholomæus Anglicus De Proprietatibus Rerum*, ed. by M.C. Seymour and others, 3 vols (Oxford: Clarendon Press, 1975–88)
Vinsauf, Geoffrey of, *Poetria Nova*, trans. by Margaret F. Nims, rev. edn (Toronto: Pontifical Institute of Medieval Studies, 2010)
Von Staden, Heinrich, ed. and trans., *Herophilus: The Art of Medicine in Early Alexandria: Edition, Translation and Essays* (Cambridge: Cambridge University Press, 1989)
Walton, John, *Boethius: De Consolatione Philosophiae*, ed. by Mark Science, EETS os 170 (London: Oxford University Press, 1927)
Watson, Nicholas and Jacqueline Jenkins, eds, *The Writings of Julian of Norwich* (Philadelphia, PA: Pennsylvania University Press, 2006)
Windeatt, Barry, ed., *The Book of Margery Kempe* (Cambridge: Brewer, 2004)
Wogan Browne, Jocelyn, ed., *The Idea of the Vernacular: An Anthology of Middle English Literary Theory* (Exeter: Exeter University Press, 1995)
Wülfing, Ernst, ed., *Laud Troy Book*, EETS, os 121 (London: Kegan Paul, Trench, Trübner & Co, 1902)

Zupitza, Julius, ed., *The Romance of Guy of Warwick: The Second or Fifteenth-Century Version: Part One*, EETS es 25 (London: N. Trübner, 1875)

Secondary Works

Abdalla, Laila, '"My body to warente...": Linguistic Corporeality in Chaucer's Pardoner', in *Rhetorics of Bodily Disease and Health in Medieval and Early Modern England*, ed. by Jennifer C. Vaught (Farnham: Ashgate, 2010), pp. 65–84

Abdel-Halim, Rabie E., 'Medicine and Health in Medieval Arabic Poetry: An Historical Review', *International Journal of the History and Philosophy of Medicine*, 3 (2013), 1–7

Agrimi, Jole and Chiara Crisciani, 'The Science and Practice of Medicine in the Thirteenth Century According to Guglielmo de Saliceto, Italian Surgeon', in *Practical Medicine from Salerno to the Black Death*, ed. by Luis Garcia Ballester (Cambridge: Cambridge University Press, 1994), pp. 60–87

Akbari, Suzanne Conklin, *Seeing Through the Veil: Optical Theory and Medieval Allegory* (Toronto: University of Toronto Press, 2004)

Alexander, Gavin, 'Prosopopoeia: The Speaking Figure', in *Renaissance Figures of Speech*, ed. by Sylvia Adamson and others (Cambridge: Cambridge University Press, 2007), pp. 97–112

Alonso-Almeida, Francisco, 'Genre Conventions in English Recipes, 1600–1800', in *Reading and Writing Recipe Books 1550–1800*, ed. by Michelle DiMeo and Sara Pennell (Manchester: Manchester University Press, 2013), pp. 68–90

Anderson, Frank J., *An Illustrated History of the Herbals* (New York: Columbia University Press, 1977)

Appelbaum, Robert, 'Rhetoric and Epistemology in Early Printed Recipe Collections', *Journal for Early Modern Cultural Studies*, 3 (2003), 1–35

Appleford, Amy, *Learning to Die in London, 1380–1540* (Philadelphia, PA: University of Pennsylvania Press, 2015)

Arberry, Arthur J., 'Fārābī's Canons of Poetry', *Rivista degli studi orientali*, 17 (1937), 266–78

Arbesmann, R., 'The Concept of "Christus Medicus" in St. Augustine', *Traditio*, 10 (1954), 1–20

Archer, Jayne Elisabeth, '"The Quintessence of Wit": Poems and Recipes in Early Modern Women's Writing', in *Reading and Writing Recipe Books 1550–1800*, ed. by Michelle DiMeo and Sara Pennell (Manchester: Manchester University Press, 2013), pp. 114–34

Astell, Ann W., 'On the Usefulness and Use Value of Books: A Medieval and Modern Inquiry', in *Medieval Rhetoric: A Casebook*, ed. by Scott D. Troyan (London: Routledge, 2004), pp. 41–62

Atkinson, Stephen, '"They...toke their shyldys before them and drew oute their swerdys...": Inflicting and Healing Wounds in Malory's *Morte Darthur*', in *Wounds and Wound Repair in Medieval Culture*, ed. by Larissa Tracy and Kelly DeVries (Leiden: Brill, 2015), pp. 519–43

Attridge, Derek, *Peculiar Language: Literature as Difference from the Renaissance to James Joyce*, 2nd edn (London: Routledge, 2004)
Attridge, Derek, *The Singularity of Literature* (London: Routledge, 2004)
Auerbach, Erich, *Mimesis: The Representation of Reality in Western Literature*, 50th anniversary edn (Princeton, NJ: Princeton University Press, 2003)
Bahr, Arthur, *Fragments and Assemblages: Forming Compilations of Medieval London* (Chicago, IL: University of Chicago Press, 2015)
Bahr, Arthur and Alexandra Gillespie, 'Medieval English Manuscripts: Form, Aesthetics, and the Literary Text', *Chaucer Review*, 47 (2013), 346–60
Bailey, Michael D., *Fearful Spirits, Reasoned Follies: The Boundaries of Superstition in Late Medieval Europe* (Ithaca, NY: Cornell University Press, 2013)
Bakhtin, M., *Rabelais and His World*, trans. by Hélène Iswolsky (Bloomington, IN: Indiana University Press, 1984)
Bale, Anthony, 'A Norfolk Gentlewoman and Lydgatian Patronage: Lady Sibylle Boys and Her Cultural Environment', *Medium Aevum*, 78 (2009), 394–413
Banham, Debby, 'Dun, Oxa and Pliny the Great Physician: Attribution and Authority in Old English Medical Texts', *Social History of Medicine*, 24 (2011), 57–73
Barney, Stephen A., 'Chaucer's Lists', in *The Wisdom of Poetry: Essays in English Literature in Honour of Morton W. Bloomfield*, ed. by Larry D. Benson and Siegfried Wenzel (Kalamazoo, MI: Medieval Institute Publications, 1982), pp. 189–223
Barron, Caroline, 'Telling the Time in Chaucer's London', in *'A verray parfit praktisour': Essays Presented to Carole Rawcliffe*, ed. by Linda Clark and Elizabeth Danbury (Woodbridge: Boydell, 2017), pp. 141–51
Bartlett, Robert, *The Natural and the Supernatural in the Middle Ages* (Cambridge: Cambridge University Press, 2008)
Baum, Paull F., 'Chaucer's Puns', *PMLA*, 71 (1956), 225–46
Bayless, Martha, *Parody in the Middle Ages: The Latin Tradition* (Ann Arbor, MI: University of Michigan Press, 1996)
Beale, Walter, *Learning from Language: Symmetry, Asymmetry and Literary Humanism* (Pittsburgh, PA: University of Pittsburgh Press, 2009)
Becker, Karin, 'Eustache Deschamps's Medical Poetry', in *Eustache Deschamps, French Courtier Poet: His Work and His World*, ed. by Deborah M. Sinnreich-Levi (New York: AMS Press, 1998), pp. 209–27
Bennet, H.S., 'Science and Information in English Writings of the Fifteenth Century', *The Modern Language Review*, 39 (1944), 1–8
Benskin, M., 'For a Wound in the Head: A Late Medieval View of the Brain', *Neuphilologische Mitteilungen*, 86 (1985), 199–215
Benson, Larry D., 'The "Queynte" Punnings of Chaucer's Critics', in *Contradictions: From Beowulf to Chaucer—Selected Studies of Larry D. Benson*, ed. by Theodore M. Anderson and Stephen A. Barney (Aldershot: Scolar Press, 1995), pp. 217–42
Bernau, Anke, 'Translating Form with *Patience*', in *The Medieval Literary Beyond Form*, ed. by Robert J. Meyer-Lee and Catherine Sanok (Cambridge: Brewer, 2018), pp. 161–83
Bernau, Anke, 'Figuring with Knots', *Digital Philology: A Journal of Medieval Cultures*, 10 (2021), 13–38

Biller, Peter and Joseph Ziegler, eds, *Religion and Medicine in the Middle Ages* (Woodbridge: Boydell, 2001)

Bishop, Louise, *Words, Stones and Herbs: The Healing Word in Medieval and Early Modern England* (Syracuse, NY: Syracuse University Press, 2007)

Black, Deborah L., 'The Imaginative Syllogism in Arabic Philosophy: A Medieval Contribution to the Philosophical Study of Metaphor', *Medieval Studies*, 51 (1989), 242–67

Black, Winston, '"I will add what the Arab once taught": Constantine the African in Northern European Medical Verse', in *Herbs and Healers from the Ancient Mediterranean through the Medieval West: Essays in Honor of John M. Riddle* (Farnham: Ashgate, 2012), pp. 153–85

Blair, Ann, *Too Much to Know: Managing Scholarly Information Before the Modern Age* (New Haven, CT: Yale University Press, 2010)

Blair, Ann and Peter Stallybrass, 'Mediating Information', in *This Is Enlightenment*, ed. by Clifford Siskin and William Warner (Chicago, IL: Chicago of University Press, 2010), pp. 139–63

Bloch, Howard, *Etymologies and Genealogies: A Literary Anthropology of the French Middle Ages* (Chicago, IL: University of Chicago Press, 1983)

Bloch, Howard, *The Scandal of the Fabliaux* (Chicago, IL: University of Chicago Press, 1986)

Boffey, Julia, 'Bodleian Library, MS Arch Selden B.24 and Definitions of the Household Book', in *The English Medieval Book: Studies in Memory of Jeremy Griffiths*, ed. by A.S.G. Edwards and others (London: The British Library, 2000), pp. 125–34

Boffey, Julia and A.S.G. Edwards, 'Towards a Taxonomy of Middle English Manuscript Assemblages', in *Insular Books: Vernacular Manuscript Miscellanies in Late Medieval Britain*, ed. by Margaret Connolly and Raluca Radulescu (Oxford: Oxford University Press, 2015), pp. 263–80

Bonfield, Christopher, 'The First Instrument of Medicine: Diet and Regimens of Health in Late Medieval England', in *'A verray parfit praktisour'*: *Essays Presented to Carole Rawcliffe* (Woodbridge: Boydell, 2017), pp. 99–119

Bourdieu, Pierre, *Outline of a Theory of Practice*, trans. by Richard Nice (Cambridge: Cambridge University Press, 1977)

Bower, Hannah, 'Similes We Cure By: The Poetics of Late Medieval Medical Texts', *New Medieval Literatures*, 18 (2018), 183–210

Bower, Hannah, '"Her ovn self seid me": The Function of Anecdote in Henry Daniel's *Liber Uricrisiarum*', in *Henry Daniel and the Rise of Middle English Medical Writing*, ed. by Sarah Star (Toronto: University of Toronto Press, forthcoming), pp. 133–57

Bozóky, Edina, 'Mythic Mediation in Healing Incantations', in *Health, Disease and Healing in Medieval Culture*, ed. by Sheila Campbell and others (Basingstoke: Macmillan, 1992)

Brand, Paul, 'Lawyers' Time in the Later Middle Ages', in *Time in the Medieval World*, ed. by Chris Humphrey and W.M. Ormrod (Woodbridge: Boydell, 2001), pp. 73–104

Brantley, Jessica, 'Forms of the Hours in Late Medieval England', in *The Medieval Literary Beyond Form*, ed. by Robert J. Meyer-Lee and Catherine Sanok (Cambridge: Brewer, 2018), pp. 61–84

Braswell, Laurel, 'Utilitarian and Scientific Prose', in *Middle English Prose: A Critical Guide to Major Authors and Genres*, ed. by A.S.G. Edwards (New Brunswick, NJ: Rutgers University Press, 1984), pp. 337–87

Brewer, Keagan, *Wonder and Skepticism in the Middle Ages* (London: Routledge, 2016)

Bullough, Vern, 'Medical Study at Mediaeval Oxford', *Speculum*, 36 (1961), 600–12

Burge, Amy, 'Desiring the East: A Comparative Study of Middle English Romance and Modern Popular Sheikh Romance' (unpublished doctoral thesis, University of York, 2012)

Burger, Glenn D. and Rory Critten, eds, *Household Knowledges in Late Medieval England and France* (Manchester: Manchester University Press, 2019)

Burger, Glenn D. and Holly A. Crocker, eds, *Medieval Affect, Feeling, and Emotion* (Cambridge: Cambridge University Press, 2019)

Butler, Sara M., 'Portrait of a Surgeon in Fifteenth-Century England', in *Medicine and the Law in the Middle Ages*, ed. by Wendy J. Turner and Sara M. Butler (Leiden: Brill, 2014), pp. 243–66

Camargo, Martin, *Essays on Medieval Rhetoric* (Farnham: Ashgate, 2012)

Camille, Michael, *Image on the Edge: The Margins of Medieval Art* (Cambridge, MA: Harvard University Press, 1992)

Cannon, Christopher, *The Making of Chaucer's English: A Study of Words* (Cambridge: Cambridge University Press, 1998)

Cannon, Christopher, *The Grounds of English Literature* (Oxford: Oxford University Press, 2004)

Cannon, Christopher, 'Chaucer and the Language of London', in *Chaucer and the City*, ed. by Ardis Butterfield (Cambridge: Brewer, 2006), pp. 79–95

Cannon, Christopher, 'Form', in *Twenty-First-Century Approaches to Literature: Middle English*, ed. by Paul Strohm (Oxford: Oxford University Press, 2007), pp. 177–90

Cannon, Christopher, 'Proverbs and the Wisdom of Literature: The Proverbs of Alfred and Chaucer's Tale of Melibee', *Textual Practice*, 24 (2010), 407–34

Cannon, Christopher, *From Literacy to Literature: England, 1300–1400* (Oxford: Oxford University Press, 2016)

Carrera, Elena, 'Anger and the Mind–Body Connection in Medieval and Early Modern Medicine', in *Emotions and Health 1200–1700*, ed. by Elena Carrera (Leiden: Brill, 2013), pp. 95–146

Carroll, Ruth, 'Middle English Recipes: Vernacularisation of a Text-Type', in *Medical and Scientific Writing in Late Medieval English*, ed. by Irma Taavitsainen and Päivi Pahta (Cambridge: Cambridge University Press, 2004), pp. 174–91

Carruthers, Mary, *The Book of Memory: A Study of Memory in Medieval Culture*, 2nd edn (Cambridge: Cambridge University Press, 2008)

Carruthers, Mary, ed., *Rhetoric Beyond Words: Delight and Persuasion in the Arts of the Middle Ages* (Cambridge: Cambridge University Press, 2010)

Carruthers, Mary, *The Experience of Beauty in the Middle Ages* (Oxford: Oxford University Press, 2013)

Carter, Ronald and Walter Nash, 'Language and Literariness', *Prose Studies*, 6 (1983), 123–41

Cavanaugh, Susan, 'A Study of Books Privately Owned in England 1300–1450', 2 vols (unpublished doctoral thesis, University of Pennsylvania, 1980)

Chang, Yung-Ming and others, 'Earthworms: A Potential Target for TCM (CAM) Research', in *Biology of Earthworms*, ed. by Ayten Karaca (Berlin: Springer, 2011) pp. 247–60

Chartier, Roger, *Forms and Meanings: Texts, Performances, and Audiences from Codex to Computer* (Philadelphia, PA: University of Pennsylvania Press, 1995)

Chunko-Dominguez, Betsy, 'Imagery of Illness and Abjection in the Medieval Choir', *Postmedieval*, 8 (2017), 194–201

Citrome, J.J., *The Surgeon in Medieval English Literature* (New York: Palgrave Macmillan, 2006)

Clanchy, Michael, *From Memory to Written Record: England 1066–1307*, 3rd edn (Oxford: Wiley-Blackwell, 2013)

Cohen, Ester, *The Modulated Scream: Pain in Late Medieval Culture* (Chicago, IL: University of Chicago Press, 2010)

Cohen, Jeffrey Jerome, 'On Saracen Enjoyment: Some Fantasies of Race in Late Medieval France and England', *Journal of Late Medieval and Early Modern Studies*, 31 (2001), 113–46

Coleman, Joyce, *Public Reading and the Reading Public in Late Medieval England and France* (Cambridge: Cambridge University Press, 1996)

Collins, Minta, *Medieval Herbals: The Illustrative Traditions* (London: British Library, 2000)

Cooper, Helen, *Oxford Guides to Chaucer: The Canterbury Tales*, 2nd edn (Oxford: Oxford University Press, 1996)

Cooper, Helen, 'Prose Romances', in *A Companion to Middle English Prose*, ed. by A.S.G. Edwards (Woodbridge: Brewer, 2004), pp. 215–30

Cooper, Lisa H., 'The Poetics of Practicality', in *Twenty-First-Century Approaches to Literature: Middle English*, ed. by Paul Strohm (Oxford: Oxford University Press, 2007), pp. 491–505

Cooper, Lisa H., *Artisans and Narrative Craft* (Cambridge: Cambridge University Press, 2011)

Cooper, Lisa H., 'Recipes for the Realm: John Lydgate's "Sotelties" and *The Debate of the Horse, Goose and Sheep*', in *Essays on Aesthetics and Medieval Literature in Honour of Howell Chickering*, ed. by John M. Hill, Bonnie Wheeler, and R.F. Yeager (Toronto: Pontifical Institute of Mediaeval Studies, 2014), pp. 194–214

Cooper, Lisa H. and Andrea Denny-Brown, eds, *Lydgate Matters: Poetry and Material Culture in the Fifteenth Century* (New York: Palgrave Macmillan, 2007)

Copeland, Rita, 'Horace's *Ars poetica* in the Medieval Classroom and Beyond: The Horizons of Ancient Precept', in *Answerable Style: The Idea of the Literary in Medieval England*, ed. by Frank Grady and Andrew Galloway (Columbus, OH: Ohio State University Press, 2013), pp. 15–33

Cracolici, Stefano, 'The Art of Invective', in *Petrarch: A Critical Guide to the Complete Works*, ed. by Victoria Kirkham and Armando Maggi (Chicago, IL: Chicago University Press, 2009), pp. 255–73

Crisciani, Chiara, 'History, Novelty and Progress in Scholastic Medicine', *Osiris*, 6 (1990), 118–39

Crisciani, Chiara, 'Histories, Stories, Exempla and Anecdotes: Michele Savonarola from Latin to Vernacular', in *Historia: Empiricism and Erudition in Early Modern Europe*, ed. by Gianna Pomata and Nancy G. Siraisi (Cambridge, MA: MIT Press, 2005), pp. 297–324

Crocker, Holly, 'Medieval Affects Now', *Exemplaria*, 29 (2017), 82–98

Crossley, John N., 'Old-Fashioned versus Newfangled: Reading and Writing Numbers, 1200–1500', *Studies in Medieval and Renaissance History*, 3rd series, 10 (2013), 79–109

Culler, Jonathan, *The Literary in Theory* (Stanford, CA: Stanford University Press, 2007)

D'Agata D'Ottavi, Stefania, 'Between Astronomy and Astrology: Chaucer's "Treatise on the Astrolabe" and the Measurement of Time in Late-Medieval England', in *Medieval and Early Modern Literature, Science and Medicine*, ed. by Rachel Falconer and Denis Renevey (Tübingen: Narr, 2013), pp. 49–66

Daniell, Christopher, *Death and Burial in Medieval England 1066–1550* (London: Routledge, 1997)

Daston, Lorraine and Katharine Park, *Wonders and the Order of Nature, 1150–1750* (New York: Zone Books, 1998)

Davis, Norman, 'Style and Stereotype in Early English Letters', *Leeds Studies in English*, 1 (1967), 7–17

Delaney, Sheila, *Medieval Literary Politics: Shapes of Ideology* (Manchester: Manchester University Press, 1990)

Demaitre, Luke, 'Medieval Notions of Cancer: Malignancy and Metaphor', *Bulletin of the History of Medicine*, 72 (1998), 609–37

Demaitre, Luke, *Medieval Medicine: The Art of Healing from Head to Toe* (Santa Barbara, CA: Praeger, 2013)

De Mayo, Thomas Benjamin, *The Demonology of William of Auvergne: By Fire and Sword* (New York: Mellen, 2007)

DiMeo, Michelle, 'Authorship and Medical Networks: Reading Attributions in Early Modern Manuscript Recipe Books', in *Reading and Writing Recipe Books 1550–1800*, ed. by Michelle DiMeo and Sara Pennell (Manchester: Manchester University Press, 2013), pp. 25–46

DiMeo, Michelle and Rebecca Laroche, 'On Elizabeth Isham's "Oil of Swallows": Animal Slaughter and Early Modern Women's Recipes, in *Eco-Feminist Approaches to Early Modernity*, ed. by Jennifer Munroe and Rebecca Laroche (New York: Palgrave Macmillan, 2011), pp. 87–104

Dinshaw, Carolyn, *How Soon Is Now: Medieval Texts, Amateur Readers, and the Queerness of Time* (Durham, NC: Duke University Press, 2012)

Douglas, Mary, *Purity and Danger: An Analysis of Concepts of Pollution and Taboo* (London: Routledge, 2003; first published 1966)

Duffy, Eamon, *The Stripping of the Altars: Traditional Religion in England c.1400–c.1580* (New Haven, CT: Yale University Press, 1992)

Eamon, William, *Science and the Secrets of Nature: Books of Secrets in Medieval and Early Modern Culture* (Princeton, NJ: Princeton University Press, 1994)

Eamon, William, 'How to Read a Book of Secrets', in *Secrets and Knowledge in Medicine and Science, 1500–1800*, ed. by Elaine Leong and Alisha Rankin (Farnham: Ashgate, 2011), pp. 31–50

Eco, Umberto, *Art and Beauty in the Middle Ages* (New Haven, CT: Yale University Press, 1986)

Eco, Umberto, *The Aesthetics of Thomas Aquinas* (London: Radius, 1988)

Eis, Gerhard, *Mittelalterliche Fachliteratur* (Stuttgart: Metzler, 1962)

Eisner, Sigmund and Marijane Osborn, 'Chaucer as Teacher: Chaucer's Treatise on the Astrolabe', in *Medieval Literature for Children*, ed. by Daniel T. Kline (New York: Routledge, 2003), pp. 155-87

Epstein, Steven, *Wage Labor and Guilds in Medieval Europe* (Chapel Hill, NC: University of North Carolina Press, 1991)

Eyler, Joshua R., *Disability in the Middle Ages: Reconsiderations and Reverberations* (Farnham: Ashgate, 2010)

Fein, Susanna, ed., *Interpreting MS Digby 86: A Trilingual Book from Thirteenth-Century Worcestershire* (York: York Medieval Press, 2019)

Felski, Rita, 'The Invention of Everyday Life', in *Doing Time: Feminist Theory and Postmodern Culture* (New York: New York University Press, 2000) pp. 77-98

Feros Rhys, Juanita, 'Didactic I's and the Voice of Experience in Advice from Medieval and Early-Modern Parents to Their Children', in *What Nature Does Not Teach: Didactic Literature in the Medieval and Early Modern Periods* (Turnhout: Brepols, 2008), pp. 129-62

Firth Green, Richard, *Elf Queens and Holy Friars: Fairy Beliefs and the Medieval Church* (Philadelphia, PA: University of Pennsylvania Press, 2016)

Fischer, Klaus-Dietrich, 'A Mirror for Deaf Ears? A Medieval Mystery', *The Electronic British Library Journal*, (2008), 1-16

Fish, Stanley 'How to Recognize a Poem When You See One', in *Is There A Text in This Class? The Authority of Interpretive Communities* (Cambridge, MA: Harvard University Press, 1980), pp. 322-37

Fissell, Mary, 'Readers, Texts, and Contexts: Vernacular Medical Works in Early Modern England', in *The Popularization of Medicine 1650-1850*, ed. by Roy Porter (London: Routledge, 1992), pp. 72-96

Fissell, Mary, 'Popular Medical Writing', in *Cheap Print in Britain and Ireland to 1660*, ed. by Joad Raymond (Oxford: Oxford University Press, 2011), pp. 417-30

Flannery, Mary C., 'Emotion and the Ideal Reader in Middle English Gynaecological Texts', in *Medieval and Early Modern Literature, Science and Medicine*, ed. by Rachel Falconer and Denis Renevey (Tübingen: Narr, 2013), pp. 103-13

Fleming, Juliet, *Cultural Graphology: Writing After Derrida* (Chicago, IL: University of Chicago Press, 2016)

Flood Jr., Bruce P., 'The Medieval Herbal Tradition of Macer Floridus', *Pharmacy in History*, 18 (1976), 62-6

Flood Jr., Bruce P., 'Pliny and the Medieval "Macer" Text', *Journal of the History of Medicine and Allied Sciences*, 32 (1977), 395-402

Floyd, Janet and Laurel Forster, *The Recipe Reader: Narratives, Contexts, Traditions* (Aldershot: Ashgate, 2003)

Forbes, Thomas R., *The Midwife and the Witch* (New Haven, CT: Yale University Press, 1966)

Foucault, Michel, *The Order of Things: An Archaeology of the Human Sciences* (New York: Vintage Books, 1994)

Fox, Denton, 'Henryson's "Sum Practysis"', *Studies in Philology*, 69 (1972), 453–60
Fradenburg, Aranye, 'Imagination', in *A Handbook to Middle English Studies*, ed. by Marion Turner (Chichester: Wiley-Blackwell, 2013), pp. 15–32
Frazer, James George, *The Golden Bough: A Study in Magic and Religion*, rev. edn (Oxford: Oxford University Press, 1998; first published 1890)
Freedman, Paul, *Out of the East: Spices and the Medieval Imagination* (New Haven, CT: Yale University Press, 2008)
Friedman, Jamie, 'Making Whiteness Matter: *The King of Tars*', *Postmedieval*, 6 (2015), 52–63
Friedman John B., 'Safe Magic and Invisible Writing in the *Secretum Philosophorum*', in *Conjuring Spirits: Texts and Traditions of Medieval Ritual Magic*, ed. by Claire Fanger (Philadelphia, PA: Pennsylvania University Press, 1998), pp. 76–86
Friis-Jensen, Karsten, 'The *Ars poetica* in Twelfth-Century France: The Horace of Matthew of Vendôme, Geoffrey of Vinsauf and John of Garland', in *The Medieval Horace*, ed. by Karsten Friis-Jensen and others (Rome: Edizioni Quasar, 2015), pp. 51–99
Furdell, Elizabeth Lane, *Publishing and Medicine in Early Modern England* (Woodbridge: Boydell, 2002)
Furdell, Elizabeth Lane, *Fatal Thirst: Diabetes in Britain until Insulin* (Leiden: Brill, 2009)
Gabrovsky, Alexander N., *Chaucer the Alchemist: Physics, Mutability, and the Medieval Imagination* (New York: Palgrave Macmillan, 2015)
Gallagher, Catherine, 'Formalism and Time', in *Reading for Form*, ed. by Susan J. Wolfson and Marshall Brown (Seattle, WA: University of Washington Press, 2006), pp. 305–27
Gayk, Shannon and Robyn Malo, 'Introduction: The Sacred Object', in *The Sacred Object*, ed. by Shannon Gayk and Robyn Malo as a special issue of *The Journal of Medieval and Early Modern Studies*, 44 (2014), 457–67
Getz, Faye, 'Gilbertus Anglicus Anglicized', *Medical History*, 26 (1982), 436–42
Getz, Faye, 'Charity, Translation, and the Language of Medical Learning in Medieval England', *Bulletin of the History of Medicine*, 64 (1990), 1–17
Getz, Faye, 'The Faculty of Medicine before 1500', in *The History of the University of Oxford: Volume II. Late Medieval Oxford*, ed. by J.I. Catto and T.A.R. Evans (New York: Oxford University Press, 1993), pp. 373–405
Getz, Faye, *Medicine in the English Middle Ages* (Princeton, NJ: Princeton University Press, 1998)
Gillespie, Vincent, 'Never Look a Gift Horace in the Mouth: Affective Poetics in the Middle Ages', *Litteraria Pragensia*, 10 (1995), 59–82
Gillespie, Vincent, 'Anonymous Devotional Writings', in *A Companion to Middle English Prose*, ed. by A.S.G. Edwards (Woodbridge: Brewer, 2004), pp. 127–49
Gillespie, Vincent, '"[S]he Do the Police in Different Voices": Pastiche, Ventriloquism and Parody in Julian of Norwich', in *A Companion to Julian of Norwich*, ed. by Liz Herbert McAvoy (Woodbridge: Boydell and Brewer, 2008), pp. 192–207
Gillespie, Vincent, *Looking in Holy Books: Essays in Late Medieval Religious Writing in England* (Turnhout: Brepols, 2011)

Gillespie, Vincent, 'The Senses in Literature: The Textures of Perception', in *A Cultural History of the Senses*, ed. by Richard Newhauser (London: Bloomsbury, 2014), pp. 153-73

Gillespie, Vincent, 'Ethice Subponitur: The Imaginative Syllogism and the Idea of the Poetic', in *Medieval Thought Experiments: Poetry, Hypothesis and Experience in the European Middle Ages*, ed. by Phillip Knox, Jonathan Morton, and Daniel Reeve (Turnhout: Brepols, 2018), pp. 297-327

Gillespie, Vincent and Maggie Ross, 'The Apophatic Image: The Poetics of Effacement in Julian of Norwich', in *The Medieval Mystical Tradition in England: Exeter Symposium V* (Woodbridge: Brewer, 1992), pp. 53-77

Ginzburg, Carlo and Anna Davin, 'Morelli, Freud and Sherlock Holmes: Clues and Scientific Method', *History Workshop*, 9 (1980), 5-36

Goody, Jack, *The Domestication of the Savage Mind* (Cambridge: Cambridge University Press, 1977)

Gordon, Bruce and Peter Marshall, eds, *The Place of the Dead: Death and Remembrance in Late Medieval and Early Modern Europe* (Cambridge: Cambridge University Press, 2000)

Gordon, Sarah, *Culinary Comedy in Medieval French Literature* (West Lafayette, IN: Purdue University Press, 2006)

Goulding, Robert, 'Deceiving the Senses in the Thirteenth Century: Trickery and Illusion in the *Secretum Philosophorum*', in *Magic and the Classical Tradition*, ed. by Charles Burnett and W.F. Ryan (London: Warburg Institute, 2006), pp. 135-62

Gray, Annie, '"A Practical Art": An Archaeological Perspective on the Use of Recipe Books', in *Reading and Writing Recipe Books 1550-1800*, ed. by Michelle DiMeo and Sara Pennell (Manchester: Manchester University Press, 2013), pp. 47-67

Green, Monica H., 'Obstetrical and Gynaecological Texts in Middle English', *Studies in the Age of Chaucer*, 14 (1992), 53-88

Green, Monica H., *Women's Healthcare in the Medieval West* (Aldershot: Ashgate, 2000)

Green, Monica H., *Making Women's Medicine Masculine: The Rise of Male Authority in Pre-Modern Gynaecology* (Oxford: Oxford University Press, 2008)

Griffin, Carrie, '"A Good Reder": The Middle English *Wise Book of Philosophy and Astronomy*, Instruction, Publics and Manuscripts' (unpublished doctoral thesis, National University of Ireland, 2006)

Griffin, Carrie, *The Middle English Wise Book of Philosophy and Astronomy: A Parallel Text Edition—Edited from London, British Library, MS Sloane 2453 with a Parallel Text from New York, Columbia University, MS Plimpton 260* (Heidelberg: Winter, 2013)

Griffin, Carrie, 'Reconsidering the Recipe: Materiality, Narrative and Text in Later Medieval Instructional Manuscripts and Collections', in *Manuscripts and Printed Books in Europe, 1350-1550: Packaging, Presentation and Consumption*, ed. by Emma Cayley and Susan Powell (Liverpool: Liverpool University Press, 2013), pp. 135-49

Griffin, Carrie, 'Instruction and Inspiration: Fifteenth-Century Codicological Recipes', *Exemplaria*, 30 (2018), 20-34

Griffin, Carrie, *Instructional Writing in English, 1350-1650: Materiality and Meaning* (London: Routledge, 2019)

Griffiths, Eric, 'Lists', in *If Not Critical*, ed. by Freya Johnston (Oxford: Oxford University Press, 2018), pp. 8–28

Grisby, Bryon Lee, *Pestilence in Medieval and Early Modern English Literature* (New York: Routledge, 2004)

Hanna, Ralph, 'Henry Daniel's *Liber Uricrisiarum*', in *Popular and Practical Science of Medieval England*, ed. by Lister M. Matheson (East Lansing, MI: Colleagues Press, 1994), pp. 185–218

Hanna, Ralph, 'Miscellaneity and Vernacularity: Conditions of Literary Production in Late Medieval England', in *The Whole Book: Cultural Perspectives on the Medieval Miscellany*, ed. by Stephen G. Nichols and Siegfried Wenzel (Ann Arbor, MI: University of Michigan Press, 1996), pp. 37–51

Hardman, Phillipa, 'Lydgate's Uneasy Syntax', in *John Lydgate: Poetry, Culture, and Lancastrian England*, ed. by Larry Scanlon and James Simpson (Notre Dame, IN: University of Notre Dame Press, 2006), pp. 12–35

Hargreaves, Henry, 'Some Problems in Indexing Middle English Recipes', in *Middle English Prose: Essays on Bibliographic Problems*, ed. by A.S.G. Edwards and Derek Pearsall (New York: Garland Publishing, 1981), pp. 91–113

Harris, Kate, 'Patrons, Buyers and Owners: The Evidence for Ownership and the Role of Book Owners in Book Production and the Book Trade', in *Book Production and Publishing in Britain, 1375–1475*, ed. by Jeremy Griffiths and Derek Pearsall (Cambridge: Cambridge University Press, 1989), pp. 163–99

Hartnell, Jack, *Medieval Bodies: Life, Death, and Art in the Middle Ages* (London: Profile Books, 2018)

Harvey, E. Ruth, *The Inward Wits: Psychological Theory in the Middle Ages and Renaissance* (London: The Warburg Institute, 1975)

Hawkins, Joy, 'Seeing the Light? Blindness and Sanctity in Later Medieval England', *Studies in Church History*, 47 (2011), 148–58

Hawkins, Joy, 'Sights for Sore Eyes: Vision and Health in Medieval England', in *On Light*, ed. by K.P. Clarke and S. Baccianti (Oxford: The Society for the Study of Medieval Languages and Literature, 2014), pp. 137–156

Heng, Geraldine, 'The Invention of Race in the European Middle Ages: Race Studies, Modernity, and the Middle Ages', *Literature Compass*, 8 (2011), 258–74

Heng, Geraldine, *The Invention of Race in the European Middle Ages* (Cambridge: Cambridge University Press, 2018)

Henry, John, 'The Fragmentation of Renaissance Occultism and the Decline of Magic', in John Henry, *Religion, Magic and the Origins of Science in Early Modern England* (Farnham: Ashgate, 2012), pp. 1–48

Herbert McAvoy, Liz, 'Medievalism and the Medical Humanities', *Postmedieval*, 8 (2017), 254–65

Hoepffner, Ernest, 'Une ballade d'Eustache Deschamps', *Romania*, 50 (1924), 413–26

Horden, Peregrine, 'A Non-Natural Environment: Medicine Without Doctors and the Medieval European Hospital', in *The Medieval Hospital and Medical Practice*, ed. by Barbara S. Bowers (Aldershot: Ashgate, 2007), pp. 133–45

Horden, Peregrine, *Hospitals and Healing from Antiquity to the Later Middle Ages* (Aldershot: Ashgate, 2008)

Horden, Peregrine, 'What's Wrong with Early Medieval Medicine?', *Social History of Medicine*, 24 (2011), 5–25

Hudson, Robert P. and Linda E. Voigts, 'A drynke þat men callen dwale to make a man to slepe whyle men kerven him: A Surgical Anaesthetic from Late Medieval England', in *Health, Disease and Healing in Medieval Culture*, ed. by Sheila Campbell and others (Basingstoke: Macmillan, 1992), pp. 34–56

Huizinga, Johan, *Homo Ludens: A Study of the Play Element in Culture*, trans. by R.F.C. Hull (London: Routledge, 1949)

Humphrey, Chris, 'Time and Urban Culture in Late Medieval England', in *Time in the Medieval World*, ed. by Chris Humphrey and W.M. Ormrod (Woodbridge: Boydell Press, 2001), pp. 105–17

Hunt, Tony, *Plant Names of Medieval England* (Cambridge: Brewer, 1989)

Hunt, Tony, *Popular Medicine in Thirteenth-Century England* (Cambridge: Brewer, 1990)

Hunt, Tony, 'The Poetic Vein: Phlebotomy in Middle English Verse', *English Studies*, 77 (1996), 311–22

Hunt, Tony, 'Code-Switching in Medical Texts', in *Multilingualism in Later Medieval Britain*, ed. by D.A. Trotter (Cambridge: Brewer, 2000), pp. 131–47

Hunt, Tony, 'The Languages of Medical Writing in Medieval England', in *Medieval and Early Modern Literature, Science and Medicine*, ed. by Rachel Falconer and Denis Renevey (Tübingen: Narr, 2013), pp. 79–101

Hunter, J. Paul, 'Formalism and History: Binarism and the Anglophone Couplet', in *Reading for Form*, ed. by Susan J. Wolfson and Marshall Brown (Seattle, WA: University of Washington Press, 2006), pp. 129–49

Ingham, Patricia Clare, *The Medieval New: Ambivalence in an Age of Innovation* (Philadelphia, PA: University of Pennsylvania Press, 2015)

Irvine, Martin and David Thomson, '*Grammatica* and Literary Theory', in *The Cambridge History of Literary Criticism: Volume II. The Middle Ages*, ed. by Alastair Minnis and Ian Johnson (Cambridge: Cambridge University Press, 2005), pp. 15–41

Izmirlieva, Valentina, *All the Names of the Lord: Lists, Mysticism and Magic* (Chicago, IL: University of Chicago Press, 2008)

Jacquart, Danielle, 'Medical Scholasticism', in *Western Medical Thought from Antiquity to the Middle Ages*, ed. by Mirko D. Grmek and others (Cambridge, MA: Harvard University Press, 1998), pp. 197–240

Jahner, Jennifer, 'Literary Therapeutics: Experimental Knowledge in MS Digby 86', in *Interpreting MS Digby 86: A Trilingual Book from Thirteenth-Century Worcestershire*, ed. by Susanna Fein (York: York Medieval Press, 2019), pp. 73–86

Jakobson, Roman, 'Two Aspects of Language and Two Types of Aphasic Disturbances', in *Language in Literature*, ed. by Krystyna Pomorska and Stephen Rudy (Cambridge, MA: Harvard University Press, 1987), pp. 95–114

Jarvis, Simon 'Why Rhyme Pleases', *Thinking Verse*, 1 (2011), 17–43

Johnson, Eleanor, 'Chaucer and the Consolation of *Prosimetrum*', *Chaucer Review*, 43 (2009), 455–72

Johnson, Eleanor, *Practicing Literary Theory in the Middle Ages: Ethics and the Mixed Form in Chaucer, Gower, Usk and Hoccleve* (Chicago, IL: University of Chicago Press, 2013)

Johnson, Mark and George Lakoff, *Metaphors We Live By*, rev. edn (Chicago, IL: Chicago University Press, 2003)

Jones, Claire, 'Formula and Formulation: Efficacy Phrases in Medieval English Medical Manuscripts', *Neuphilologische Mitteilungen*, 99 (1998), 199–209

Jones, Claire, 'Discourse Communities and Medical Texts', in *Medical and Scientific Writing in Late Medieval English*, ed. by Irma Taavitsainen and Päivi Pahta (Cambridge: Cambridge University Press, 2004), pp. 23–36

Justice, Steven, 'Did the Middle Ages Believe in Their Miracles?', *Representations*, 103 (2008), 1–29

Justice, Steven, 'Chaucer's History Effect', in *Answerable Style: The Idea of the Literary in Medieval England*, ed. by Frank Grady and Andrew Galloway (Columbus, OH: Ohio State University Press, 2013), pp. 169–94

Kafer, Alison, *Feminist, Queer, Crip* (Bloomington, IN: Indiana University Press, 2013)

Kärkkäinen, Pekka, 'The Senses in Philosophy and Science: Mechanics of the Body or Activity of the Soul', in *A Cultural History of the Senses*, ed. by Richard Newhauser (London: Bloomsbury, 2014), pp. 111–32

Karnes, Michelle, *Imagination, Meditation and Cognition in the Middle Ages* (Chicago, IL: University of Chicago Press, 2011)

Karnes, Michelle, 'Wonder, Marvels and Metaphor in the *Squire's Tale*', *ELH*, 82 (2015), 461–90

Kaye, Joel, *A History of Balance, 1250–1375: The Emergence of a New Model of Equilibrium and Its Impact on Thought* (Cambridge: Cambridge University Press, 2014)

Keil, Gundolf and others, eds, *Fachliteratur des Mittelalters, Festschrift für Gerhard Eis* (Stuttgart: Metzler, 1968)

Keiser, George R., 'More Light on the Life and Milieu of Robert Thornton', *Studies in Bibliography*, 36 (1983), 111–19

Keiser, George R., 'Practical Books for the Gentleman', in *The Cambridge History of the Book in Britain: Volume III*, ed. by Lotte Hellinga and J.B. Trapp (Cambridge: Cambridge University Press, 1999), pp. 470–94

Keiser, George R., 'Verse Introductions to Middle English Medical Treatises', *English Studies*, 84 (2003), 301–17

Keiser, George R., 'Robert Thornton's *Liber de Diversis Medicinis*: Text, Vocabulary, and Scribal Confusion', in *Rethinking Middle English: Linguistic and Literary Approaches*, ed. by N. Ritt and H. Schnedel (Frankfurt: Peter Lang, 2005), pp. 30–41

Keiser, George R., 'Rosemary: Not Just for Remembrance', in *Health and Healing from the Medieval Garden*, ed. by Peter Dendle and Alain Touwaide (Woodbridge: Boydell, 2008), pp. 180–204

Keiser, George R., 'Vernacular Herbals: A Growth Industry in Late Medieval England', in *Design and Distribution of Late Medieval Manuscripts in England*, ed. by Margaret Connolly and Linne R. Mooney (York: York Medieval Press, 2008), pp. 292–307

Kemal, Salim, *The Philosophical Poetics of Alfarabi, Avicenna and Averroës: The Aristotelian Reception* (London: Routledge-Curzon, 2003)

Kesling, Emily, *Medical Texts in Anglo-Saxon Literary Culture* (Cambridge: Brewer, 2020)
Kidwell, Jeremy, 'Labour in St. Augustine', in *The Oxford Guide to the Historical Reception of Augustine*, ed. by Karla Pollmann (Oxford: Oxford University Press, 2013), pp. 779–84
Kieckhefer, Richard, *Magic in the Middle Ages* (Cambridge: Cambridge University Press, 1989)
Kieckhefer, Richard, *Forbidden Rites: A Necromancer's Manual of the Fifteenth Century* (Stroud: Sutton Publishing, 1997)
King, Elizabeth, 'Clockwork Prayer: A Sixteenth-Century Mechanical Monk', in *Blackbird: An Online Journal of Literature and the Arts*, 1 (2002), n.p.
Kirkham, Anne and Cordelia Warr, eds, *Wounds in the Middle Ages* (Farnham: Ashgate, 2014)
Klaassen, Frank, *The Transformations of Magic: Illicit Learned Magic in the Later Middle Ages and Renaissance* (Philadelphia, PA: Pennsylvania State University Press, 2013)
Knapp, Ethan, *The Bureaucratic Muse: Thomas Hoccleve and the Literature of Late Medieval England* (Philadelphia, PA: University of Pennsylvania Press, 2001)
Knapp, Peggy, *Chaucer and the Social Contest* (New York: Routledge, 1990)
Knapp, Peggy, *Chaucerian Aesthetics* (New York: Palgrave Macmillan, 2008)
Knight, Jeffrey Todd, *Bound to Read: Compilations, Collections, and the Making of Renaissance Literature* (Philadelphia, PA: University of Pennsylvania Press, 2013)
Krug, Rebecca, *Reading Families: Women's Literate Practice in Late Medieval England* (Ithaca, NY: Cornell University Press, 2002)
Kumler, Aden 'Imitatio Rerum: Sacred Objects in the St Giles's Hospital Processional', in *The Sacred Object*, ed. by Shannon Gayk and Robyn Malo as a special issue of *The Journal of Medieval and Early Modern Studies*, 44 (2014), 469–502
Kwakkel, Eric, 'A New Type of Book for a New Type of Reader: The Emergence of Paper in Vernacular Book Production', *The Library*, 4 (2003), 219–48
Lacey, Simon, Randall Stilla, and K. Sathian, 'Metaphorically Feeling: Comprehending Textural Metaphors Activates Somatosensory Cortex', *Brain and Language*, 120 (2012), 416–21
Lakoff, George, 'The Neural Theory of Metaphor', in *The Cambridge Handbook of Metaphor and Thought*, ed. by Raymond W. Gibbs Jr. (Cambridge: Cambridge University Press, 2008), pp. 17–38
Lakoff, George, 'Mapping the Brain's Metaphor Circuitry: Metaphorical Thought in Everyday Reason', *Frontiers in Human Neuroscience*, 8 (2014), 1–14
Langum, Virginia, 'Medicine, Passion and Sin in Gower', in *Medieval and Early Modern Literature, Science and Medicine*, ed. by Rachel Falconer and Denis Renevey (Tübingen: Narr, 2013), pp. 117–30
Langum, Virginia, '"The Wounded Surgeon": Devotion, Compassion and Metaphor in Medieval England', in *Wounds and Wound Repair in Medieval Culture*, ed. by Larissa Tracy and Kelley Devries (Leiden: Brill, 2015), pp. 269–90
Langum, Virginia, *Medicine and the Seven Deadly Sins in Late Medieval Literature and Culture* (New York: Palgrave Macmillan, 2016)

Laroche, Rebecca, *Medical Authority and English Women's Herbal Texts, 1550–1650* (Farnham: Ashgate, 2009)

Latour, Bruno, *We Have Never Been Modern*, trans. by Catherine Porter (Cambridge, MA: Harvard University Press, 1993)

Lawrence, Tom, 'Infectious Fear: The Rhetoric of Pestilence in Middle English Didactic Texts on Death', *English Studies*, 98 (2017), 866–80

Lawton, David, *Chaucer's Narrators* (Cambridge: Brewer, 1985)

Lawton, David, 'Dullness and the Fifteenth Century', *English Literary History*, 54 (1987), 761–99

Lawton, David, 'Voice After Arundel', in *After Arundel*, ed. by Vincent Gillespie and Kantik Ghosh (Turnhout: Brepols, 2011), pp. 133–52

Lawton, David, 'Voice and Public Interiorities: Chaucer, Orpheus, Machaut', in *Answerable Style: The Idea of the Literary in Medieval England*, ed. by Frank Grady and Andrew Galloway (Columbus, OH: Ohio State University Press, 2013), pp. 284–306

Lawton, David, *Voice in Later Medieval English Literature: Public Interiorities* (Oxford: Oxford University Press, 2017)

Leahy, Michael, '"To Speke of Phisik": Medical Discourse in Late Medieval English Culture' (unpublished doctoral thesis, Birkbeck College, University of London, 2015)

Leahy, Michael, 'Domestic Ideals: Healing, Reading, and Perfection in the Late Medieval Household', in *Household Knowledges in Late Medieval England and France*, ed. by Glenn Burger and Rory Critten (Manchester: Manchester University Press, 2019), n.p., accessed online at www.perlego.com/home

Le Goff, Jacques, *Time, Work and Culture in the Middle Ages*, trans. by Arthur Goldhammer (Chicago, IL: University of Chicago Press, 1980)

Le Goff, Jacques, *The Medieval Imagination*, trans. by Arthur Goldhammer (Chicago, IL: University of Chicago Press, 1985)

Lehmann, Gilly, 'Reading Recipe Books and Culinary History: Opening a New Field', in *Reading and Writing Recipe Books 1550–1800*, ed. by Michelle DiMeo and Sara Pennell (Manchester: Manchester University Press, 2013), pp. 93–113

Leonardi, Susan, 'Recipes for Reading: Summer Pasta, Lobster a'la Riseholme, and Key Lime Pie', *PMLA*, 104 (1989), 340–7

Leong, Elaine, 'Medical Recipe Collections in Seventeenth-Century England: Knowledge, Text, and Gender' (unpublished doctoral thesis, University of Oxford, 2005)

Leong, Elaine, 'Making Medicines in the Early Modern Household', *Bulletin of the History of Medicine*, 82 (2008), 145–68

Leong, Elaine, 'Collecting Knowledge for the Family: Recipes, Gender and Practical Knowledge in the Early Modern English Household', *Centaurus*, 55 (2013), 81–103

Leong, Elaine, '"Herbals She Peruseth": Reading Medicine in Early Modern England', *Renaissance Studies*, 28 (2014), 556–78

Leong, Elaine, *Recipes and Everyday Knowledge: Medicine, Science and the Household in Early Modern England* (Chicago, IL: University of Chicago Press, 2018)

Lerer, Seth, 'Medieval English Literature and the Idea of the Anthology', *PMLA*, 118 (2003), 1251–67

Levine, Caroline, *Forms: Whole, Rhythm, Hierarchy, Network* (Princeton, NJ: Princeton University Press, 2015)
Levinson, Marjorie, 'What Is New Formalism?', *PMLA*, 122 (2007), 558–69
Levinson, Stephen C., *Pragmatics* (Cambridge: Cambridge University Press, 1983)
Lévi-Strauss, Claude, *The Elementary Structures of Kinship*, trans. by James Harle Bell and others (Boston, MA: Beacon Press, 1969)
Lochrie, Karma, *Covert Operations: The Medieval Uses of Secrecy* (Philadelphia, PA: University of Pennsylvania Press, 1999)
Long, Pamela O., *Openness, Secrecy, Authorship: Technical Arts and the Culture of Knowledge from Antiquity to the Renaissance* (Baltimore, MD: Johns Hopkins University Press, 2001)
Macnaughton, Jane, 'The Past, Present, and Future of Medical Humanities', *Postmedieval*, 8 (2017), 234–9
Mäkinen, Martti, 'Herbal Recipes and Recipes in Herbals: Intertextuality in Early English Medical Writing', in *Medical and Scientific Writing in Late Medieval English*, ed. by Irma Taavitsainen and Päivi Pahta (Cambridge: Cambridge University Press, 2004), pp. 144–73
Marsh, David, 'Petrarch's Adversaries: The Invectives', in *The Cambridge Companion to Petrarch*, ed. by Albert Russell Ascoli and Unn Falkeid (Cambridge: Cambridge University Press, 2015), pp. 167–76
Marshall, Helen and Peter Buchanan, 'New Formalism and the Forms of Middle English Literary Texts', *Literature Compass*, 8 (2011), 164–72
McCann, Daniel, 'Medicine of Words: Purgative Reading in Richard Rolle's Meditations on the Passion', *The Medieval Journal*, 5 (2015), 53–83
McCann, Daniel, *Soul Health: Therapeutic Reading in Later Medieval England* (Cardiff: University of Wales Press, 2018)
McCartney, Eugene S., 'Verbal Homeopathy and the Etymological Story', *The American Journal of Philology*, 48 (1927), 326–43
McDonald, Nicola, 'Eating People and the Alimentary Logic of *Richard Coeur de Lion*', in *Pulp Fictions of Medieval England: Essays in Popular Romance*, ed. by Nicola McDonald (Manchester: Manchester University Press, 2004), pp. 124–50
McDonald, Nicola, 'Desire Out of Order and Undo Your Door', *Studies in the Age of Chaucer*, 34 (2012), 247–75
McGavin, John J., *Chaucer and Dissimilarity: Literary Comparisons in Chaucer and other Late Medieval Writing* (Madison, WI: Fairleigh Dickinson University Presses, 2000)
McGuiness, Daniel, 'Purple Hearts and Coronets: Caring for Wounds in Malory', *Arthurian Interpretations*, 4 (1989), 43–54
McLeod, Judyth, *In a Unicorn's Garden: Recreating the Magic and Mystery of Medieval Gardens* (London: Murdoch, 2008)
McNamer, Sarah, 'Feeling', in *Twenty-First-Century Approaches to Literature: Middle English*, ed. by Paul Strohm (Oxford: Oxford University Press, 2007), pp. 241–57
McVaugh, Michael, 'The Nature and Limits of Medical Certitude at Early Fourteenth-Century Montpellier', *Osiris*, 6 (1990), 62–84
McVaugh, Michael, *The Rational Surgery of the Middle Ages* (Tavarnuzze: SISMEL Edizioni del Galluzzo, 2006)

Meale, Carol, 'Patrons, Buyers and Owners: Book Production and Social Status', in *Book Production and Publishing in Britain, 1375–1475*, ed. by Jeremy Griffiths and Derek Pearsall (Cambridge: Cambridge University Press, 1989), pp. 201–38

Meale, Carol, '"alle the bokes that I haue of latyn, englisch, and frensch": Laywomen and Their Books in Late Medieval England', in *Women and Literature in Britain 1150–1500*, ed. by Carol Meale (Cambridge: Cambridge University Press, 1993), pp. 128–58

Meale, Carol, 'Amateur Book Production and the Miscellany in Late Medieval East Anglia', in *Insular Books: Vernacular Manuscript Miscellanies in Late Medieval Britain*, ed. by Margaret Connolly and Raluca Radulescu (Oxford: Oxford University Press, 2015), pp. 157–73

Melancon, Lisa Kay, 'Rhetoric, Remedies, Regimen' (unpublished doctoral thesis, University of South Carolina, 2005)

Metzler, Irina, *Disability in Medieval Europe: Thinking about Physical Impairment during the High Middle Ages, c. 1100–1400* (London: Routledge, 2006)

Metzler, Irina, 'Disability in the Middle Ages: Impairment at the Intersection of Historical Inquiry and Disability Studies', *History Compass*, 9 (2011), 45–60

Meyer-Lee, Robert J., 'The Vatic Penitent: John Audelay's Self Representation', in *My Wyl and My Wrytyng: Essays on John the Blind Audelay*, ed. by Susanna Fein (Kalamazoo, MI: Medieval Institute Publications, 2009), pp. 54–85

Meyer-Lee, Robert J., 'The Emergence of the Literary in John Lydgate's Life of Our Lady', *Journal of English and Germanic Philology*, 109 (2010), 322–48

Meyer-Lee, Robert J. and Catherine Sanok, eds, *The Medieval Literary Beyond Form* (Cambridge: Brewer, 2018)

Minnis, Alastair, *Medieval Theory of Authorship: Scholastic Literary Attitudes in the Late Middle Ages* (London: Scolar Press, 1984)

Minnis, Alastair, 'Nolens Auctor Sed Compilator Reputari: The Late Medieval Discourse of Compilatio', in *La méthode critique au Moyen Âge*, ed. by Mireille Chazan and Gilbert Dahan (Turnhout: Brepols, 2006), pp. 47–63

Minnis, Alastair, 'Medieval Imagination and Memory', in *The Cambridge History of Literary Criticism: Volume II. The Middle Ages* (Cambridge: Cambridge University Press, 2008), pp. 237–74

Minnis, Alastair and A.B. Scott, eds, *Medieval Literary Theory and Criticism c. 1100–c. 1375: The Commentary Tradition*, rev. edn (Oxford: Clarendon Press, 1991)

Mitchell, Laura T., 'Cultural Uses of Magic in Fifteenth-Century England' (unpublished doctoral thesis, University of Toronto, 2011)

Mitchell, Piers D., *Medicine in the Crusades: Warfare, Wounds and the Medieval Surgeon* (Cambridge: Cambridge University Press, 2004)

Mooney, Linne R., 'A Middle English Compendium of Astrological Medicine', *Medical History*, 28 (1984), 406–19

Mooney, Linne R., 'The Cock and the Clock: Telling Time in Chaucer's Day', *Studies in the Age of Chaucer*, 15 (1993), 91–109

Mooney, Linne R., 'Manuscript Evidence for the Use of Medieval Scientific and Utilitarian Texts', in *Interstices: Studies in Middle English and Anglo-Latin Texts in Honour of A.G. Rigg* (Toronto: University of Toronto Press, 2004), pp. 184–202

Morrison, Susan Signe, *Excrement in the Late Middle Ages: Sacred Filth and Chaucer's Fecopoetics* (New York: Palgrave Macmillan, 2008)
Morse, Ruth, *Truth and Convention in the Middle Ages: Rhetoric, Representation, and Reality* (Cambridge: Cambridge University Press, 1991)
Morse, Ruth, *The Medieval Medea* (Cambridge: Brewer, 1996)
Mount, Toni, *Dragon's Blood and Willow Bark: The Mysteries of Medieval Medicine* (Stroud: Amberly, 2015)
Murphy, James Jerome, *Rhetoric in the Middle Ages: A History of Rhetorical Theory from Saint Augustine to the Renaissance* (Berkeley, CA: University of California Press, 1974)
Murphy, James Jerome, *Medieval Eloquence: Studies in the Theory and Practice of Medieval Rhetoric* (Berkeley, CA: University of California Press, 1978)
Murphy, James Jerome, 'The Arts of Poetry and Prose', in *The Cambridge History of Literary Criticism: Volume II. The Middle Ages*, ed. by Alastair Minnis and Ian Johnson (Cambridge: Cambridge University Press, 2005) pp. 42–67
Murray Jones, Peter, *Medieval Medical Miniatures* (London: British Library, 1984)
Murray Jones, Peter, 'Four Middle English Translations of John of Arderne', in *Latin and Vernacular Studies in Late Medieval Manuscripts*, ed. by A.J. Minnis (Cambridge: Brewer, 1989), pp. 61–89
Murray Jones, Peter, 'Information and Science', in *Fifteenth-Century Attitudes: Perceptions of Society in Late Medieval England*, ed. by Rosemary Horrox (Cambridge: Cambridge University Press, 1994), pp. 97–111
Murray Jones, Peter, 'Book Ownership and the Lay Culture of Medicine in Tudor Cambridge', in *The Task of Healing: Medicine, Religion, and Gender in England and the Netherlands, 1485–1800*, ed. by Hilary Marland and Margaret Pelling (Rotterdam: Erasmus, 1996), pp. 49–68
Murray Jones, Peter, 'Medicine', in *Medieval Latin: An Introduction and Bibliographical Guide*, ed. by Frank Anthony Carl Mantello and A.G. Rigg (Washington, DC: Catholic University of America Press, 1996), pp. 416–21
Murray Jones, Peter, 'Medicine and Science', in *The Cambridge History of the Book in Britain: Volume III*, ed. by Lotte Hellinga and J.B. Trapp (Cambridge: Cambridge University Press, 1999), pp. 433–48
Murray Jones, Peter, 'Image, Word, and Medicine in the Middle Ages', in *Visualizing Medieval Medicine and Natural History 1200–1500*, ed. by Jean A. Givens and others (Aldershot: Ashgate, 2006), pp. 1–24
Murray Jones, Peter, 'Herbs and the Medieval Surgeon', in *Health and Healing in the Medieval Garden*, ed. by Peter Dendle and Alain Touwaide (Woodbridge: Boydell and Brewer, 2008)
Murray Jones, Peter, 'The Surgeon as Story-Teller', *Poetica*, 72 (2009), 77–91
Murray Jones, Peter, 'Complexio and Experimentum: Tensions in Late Medieval Medical Practice', in *The Body in Balance: Humoral Medicines in Practice*, ed. by Peregrine Horden and Elisabeth Hus (New York: Berghahn Books, 2013), pp. 107–28
Murray Jones, Peter, 'Language and Register in English Medieval Surgery', in *Language in Medieval Britain: Networks and Exchanges—Proceedings of the 2013 Harlaxton Symposium* (Donington: Shaun Tyas, 2015), pp. 74–89

Murray Jones, Peter, '*Experimenta*, Compilation and Construction in Two Medieval Books', *Poetica*, 91 and 92 (2019), 61–80

Nauert Jr., Charles G., 'Humanists, Science, and Pliny: Changing Approaches to a Classical Author', *American Historical Review*, 84 (1979), 72–85

Nelson, Ingrid, 'Form's Practice: Lyrics, Grammars, and the Medieval Idea of the Literary', in *The Medieval Literary Beyond Form*, ed. by Robert J. Meyer-Lee and Catherine Sanok (Cambridge: Brewer, 2018), pp. 35–60

Newhauser, Richard G., 'Introduction: The Sensual Middle Ages', in *A Cultural History of the Senses*, ed. by Richard Newhauser (London: Bloomsbury, 2014), pp. 1–22

Nolan, Maura, 'Making the Aesthetic Turn: Adorno, the Medieval and the Future of the Past', *Journal of Medieval and Early Modern Studies*, 34 (2004), 549–75

Nolan, Maura, *John Lydgate and the Making of Public Culture* (Cambridge: Cambridge University Press, 2005)

Nolan, Maura, 'Lydgate's Worst Poem', in *Lydgate Matters*, ed. by Lisa H. Cooper and Andrea Denny-Brown (New York: Palgrave Macmillan, 2007), pp. 71–87

Nolan, Maura, 'Aesthetics', in *A Handbook to Middle English Studies*, ed. by Marion Turner (Chichester: Wiley-Blackwell, 2013), pp. 223–38

Nolan, Maura, 'The Biennial Chaucer Lecture: The Invention of Style', *Studies in the Age of Chaucer*, 41 (2019), 33–71

Norri, Juhani, 'Entrances and Exits in English Medical Vocabulary, 1400–1550', in *Medical and Scientific Writing in Late Medieval English*, ed. by Irma Taavitsainen and Päivi Pahta (Cambridge: Cambridge University Press, 2004), pp. 100–43

Olsan, Lea T., 'Latin Charms of Medieval England: Verbal Healing in a Christian Oral Tradition', *Oral Tradition*, 7 (1992), 116–42

Olsan, Lea T., 'Charms and Prayers in Medieval Medical Theory and Practice', *Social History of Medicine*, 16 (2003), 344–66

Olsan, Lea T., 'Charms in Medieval Memory', in *Charms and Charming in Europe*, ed. by Jonathan Roper (Basingstoke: Palgrave Macmillan, 2004), pp. 59–88

Olson, Glending, 'Making and Poetry in the Age of Chaucer', *Comparative Literature*, 31 (1979), 272–90

Olson, Glending, *Literature as Recreation in the Later Middle Ages* (Ithaca, NY: Cornell University Press, 1982)

Orlemanski, Julie, 'Physiognomy and Otiose Practicality', *Exemplaria*, 23 (2011), 194–218

Orlemanski, Julie, 'Jargon and the Matter of Medicine in Middle English', *Journal of Medieval and Early Modern Studies*, 42 (2012), 395–420

Orlemanski, Julie, 'Thornton's Remedies and the Practices of Medical Reading', in *Robert Thornton and His Books: Essays on the Lincoln and London Thornton Manuscripts*, ed. by Susanna Fein and Michael Johnston (York: York Medieval Press, 2014), pp. 235–57

Orlemanski, Julie, 'Margery's "Noyse" and Distributed Expressivity', in *Voice and Voicelessness in Medieval Europe*, ed. by Irit Ruth Kleiman (Basingstoke: Palgrave Macmillan, 2015), pp. 123–38

Orlemanski, Julie, *Symptomatic Subjects: Bodies, Medicine and Causation in the Literature of Late Medieval England* (Philadelphia, PA: University of Pennsylvania Press, 2019)

Orme, Nicholas, *Medieval Schools: From Roman Britain to Renaissance England* (New Haven, CT: Yale University Press, 2006)
Page, Sophie, *Astrology in Medieval Manuscripts* (London: British Library, 2002)
Page, Sophie, *Magic in Medieval Manuscripts* (London: British Library, 2004)
Page, Sophie, *Magic in the Cloister: Pious Motives, Illicit Interests and Occult Approaches to the Medieval Universe* (Philadelphia, PA: Pennsylvania State University Press, 2013)
Pahta, Päivi, 'On Structures of Code-Switching in Medical Texts from Medieval England', *Neuphilologische Mitteilungen*, 104 (2003), 197–210
Pahta, Päivi, 'Code Switching in Medieval Medical Writing', in *Medical and Scientific Writing in Late Medieval English*, ed. by Irma Taavitsainen and Päivi Pahta (Cambridge: Cambridge University Press, 2004), pp. 73–99
Park, Katharine, 'The Criminal and the Saintly Body: Autopsy and Dissection in Renaissance Italy', *Renaissance Quarterly*, 47 (1994), 1–33
Park, Katharine, *Secrets of Women: Gender, Generation and the Origins of Human Dissection* (New York: Zone Books, 2006)
Parkes, Malcolm, 'The Literacy of the Laity', in *Literature and Western Civilisation: The Medieval World*, ed. by David Daiches and Anthony Thorlby (London: Aldus Books, 1973), pp. 555–77
Parkes, Malcolm, *Scribes, Scripts and Readers: Studies in the Communication, Presentation and Dissemination of Medieval Texts* (London: The Hambledon Press, 1991)
Parkes, Malcolm, *Pause and Effect: An Introduction to the History of Punctuation in the West* (Aldershot: Scolar Press, 1992)
Pearsall, Derek, *John Lydgate* (London: Routledge, 1970)
Pearsall, Derek, *The Canterbury Tales* (London: Routledge, 1985)
Pearsall, Derek, 'The Wife of Bath's "Experience": Some Lexicographical Reflections', in *Readings in Medieval Textuality: Essays in Honour of AC Spearing*, ed. by Cristina Maria Cervone and D. Vance Smith (Cambridge: Brewer, 2016), pp. 3–16
Pender, Stephen and Nancy Struever, eds, *Rhetoric and Medicine in Early Modern Europe* (Farnham: Ashgate, 2012)
Penn, Stephen, 'Literary Nominalism and Medieval Sign Theory', in *Nominalism and Literary Discourse: New Perspectives*, ed. by Christoph Bode, Hugo Keiper, and Richard J. Utz (Amsterdam: Rodopi, 1997), pp. 157–89
Pennell, Sara, 'Mundane Materiality, or Should Small Thing Still Be Forgotten? Material Culture, Micro-Histories and the Problem of Scale', in *History and Material Culture*, ed. by K. Harvey, 2nd edn (London: Routledge, 2017), pp. 221–31
Pennell, Sara and Elaine Leong, 'Recipe Collections and the Currency of Medical Knowledge in the Early Modern "Medical Marketplace"', in *Medicine and the Market in England and Its Colonies c.1450–c.1850*, ed. by Mark S.R. Jenner and Patrick Wallis (Basingstoke: Palgrave Macmillan, 2007), pp. 133–52
Pereira, Michela, 'Alchemy and the Use of Vernacular Languages in the Late Middle Ages', *Speculum*, 74 (1999), 336–56
Petit, Caroline, 'Galen, Pharmacology and the Boundaries of Medicine: A Reassessment', in *Collecting Recipes: Byzantine and Jewish Pharmacology in*

Dialogue, ed. by Lennart Lehmhaus and Matteo Martelli (Berlin: De Gruyter, 2017), pp. 51–79

Plummer, John F., 'Style', in *A Companion to Chaucer*, ed. by Peter Brown (Oxford: Blackwell, 2000), pp. 414–27

Pope, Nancy, 'A Middle English Satirical Letter in Brogyntyn MS II.1', *American Notes and Queries*, 18 (2005), 38–42

Pouchelle, Marie-Christine, *The Body and Surgery in the Middle Ages*, trans. by Rosemary Morris (New Brunswick, NJ: Rutgers University Press, 1990)

Pounds, N.J.G., *A History of the English Parish: The Culture of Religion from Augustine to Victoria* (Cambridge: Cambridge University Press, 2000)

Prendergast, Thomas, 'Canon Formation', in *A Handbook to Middle English Studies*, ed. by Marion Turner (Chichester: Wiley-Blackwell, 2013), pp. 239–52

Prioreschi, Plinio, *A History of Medicine, Volume V: Medieval Medicine* (Omaha, NE: Horatius Press, 2003)

Pye, David, *The Nature and Aesthetics of Design: A Design Handbook* (London: Herbert Press, 1978)

Raine, Melissa, 'Searching for Emotional Communities in Late Medieval England', in *Emotions and Social Change: Historical and Sociological Perspectives*, ed. by David Lemmings and Ann Brooks (New York: Routledge, 2014), pp. 65–81

Rankin, Alisha, *Panaceia's Daughters: Noblewomen as Healers in Early Modern Germany* (Chicago, IL: University of Chicago Press, 2013)

Rawcliffe, Carole, *Medicine and Society in Later Medieval England* (Stroud: Sutton, 1995)

Rawcliffe, Carole, trans., *Sources for the History of Medicine in Late Medieval England* (Kalamazoo, MI: Medieval Institute Publications, 1995)

Rawcliffe, Carole, 'Curing Bodies and Healing Souls: Pilgrimage and the Sick in Medieval East Anglia', in *Pilgrimage: The English Experience from Becket to Bunyan*, ed. by Colin Morris and Peter Roberts (Cambridge: Cambridge University Press, 2002), pp. 108–40

Rawcliffe, Carole, *Leprosy in Medieval England* (Woodbridge: Boydell, 2006)

Rawski, Conrad H., 'Notes on the Rhetoric in Petrarch's *Invective contra medicum*', in *Francis Petrarch, Six Centuries Later: A Symposium*, ed. by Aldo Scaglione (Chicago, IL: University of North Carolina, 1975), pp. 249–77

Redfern, Walter, *Puns: More Senses Than One*, rev. edn (London: Penguin, 2000)

Reynolds, Suzanne, *Medieval Reading: Grammar, Rhetoric and the Classical Text* (Cambridge: Cambridge University Press, 1996)

Richards, Jennifer, 'Useful Books: Reading Vernacular Regimens in Sixteenth-Century England', *Journal of the History of Ideas*, 73 (2012), 247–71

Richardson, Malcolm, 'The *Ars dictaminis*, the Formulary, and Medieval Epistolary Practice', in *Letter Writing Manuals and Instruction from Antiquity to the Present*, ed. by Carol Poster and Linda C. Mitchell (Columbia, SC: University of South California Press, 2007), pp. 52–66

Richardson, Malcolm, *Middle Class Writing in Late Medieval London* (London: Pickering & Chatto, 2011)

Riddle, John M., 'Theory and Practice in Medieval Medicine', *Viator*, 5 (1974), 157–84

Rider, Catherine, *Magic and Impotence in the Middle Ages* (Oxford: Oxford University Press, 2006)

Rider, Catherine, *Magic and Religion in Medieval England* (London: Reaktion Books, 2012)

Rider, Catherine, 'Demons and Mental Disorder in Late Medieval Medicine', in *Mental (Dis)order in Later Medieval Europe*, ed. by Sara Katajala-Peltomaa and Susanna Niiranen (Leiden: Brill, 2014), pp. 47-69

Rider, Catherine, 'Common Magic', in *The Cambridge History of Magic and Witchcraft in the West: From Antiquity to the Present*, ed. by David J. Collins (Cambridge: Cambridge University Press, 2015), pp. 303-31

Rimmon-Kenan, Shlomith, 'What Can Narrative Theory Learn from Illness Narratives?', *Literature and Medicine*, 25 (2006), 241-54

Rivard, Derek A., *Blessing the World: Ritual and Lay Piety in Medieval Religion* (Washington, DC: Catholic University of America Press, 2009)

Robbins, Rossell Hope, 'A Note on the Singer Survey of Medical Manuscripts in the British Isles', *Chaucer Review*, 4 (1969), 66-70

Robbins, Rossell Hope, 'Medical Manuscripts in Middle English', *Speculum*, 45 (1970), 393-415

Robertson, Kellie, *The Labourer's Two Bodies: Literary and Legal Productions in Britain 1350-1500* (Basingstoke: Palgrave Macmillan, 2006)

Robertson, Kellie, 'Medieval Things: Materiality, Historicism, and the Premodern Object', *Literature Compass*, 5 (2008), 1060-80

Rogers, William, 'Old Words Made New: Medea's Magic and Gower's Textual Healing', *South Atlantic Review*, 79 (2014), 105-17

Rosenwein, Barbara, *Emotional Communities in the Early Middle Ages* (Ithaca, NY: Cornell University Press, 2006)

Ryle, Gilbert, 'Knowing How and Knowing That: The Presidential Address', *Proceedings of the Aristotelian Society*, 46 (1945-6), 1-16

Sadlek, Gregory M., 'Otium, Negotium, and the Fear of Acedia in the Writings of England's Late Medieval Ricardian Poets', in *Idleness, Indolence and Leisure in Literature*, ed. by Monika Fludernik and Miriam Nandi (London: Palgrave Macmillan, 2014), pp. 17-39

Samuels, Ellen. 'Six Ways of Looking at Crip Time', *Disability Studies Quarterly*, 37 (2017), n.p.

Saul, Nigel, 'Sir John Clanvow', in *Oxford Dictionary of National Biography*, accessed online at https://doi.org/10.1093/ref:odnb/37286 [accessed 01/11/2020]

Saunders, Corinne, 'Bodily Narratives: Illness, Medicine and Healing in Middle English Romance', in *Boundaries in Medieval Romance*, ed. by Neil Cartlidge (Woodbridge: Boydell and Brewer, 2008), pp. 175-90

Saunders, Corrine and Jamie McKinstry, 'Introduction: Medievalism and the Medical Humanities', *Postmedieval*, 8 (2017), 139-46

Sawyer, Daniel, 'Codicological Evidence of Reading in Late Medieval England, with Particular Reference to Practical Pastoral Verse' (unpublished doctoral thesis, University of Oxford, 2016)

Sawyer, Daniel, *Reading English Verse in Manuscript, c. 1350-1500* (Oxford: Oxford University Press, 2020)

Scanlon, Larry and James Simpson, eds, *John Lydgate: Poetry, Culture, and Lancastrian England* (Notre Dame, IN: University of Notre Dame Press, 2006)

Schmidt, Kari Anne Rand, 'The *Index of Middle English Prose* and Late Medieval English Recipes', *English Studies*, 75 (1994), 423–9

Schuler, Robert M., 'Theory and Criticism of the Scientific Poem in Elizabethan England', *English Literary Renaissance*, 15 (1985), 3–41

Sennet, Richard, *The Craftsman* (New Haven, CT: Yale University Press, 2008)

Shehada, Housni Alkhateeb, *Mamluks and Animals: Veterinary Medicine in Medieval Islam* (Leiden: Brill, 2013)

Sherman, William H., 'What Did Renaissance Readers Write in Their Books?', in *Books and Readers: Material Studies*, ed. by Jennifer Andersen and others (Philadelphia, PA: University of Pennsylvania Press, 2002), pp. 42–79

Sherman, William H., *Used Books: Marking Readers in Renaissance England* (Philadelphia, PA: University of Pennsylvania Press, 2008)

Silva, Chelsea, 'Opening the Medieval Folding Almanac', *Exemplaria*, 30 (2018), 49–65

Sinclair Rohde, Eleanour, *The Old English Herbals* (London: Minerva, 1972)

Singer, Julie, *Blindness and Therapy in Late Medieval French and Italian Poetry* (Cambridge: Brewer, 2011)

Siraisi, Nancy, *Medieval and Early Renaissance Medicine: An Introduction to Knowledge and Practice* (Chicago, IL: University of Chicago Press, 1990)

Skemer, Don, *Binding Words: Textual Amulets in the Middle Ages* (Philadelphia, PA: University of Pennsylvania Press, 2006)

Slack, Paul, 'Mirrors of Health and Treasures of Poor Men: The Uses of the Vernacular Medical Literature of Tudor England', in *Health, Medicine and Mortality in the Sixteenth Century*, ed. by Charles Webster (Cambridge: Cambridge University Press, 1979), pp. 237–73

Smith, D. Vance, 'Medieval Forma: The Logic of the Work', in *Reading for Form*, ed. by Susan J. Wolfson and Marshall Brown (Seattle, WA: University of Washington Press, 2015), pp. 66–79

Smith, Kirk L., 'False Care and the Canterbury Cure: Chaucer Treats the New Galen', *Literature and Medicine*, 27 (2008), 61–81

Smith, Pamela H., 'What Is a Secret? Secrets and Craft Knowledge in Early Modern Europe', in *Secrets and Knowledge in Medicine and Science, 1500–1800*, ed. by Elaine Leong and Alisha Rankin (Farnham: Ashgate, 2011), pp. 51–67

Solomon, Michael, *Fictions of Well-Being: Sickly Readers and Vernacular Medical Writing in Late Medieval and Early Modern Spain* (Philadelphia, PA: University of Pennsylvania Press, 2010)

Sonntag, Susan, 'Illness as Metaphor', in Susan Sonntag, *Essays of the 1960s and 1970s*, ed. by David Rieff (New York: Library of America, 2013), pp. 675–729

Spearing, A.C., *Textual Subjectivity: The Encoding of Subjectivity in Medieval Narratives and Lyrics* (Oxford: Oxford University Press, 2005)

Spearing, A.C., *Medieval Autographies: The 'I' of the Text* (Notre Dame, IN: University of Notre Dame Press, 2012)

Spiegel, Gabrielle, *Romancing the Past: The Rise of Vernacular Prose Historiographies in Thirteenth-Century France* (Berkeley, CA: University of California Press, 1993)

Sponsler, Claire, 'The Culture of the Spectator: Conformity and Resistance to Medieval Performances', *Theatre Journal*, 44 (1992), 15–29

Sponsler, Claire, 'Eating Lessons: Lydgate's "Dietary" and Consumer Conduct', in *Medieval Conduct*, ed. by Kathleen Ashley and Robert L.A. Clark (Minneapolis, MN: University of Minnesota Press, 2011), pp. 1–22

Sponsler, Claire, *The Queen's Dumbshows: John Lydgate and the Making of Early Theater* (Philadelphia, PA: University of Pennsylvania Press, 2014)

Stadolnik, Joe, 'Gower's Bedside Medicine', *New Medieval Literatures*, 17 (2017), 150–74

Stallybrass, Peter and Allon White, *The Politics and Poetics of Transgression* (London: Methuen, 1986)

Stannard, Jerry, 'Magiferous Plants and Magic in Medieval Medical Botany', in *Herbs and Herbalism in the Middle Ages and Renaissance*, ed. by Katherine E. Stannard and Richard Kay (Aldershot: Ashgate, 1999), pp. 33–46

Star, Sarah, '*Anima Carnis in Sanguine Est*: Blood, Life and *The King of Tars*', *Journal of English and Germanic Philology*, 115 (2016), 442–62

Star, Sarah, 'Henry Daniel, Medieval English Medicine, and Linguistic Innovation: A Lexicographic Study of Huntington MS HM 505', *Huntington Library Quarterly*, 81 (2018), 63–105

Star, Sarah, 'The Textual Worlds of Henry Daniel', *Studies in the Age of Chaucer*, 40 (2018), 191–216

Steiner, Emily, *Documentary Culture and the Making of Medieval English Literature* (Cambridge: Cambridge University Press, 2003)

Steiner, Emily, 'Compendious Genres: Higden, Trevisa and the Medieval Encyclopedia', *Exemplaria*, 27 (2015), 73–92

Strohm, Paul, *Social Chaucer* (Cambridge, MA: Harvard University Press, 1989)

Strohm, Paul, *Hochon's Arrow: The Social Imagination of Fourteenth-Century Texts* (Princeton, NJ: Princeton University Press, 1992)

Strohm, Paul, *Theory and the Pre-Modern Text* (Minneapolis, MN: University of Minnesota Press, 2000)

Strohm, Paul, 'Writing and Reading', in *A Social History of England 1200–1500*, ed. by Rosemary Horrox and W.M. Ormrod (Cambridge: Cambridge University Press, 2006), pp. 454–72

Struever, Nancy, 'Petrarch's *Invective contra medicum*: An Early Confrontation of Rhetoric and Medicine', *Modern Language Notes*, 108 (1993), 659–79

Sugg, Richard, *Mummies, Cannibals, and Vampires: The History of Corpse Medicine from the Renaissance to the Victorians* (London: Routledge, 2011)

Swann, Alaya, '"By Expresse Experiment": The Doubting Midwife Salome in Late Medieval England', *Bulletin of the History of Medicine*, 89 (2015), 1–24

Swanson, Heather, *Medieval Artisans: An Urban Class in Late Medieval England* (Oxford: Basil Blackwell, 1989)

Taavitsainen, Irma, 'The Identification of Middle English Lunary MSS', *Neuphilologische Mitteilungen*, 88 (1987), 18–26

Taavitsainen, Irma, 'Middle English Recipes: Genre Characteristics, Text Type Features and Underlying Traditions of Writing', *Journal of Historical Pragmatics*, 2 (2001), 85–113

Taavitsainen, Irma, 'Scriptorial "House-Styles" and Discourse Communities', in *Medical and Scientific Writing in Late Medieval English*, ed. by Irma Taavitsainen and Päivi Pahta (Cambridge: Cambridge University Press, 2004), pp. 209–40

Taavitsainen, Irma, 'Genres and the Appropriation of Science: Loci Communes in English in the Late Medieval and Early Modern Period', in *Opening Windows on the Past*, ed. by Janne Skaffari and others (Philadelphia, PA: John Benjamins Publishing, 2005), pp. 179–96

Taavitsainen, Irma and Päivi Pahta, 'Vernacularisation of Scientific and Medical Writing in Its Sociohistorical Context', in *Medical and Scientific Writing in Late Medieval English*, ed. by Irma Taavitsainen and Päivi Pahta (Cambridge: Cambridge University Press, 2004), pp. 1–22

Tabak, Jessica, '"O Multiplied Misery!": The Disordered Medical Narrative of John Donne's Devotions', in *Medical Discourse in Premodern Europe*, ed. by Marion Turner as a special issue of *The Journal of Medieval and Early Modern Studies*, 46 (2016), 167–88

Talbot, C.H. and Eugene Ashby Hammond, *The Medical Practitioners in Medieval England: A Biographical Register* (London: Wellcome History Medical Library, 1985)

Tavormina, M. Teresa, 'The Twenty Jordan Series: An Illustrated Middle English Uroscopy Text', *American Notes and Queries*, 18 (2005), 43–67

Tavormina, M. Teresa, 'Three Middle English Verse Uroscopies', *English Studies*, 91 (2010), 591–622

Tavormina, M. Teresa, 'Uroscopy in Middle English: A Guide to the Texts and Manuscripts', *Studies in Medieval and Renaissance History*, 11 (2014), 1–154

Tebeaux, Elizabeth, *The Emergence of a Tradition: Technical Writing in the English Renaissance, 1475–1650* (Amityville, NY: Baywood Publishers, 1997)

Thrupp, Sylvia L., *The Merchant Class of Medieval London, 1300–1500* (Chicago, IL: University of Chicago Press, 1948)

Timmermann, Anke, 'Scientific and Encyclopaedic Verse', in *A Companion to Fifteenth-Century English Poetry*, ed. by Julia Boffey and A.S.G. Edwards (Woodbridge: Brewer, 2013), pp. 199–211

Timmermann, Anke, *Verse and Transmutation: A Corpus of Middle English Alchemical Poetry* (Leiden: Brill, 2013)

Toohey, Peter, *Epic Lessons: An Introduction to Ancient Didactic Poetry* (London: Routledge, 1996)

Trapp, J.B., 'Literacy, Books and Readers', in *The Cambridge History of the Book in Britain: Volume III*, ed. by Lotte Hellinga and J.B. Trapp (Cambridge: Cambridge University Press, 1999), pp. 31–43

Trease, G.E., 'The Spicers and Apothecaries of the Royal Household in the Reigns of Henry III, Edward I and Edward II', *Nottingham Medieval Studies*, 3 (1959), 19–52

Trigg, Stephanie, 'Weeping Like a Beaten Child: Figurative Language and the Emotions in Chaucer and Malory', in *Medieval Affect, Feeling, and Emotion*, ed. by Glenn D. Burger and Holly A. Crocker (Cambridge: Cambridge University Press, 2019), pp. 25–46

Truitt, Elly Rachel, *Medieval Robots: Mechanism, Magic, Nature, and Art* (Philadelphia, PA: University of Pennsylvania Press, 2015)

Turner, Marion, 'The Carnivalesque', in *Chaucer: An Oxford Guide*, ed. by Steve Ellis (Oxford: Oxford University Press, 2004), pp. 384–99

Turner, Marion, *Chaucerian Conflict: Languages of Antagonism in Late Fourteenth-Century London* (Oxford: Clarendon Press, 2007)
Turner, Marion, 'Thomas Usk and John Arderne', *Chaucer Review*, 47 (2012), 95–105
Turner, Marion, 'Imagining Polities', in *Medieval Literature: Criticism and Debates*, ed. by Holly Crocker and D. Vance Smith (Abingdon: Routledge, 2014), pp. 398–406
Turner, Marion, 'Illness Narratives in the Later Middle Ages: Arderne, Chaucer and Hoccleve', in *Medical Discourse in Premodern Europe*, ed. by Marion Turner as a special issue of *The Journal of Medieval and Early Modern Studies*, 46 (2016), 61–87
Turner, Marion, *Chaucer: A European Life* (Princeton, NJ: Princeton University Press, 2019)
Turner, Marion, 'The Senses', in *A New Companion to Chaucer*, ed. by Peter Brown (Hoboken, NJ: Wiley-Blackwell, 2019), pp. 395–408
Turner, Wendy J. and Sara M. Butler, 'Medicine and Law: The Confluence of Art and Science in the Middle Ages', in *Medicine and the Law in the Middle Ages*, ed. by Wendy J. Turner and Sara M. Butler (Leiden: Brill, 2014), pp. 1–22
Ussery, Huling E., *Chaucer's Physician: Medicine and Literature in Fourteenth-Century England* (New Orleans, LA: Tulane University, 1971)
Van Arsdall, Anne, 'Reading Medieval Medical Texts with an Open Mind', in *Textual Healing: Essays on Medieval and Early Modern Medicine*, ed. by Elizabeth Lane Furdell (Leiden: Brill, 2005), pp. 9–29
Van Arsdall, Anne, 'Challenging the "Eye of Newt" Image of Medieval Medicine', in *The Medieval Hospital and Medical Practice*, ed. by Barbara S. Bowers (Aldershot: Ashgate, 2007), pp. 195–205
Van der Lugt, Maaike, '"Abominable Mixtures": The *Liber Vaccae* in the Medieval West, or the Dangers and Attractions of Natural Magic', *Traditio*, 64 (2009), 229–77
Van Winter, J.M., *Spices and Comfits: Collected Papers on Medieval Food* (Totnes: Prospect, 2007)
Varila, Mari-Liisa, 'In Search of Textual Boundaries: A Case Study on the Transmission of Scientific Writing in 16th-Century England' (unpublished doctoral thesis, University of Turku, 2016)
Vaugt, Jennifer, *Literary and Scientific Cultures of Early Modernity: Rhetoric of Bodily Disease and Health in Medieval and Early Modern England* (Farnham: Ashgate, 2010)
Ventura, Iolanda, 'Il "Circa instans" attribuito a Platearius: trasmissione manoscritta, redazioni, criteri di costruzione di un'edizione critica', *Revue d'Histoire des Textes*, 10 (2015), 249–362
Voigts, Linda E., 'Medical Prose', in *Middle English Prose: A Critical Guide to Major Authors and Genres*, ed. by A.S.G. Edwards (New Brunswick, NJ: Rutgers University Press, 1984), pp. 315–35
Voigts, Linda E., 'Scientific and Medical Books', in *Book Production and Publishing in Britain, 1375–1475*, ed. by Jeremy Griffiths and Derek Pearsall (Cambridge: Cambridge University Press, 1989), pp. 345–402
Voigts, Linda E., 'The "Sloane Group": Related Scientific and Medical Manuscripts from the Fifteenth Century in the Sloane Collection', *The British Library Journal*, 16 (1990), 26–57

Voigts, Linda E., 'Multitudes of Middle English Medical Manuscripts, or the Englishing of Science and Medicine', in *Manuscript Sources of Medieval Medicine*, ed. by Margaret R. Schleissner (New York: Garland, 1995), pp. 183-95

Voigts, Linda E., 'What's the Word? Bilingualism in Late-Medieval England', *Speculum*, 71 (1996), 813-26

Voigts, Linda E., 'The Master of the King's Stillatories', in *Proceedings of the 2001 Harlaxton Symposium: The Lancastrian Court*, ed. by Jenny Stratford (Donington: Shaun Tyas, 2003), pp. 233-52

Voigts, Linda E., 'Fifteenth-Century English Banns Advertising the Services of an Itinerant Doctor', in *Between Text and Patient: The Medical Enterprise in Medieval and Early Modern Europe*, ed. by Florence Eliza Glaze and Michael M.R. McVaugh (Firenze: SIMEL Edizioni del Galluzzo, 2011), pp. 245-78

Voigts, Linda E., 'Herbs and Herbal Healing Satirized in Middle English Texts', in *Herbs and Healers from the Ancient Mediterranean through the Medieval West: Essays in Honor of J. M. Riddle*, ed. by Anne Van Arsdall and Timothy Graham (Farnham: Ashgate, 2012), pp. 217-30

Voigts, Linda E., 'Rhetorical and Random Language Mixing in a Fifteenth-Century Medical Manuscript (BL MS Harley 2390)', in *Language in Medieval Britain: Networks and Exchanges—Proceedings of the 2013 Harlaxton Symposium* (Donington: Shaun Tyas, 2015), pp. 90-103

Wack, Mary, *Lovesickness in the Middle Ages: The Viaticum and Its Commentaries* (Philadelphia, PA: University of Pennsylvania Press, 1990)

Wakelin, Daniel, 'William Worcester Writes a History of His Reading', *New Medieval Literatures*, 7 (2005), 53-71

Wakelin, Daniel, 'Instructing Readers in Fifteenth-Century Poetic Manuscripts', *Huntington Library Quarterly*, 73 (2010), 433-52

Wakelin, Daniel, 'Writing the Words', in *The Production of Books in England 1350-1500*, ed. by Daniel Wakelin and Alexandra Gillespie (Cambridge: Cambridge University Press, 2011), pp. 34-58

Wakelin, Daniel, 'Classical and Humanist Translations', in *A Companion to Fifteenth-Century English Poetry*, ed. by Julia Boffey and A.S.G. Edwards (Woodbridge: Brewer, 2013), pp. 171-85

Wakelin, Daniel, *Scribal Correction and Literary Craft: English Manuscripts 1375-1510* (Cambridge: Cambridge University Press, 2014)

Wakelin, Daniel, 'When Scribes Won't Write: Gaps in Middle English Books', *Studies in the Age of Chaucer*, 36 (2014), 249-78

Walker Bynum, Caroline, *The Resurrection of the Body in Western Christianity, 200-1336* (New York: Columbia University Press, 1995)

Walker Bynum, Caroline, 'Why All the Fuss about the Body? A Medievalist's Perspective', *Critical Inquiry*, 22 (1995), 1-33

Walker Bynum, Caroline, 'Wonder', *American Historical Review*, 102 (1997), 1-26

Walker Bynum, Caroline, *Metamorphosis and Identity* (New York: Zone Books, 2001)

Wall, Wendy, *Recipes for Thought: Knowledge and Taste in the Early Modern English Kitchen* (Philadelphia, PA: University of Pennsylvania Press, 2016)

Wallis, Faith, 'Signs and Senses: Diagnosis and Prognosis in Early Medieval Pulse and Urine Texts', *Social History of Medicine*, 13 (2000), 265-78

Wallis, Faith, ed., *Medieval Medicine: A Reader* (Toronto: University of Toronto Press, 2010)

Wallis, Faith, 'Medicine and the Senses: Feeling the Pulse, Smelling the Plague and Listening for the Cure', in *A Cultural History of the Senses*, ed. by Richard Newhauser (London: Bloomsbury, 2014), pp. 133–52

Walsh Morrissey, Jake, 'An Unnoticed Fragment of *A Tretys of Diverse Herbis* in British Library, MS Sloane 2460, and the Middle English Career of Pseudo-Albertus Magnus' *De Virtutibus Herbarum*', *Neuphilologische Mitteilungen*, 115 (2014), 153–61

Walsh Morrissey, Jake, 'Unpublished Verse Rubrics in a Middle English *Receptarium* (British Library, MS Sloane 2457/2458)', *Notes and Queries*, 61 (2014), 13–15

Walsh Morrissey, Jake, '"To al Indifferent": The Virtues of Lydgate's "Dietary"', *Medium Aevum*, 84 (2015), 258–78

Waters, Claire M., 'What's the Use? Marian Miracles and the Working of the Literary', in *The Medieval Literary Beyond Form*, ed. by Robert J. Meyer-Lee and Catherine Sanok (Cambridge: Brewer, 2018), pp. 15–34

Weiss Adamson, Melitta, 'The Games Cooks Play: Non-Sense Recipes and Practical Jokes in Medieval Literature', in *Food in the Middle Ages: A Book of Essays*, ed. by Melitta Weiss Adamson (New York: Garland, 1995), pp. 177–95

Weiss Adamson, Melitta, *Food in Medieval Times* (Westport, CT: Greenwood Press, 2004)

Wenzel, Siegfried, 'The Arts of Preaching', in *The Cambridge History of Literary Criticism: Volume II. The Middle Ages*, ed. by Alastair Minnis and Ian Johnson (Cambridge: Cambridge University Press, 2005), pp. 84–96

Wheatley, Edward, *Stumbling Blocks Before the Blind: Medieval Constructions of Disability* (Ann Arbor, MI: University of Michigan Press, 2010)

White, Hayden, 'The Value of Narrativity in the Representation of Reality', *Critical Inquiry*, 7 (1980), 5–27

White, Hayden, *The Content of the Form: Narrative Discourse and Historical Representation* (Baltimore, MD: Johns Hopkins University Press, 1987)

Witherden, Sian, 'Balancing Form, Function, and Aesthetic: A Study of Ruling Patterns for Zodiac Men in Astro-Medical Manuscripts of Late Medieval England', *The Journal for the Early Book Society for the Study of Manuscripts and Printing History*, 20 (2017), 79–109

Witt, Ronald G., 'The Arts of Letter-Writing', in *The Cambridge History of Literary Criticism: Volume II. The Middle Ages*, ed. by Alastair Minnis and Ian Johnson (Cambridge: Cambridge University Press, 2005), pp. 68–83

Woolf, Virginia, *On Being Ill* (Ashfield, MA: Paris Press, 2002; first published 1926)

Woolgar, C.M., *The Senses in Late Medieval England* (New Haven, CT: Yale University Press, 2006)

Woolgar, C.M., 'The Social Life of the Senses: Experiencing the Self, Others and Environments', in *A Cultural History of the Senses*, ed. by Richard Newhauser (London: Bloomsbury Academic, 2014), pp. 23–43

Woolgar, C.M., 'The Language of Food and Cooking', in *Language in Medieval Britain: Networks and Exchanges—Proceedings of the 2013 Harlaxton Symposium* (Donington: Shaun Tyas, 2015), pp. 33–47

Yoshikawa, Naoë Kukita, ed., *Medicine, Religion and Gender in Medieval Culture* (Cambridge: Brewer, 2015)

Zeeman, Nicolette, 'Imaginative Theory', in *Twenty-First-Century Approaches to Literature: Middle English*, ed. by Paul Strohm (Oxford: Oxford University Press, 2007), pp. 222–40

Zemon Davis, Natalie, *Fiction in the Archives: Pardon Tales and Their Tellers in Sixteenth-Century France* (Cambridge: Polity Press, 1988)

Ziegler, Joseph, *Medicine and Religion c. 1300: The Case of Arnau de Vilanova* (Oxford: Clarendon Press, 1998)

Zimmerman, Kees, ed., *One Leg in the Grave Revisited: The Miracle of the Transplantation of the Black Leg by the Saints Cosmas and Damian* (Groningen: Barkhuis, 2013)

Zumthor, Paul, *Toward a Medieval Poetics*, trans. by Phillip E. Bennet (Minneapolis, MN: University of Minnesota Press, 1922)

Zumthor, Paul, 'The Text and the Voice', trans. by Marilyn C. Engelhardt, *New Literary History*, 16 (1984), 67–92

Conference Papers

Cooper, Lisa, '"Out of this prosis blake": Farming, Feeling and Form in On Husbondrie', online podcast recording of a paper presented at The Provocative Fifteenth-Century Conference, Huntington Library, California, 16 October 2015, accessed online at https://itunes.apple.com/gb/itunes-u/provocative-fifteenth-century/id1052642181?mt=10 [accessed 01/11/2015]

Langum, Virginia, 'Metaphor as Medicine in Medieval Surgical Manuals', paper presented at the Metaphor Festival, Stockholm University, 2013, accessed online at www.academia.edu/19502646/Metaphor_as_Medicine_in_Medieval_Surigcal_Manuals [accessed 01/07/2016]

Nolan, Maura, 'The Invention of Style', biennial lecture presented at the New Chaucer Society Congress, University of Toronto, 14 July 2018

Nuttall, Jenni, 'Poesie and Poetrie', paper presented at the Middle English Literary Theory Workshop: Keywords and Methodologies, Centre for Early Modern and Medieval Studies at the University of Sussex, 16 June 2016, pp. 1–5, accessed online at http://stylisticienne.com/middle-english-literary-theory [accessed 28/02/2018]

Catalogues

Boffey, Julia and A.S.G. Edwards, eds, *A New Index of Middle English Verse* (London: The British Library, 2005)

Braswell, Laurel, ed., *The Index of Middle English Prose: Handlist IV. Manuscripts in the Douce Collection, Bodleian Library, Oxford* (Cambridge: Brewer, 1987)

Brown, Peter and Elton D. Higgs, eds, *The Index of Middle English Prose: Handlist V. Manuscripts in the Additional Collection 10001–14000, British Library, London* (Cambridge: Brewer, 1988)

Connolly, Margaret, ed., *The Index of Middle English Prose: Handlist XIX. Manuscripts in the University Library, Cambridge (Dd–Oo)* (Woodbridge: Brewer, 2009)

Dutschke, C.W. and Richard Rouse, *Guide to Medieval and Renaissance Manuscripts in the Huntington Library* (San Marino: Huntington Library, 1989)

Eldredge, L.M., ed., *The Index of Middle English Prose: Handlist IX. Manuscripts in the Ashmole Collection, Bodleian Library* (Cambridge: Brewer, 1992)

Hanna, Ralph, ed., *The Index of Middle English Prose: Handlist XII. Manuscripts in Smaller Bodleian Collections* (Cambridge: Brewer, 1997)

Horner, Patrick J., ed., *The Index of Middle English Prose: Handlist III. Manuscripts in the Digby Collection, Bodleian Library, Oxford* (Cambridge: Brewer, 1986)

Horner, Patrick J., ed., *The Index of Middle English Prose: Handlist XXI. Manuscripts in the Hatton and e Museo Collections, Bodleian Library, Oxford* (Cambridge: Brewer, 2014)

Keiser, George R., *A Manual of the Writings in Middle English 1050–1500: Volume 10. Works of Science and Information*, ed. by J.B. Severs and A.E. Hartung (New Haven, CT: The Connecticut Academy of Arts and Sciences, 1998)

Kibre, Pearl and Lynn Thorndike, eds, *A Catalogue of Incipits of Mediaeval Scientific Writings in Latin*, rev. edn (Cambridge, MA: The Mediaeval Academy of America, 1963); https://indexcat.nlm.nih.gov

Kurtz, Patricia and Linda E. Voigts, eds, *Scientific and Medical Writings in Old and Middle English: An Electronic Reference*, accessed online at https://indexcat.nlm.nih.gov/vivisimo/cgi-bin/query-meta?v%3aproject=indexcat&v%3asources=etkevk2& and https://cctr1.umkc.edu/search

Marx, William, ed., *The Index of Middle English Prose: Handlist XIV. Manuscripts in the National Library of Wales (Llyfrgell Genedlaethol Cymru), Aberystwyth* (Woodbridge: Brewer, 1999)

Mooney, Linne R., *The Index of Middle English Prose: Handlist XI. Manuscripts in the Library of Trinity College, Cambridge* (Cambridge: Brewer, 1995)

Mooney, Linne R. and others, eds, *Digital Index of Middle English Verse*, accessed online at www.dimev.net

Ogilvie-Thomson, Sarah, ed., *The Index of Middle English Prose: Handlist VIII. Manuscripts Containing Middle English Prose in Oxford College Libraries* (Cambridge: Brewer, 1991)

Ogilvie-Thomson, Sarah, ed., *The Index of Middle English Prose: Handlist XVI. The Laudian Collection, Bodleian Library, Oxford* (Woodbridge: Brewer, 2000)

Ogilvie-Thomson, Sarah, ed., *The Index of Middle English Prose: Handlist XXII. The Rawlinson Collection, Bodleian Library, Oxford* (Cambridge: Brewer, 2017)

Pickering, O.S. and Susan Powell, eds, *The Index of Middle English Prose: Handlist VI. Manuscripts Containing Middle English Prose in Yorkshire Libraries and Archives* (Cambridge: Brewer, 1989)

Ramsay, Nigel and James M.W. Willoughby, eds, *Hospitals, Towns and the Professions*, Corpus of British Medieval Library Catalogues, 14 (London: The British Library, 2009)

Rand Schmidt, Kari Anne, ed., *The Index of Middle English Prose: Handlist XVII. Manuscripts in the Library of Gonville and Caius College, Cambridge* (Woodbridge: Brewer, 2001)

Robinson, P.R., ed., *Catalogue of Dated and Datable Manuscripts*, 2 vols (London: British Library, 2003)

Thomson, Rodney M., ed., *The University and College Libraries of Oxford: Volume I, Corpus of British Medieval Library Catalogues*, 16 (London: The British Library, 2015)

Thorndike, Lynn, ed., *A History of Magic and Experimental Science*, 8 vols (New York: Columbia University Press, 1923–58)

Dictionaries and Works of Reference

Benskin, M. and others, *An Electronic Version of a Linguistic Atlas of Late Medieval English*, accessed online at www.lel.ed.ac.uk/ihd/elalme/elalme_frames.html

The Dictionary of the Older Scottish Tongue, accessed online at www.dsl.ac.uk

Given-Wilson, C. and others, eds, *The Parliament Rolls of Medieval England*, accessed online at www.sd-editions.com/PROME/home.html

Glick, Thomas F., Steven J. Livesey, and Faith Wallis, eds, *Medieval Science, Technology, and Medicine: An Encyclopaedia* (London: Routledge, 2005)

Latham, R.E., David Howlett, and Richard Ashdowne, eds, *Dictionary of Medieval Latin from British Sources*, accessed online at http://clt.brepolis.net/dmlbs/Default.aspx

Lewis, Robert and others, eds, *The Middle English Dictionary* (Ann Arbor, MI: University of Michigan Press, 1952–2001), accessed online at https://quod.lib.umich.edu/m/med

McSparran, Frances and others, eds, *The Middle English Compendium* (Ann Arbor, MI, 2000–18), accessed online at http://quod.lib.umich.edu/m/middle-english-dictionary

Norri, Juhani, *Dictionary of Medical Vocabulary in English, 1375–1550: Body Parts, Sicknesses, Instruments and Medicinal Preparations* (London: Routledge, 2016)

Simpson, John and others, eds, *The Oxford English Dictionary*, accessed online at www.oed.com

Walsh, Michael, *A Dictionary of Devotions* (Tunbridge Wells: Burns & Oates, 1993)

Whiting, Bartlett Jere, *Proverbs, Sentences and Proverbial Phrases: From English Writings Mainly Before 1500* (London: Oxford University Press, 1968)

Index of Manuscripts

This index refers to manuscripts cited explicitly in the text or footnotes. Citations referring to tables are indicated by an italic *t*. A full list of manuscripts consulted is included within the Bibliography.

For the benefit of digital users, indexed terms that span two pages (e.g., 52–53) may, on occasion, appear on only one of those pages.

Aberystwyth, National Library of Wales
   MS 572 187n.31

Cambridge, Cambridge University Library
   MS Dd.10.44 187
   MS Ee.1.15 135–6, 173, 183–4
   MS KK.6.33 47n.56, 51–2, 209–12

Cambridge, Gonville and Caius College
   MS 176/97 10

Cambridge, Magdalene College, Pepys Library
   MS 1236 74n.17, 80n.45
   MS 1661 99n.101, 100n.104

Cambridge, Trinity College
   MS O.1.13 47–8, 51, 67n.139, 151n.31, 155n.45
   MS O.1.65 47–8, 51–3, 58–9, 152n.37, 187n.29
   MS O.2.13 145n.15, 185–6
   MS R.14.32 92, 100–1, 126n.67, 164–5, 215*t*
   MS R.14.39 46–7, 76n.27, 131, 145n.16, 151n.31, 155n.45, 169, 190–200
   MS R.14.51 32n.5, 76n.27, 100n.104, 115n.36, 187
   MS R.14.52 188–90

Edinburgh, National Library of Scotland
   MS Advocates' 19.2.1 (Auchinleck) 167–70

Lincoln, Lincoln Cathedral Library
   MS 91 75n.24

London, British Library
   MS Additional 12195 188–9
   MS Additional 17866 76n.27, 100n.104
   MS Additional 19674 40, 209–12, 215*t*
   MS Additional 33996 40n.31, 133–5, 197, 215*t*
   MS Additional 34111 93–4, 96–8
   MS Additional 34210 184–5, 215*t*
   MS Harley 1602 40n.31, 215*t*
   MS Harley 2378 40n.31, 51n.70, 116n.39, 215*t*
   MS Harley 2390 189n.43
   MS Lansdowne 680 116–18, 215*t*
   MS Royal 17 D.i 59n.99
   MS Sloane 7 56–7
   MS Sloane 147 92, 99n.101
   MS Sloane 213 3, 162–3
   MS Sloane 340 2, 79–80, 207
   MS Sloane 347 165n.80
   MS Sloane 468 115n.36, 215*t*
   MS Sloane 1315 201n.95, 202n.98, 215*t*
   MS Sloane 1571 92, 100n.104
   MS Sloane 2457/2458 98–9, 100n.104
   MS Sloane 3160 84n.57
   MS Sloane 3466 84n.57
   MS Sloane 3866 185n.22, 215*t*

London, Wellcome Trust
   MS Wellcome 136 36, 51n.70, 116n.38, 215*t*
   MS Wellcome 542 9, 215*t*
   MS Wellcome 5262 117n.43, 121n.56, 215*t*

New Haven, Beinecke Rare Book and Manuscript Library
   MS Takamiya 46 75n.24, 76n.27, 99n.101, 100n.104

New York, Pierpont Morgan Library
   MS Bühler 21 76n.27

254 INDEX OF MANUSCRIPTS

Oxford, Bodleian Library
   Ms Ashmole 750 116n.38, 151–2, 155n.45, 215*t*
   MS Ashmole 1389 122–4, 127, 160–1, 197–8, 200–5, 215*t*
   MS Ashmole 1393 56–7, 203n.103
   MS Ashmole 1413 160–1
   MS Ashmole 1432 164–5
   MS Ashmole 1434 158n.55
   MS Ashmole 1438 12–15, 67n.136, 127–8, 145n.16, 150, 152–3, 190–200, 201n.95, 212–13, 215*t*
   MS Ashmole 1443 67n.135, 67n.137, 111–15, 126n.67, 133–4, 155–6, 168n.84, 190–200, 215*t*
   MS Ashmole 1444 11–12, 40n.31, 47–8, 51
   MS Ashmole 1477 67n.139, 68, 107, 151n.31, 187
   MS Douce 78 42–4, 145n.15, 169, 173–9
   MS Douce 84 40n.31, 42, 160–1, 215*t*
   MS e. Museo 52 202n.98
   MS Hatton 29 40n.31, 215*t*
   MS Laud misc. 553 67–9, 85, 144–5, 150, 164, 190–200, 215*t*
   MS Laud misc. 685 84–5, 126n.67, 149–51
   MS Radcliffe Trust, e. 10 69, 115n.36, 202n.98
   MS Rawlinson C.506 10n.36, 67n.136, 118–22, 136n.102, 164, 184n.13, 190–200, 215*t*
   MS Selden Supra 70 215*t*
Oxford, Corpus Christi College
   MS 125 192n.64

San Marino, Huntington Library
   MS HM 58 40n.31, 51–2, 51n.70, 147–8, 182
   MS HM 64 40–1, 51n.70, 55–6, 76n.27, 82–3, 87–9, 93–6, 116n.39, 162, 168, 215*t*
   MS HM 505 45, 56–7, 143–4
   MS HM 1336 116n.39, 215*t*
   MS HM 19079 40n.31, 51n.70
Stockholm, Kungliga Biblioteket
   MS X.90 76n.27, 99–100, 100n.104

York, York Minster
   MS XVI.E.32 38–9, 116nn.38–9, 124–6, 203n.104, 215*t*

General Index

For the benefit of digital users, indexed terms that span two pages (e.g., 52–53) may, on occasion, appear on only one of those pages.

accrual 107–37
accumulation 107–37
adulteration 33–7, 186
aesthetic 26–7, 136, 150, 160–1, 205, 209–12
aetiology 20–1
affect 26–7, 110–11, 123–4, 172, 183, 212–13
Agnus Castus 76–7, 117–18, 147
alchemy 37–8, 73, 159–60
Al-Farabi 6–7, 62–4
amateur healers 4, 11–15
amplification 49–50
analgesics 164–6, 169–70
anatomy 194
annotation 107–8, 117–18
apothecaries 4, 152–3, 188
Appelbaum, Robert 18–19
Aquinas, Thomas 63–4, 80
Arabic medical writing 5–8, 62–4, 71, 192–3
Archer, Jayne Elisabeth 18–19
Arderne, John 20–1, 158–60, 163–6
Aristotle 22–3, 141–2
ars moriendi 151–3
artes dictaminis 24–5
artes poetriae 24, 32, 37, 49–50, 53–5
artes praedicandi 24–5
artisans 23–4
astrology 4, 88–9, 118, 143–5, 152–3, 161, 180–1
atthomi 58–9
Attridge, Derek 86–7
Auchinleck manuscript 167–70
Augustine, St 32–3, 141–2, 145–6, 178, 180–1, 188
Avicenna 6–7, 32–3, 62–4, 114–15, 192

Bahr, Arthur 27–8, 108–9, 136–7, 146–7
Bakhtin, Mikhail 199–200
balsam 171
barbers 4, 10, 23–4, 34

Barron, Caroline 145–6
Bartholomew the Englishman
   De proprietatibus rerum 45–6, 48, 55, 63–6, 100–1
Bevis of Hampton 167–70
Bishop, Louise 41
Black, Deborah 62–3
Black, Winston 77–8
Bloch, Howard 198–9
bloodletting 10, 75–7, 88–9, 98
Boethius
   De consolatione philosophiae 81–2
bones 184–5, 190–200
Bonfield, Christopher 188
book-making recipes 51–2
books of secrets 109–10, 200–5
boundaries 25–6, 180–206
Bourdieu, Pierre 23, 153, 160
Brand, Paul 145–6
Buchanan, Peter 108–9
Burge, Amy 169
burial 193–4, 197–8

Cambridge 6–7
Cannon, Christopher 59–60, 81–2
carnivalesque 199–200, 202
Carruthers, Mary 72
Cavanaugh, Susan 11
charms 4, 40–1, 77, 180–2, 186–7, 191–2
Chaucer, Geoffrey
   Boece 81–2
   Canon's Yeoman's Tale 37–8, 75, 159–60
   Canterbury Tales (as a collection) 2, 60, 126–7
   General Prologue 160
   House of Fame 50–1, 75–6, 101–2, 126–7
   Knight's Tale 128–9
   Legend of Good Women 126–7
   Miller's Tale 202–3

Chaucer, Geoffrey (*cont.*)
   Pardoner's Tale 188
   Reeve's Tale 202–3
   Tale of Sir Thopas 89–90
   Treatise on the Astrolabe 55, 169–70
   Troilus and Criseyde 34–5, 37, 75–6, 94–5, 97–8
   Wife of Bath's Tale 59
Christus medicus 160–1
chronic illness 162–4
churchyards 193–4, 197–8, 205
Circa Instans 76–7, 111–12
clocks 144–5
code 168
cognition 44–7, 79–81, 83, 95–6, 102–3
collections
   dynamics of 20, 146–7, 173–208
   impulses behind 107–37, 180–206
commonplaces 58–62, 184
compilation 8–10, 20–1, 107–37, 146–7, 173–208
Constantine the African 77–8, 194
contents pages 111–12, 115–23
Cooper, Lisa 19, 21, 91–2, 144
Cosmas and Damian 193–4, 196–7
cosmetics 136
couplets 83, 87–96
craft 23–5, 53–5
craftsmen 23–4
crip time 142
Crisciani, Chiari 109–10, 130
critical days 161
Crocker, Holly 110–11
culinary
   recipes 9–10, 16, 51–2, 155–6, 184
   similes 51–2, 61, 155–6, 183–4

Dane Hew, Munk of Leicestre 198
Daniel, Henry
   Herbal 76–7
   Liber Uricrisiarum 20–1, 45, 52–3, 56–9, 109–10, 143–4
decorum 136
demonic magic 118–21, 155, 180–2, 188–9, 191–2, 194
devotional writings 11, 21–2, 59–61, 64, 102–3, 123, 151–3, 173–9
diagnosis 53, 141–4
DiMeo, Michelle 18–19
Dinshaw, Carolyn 142–3, 177

disability 142, 162–3
disability studies 142, 162–3
Dives and Pauper 181–2
domestic space 187, 202–3
doublets 41–2

early modern recipes 18–19, 212–13
efficacy
   lack of 133
   nature of 23
   statements of 112–15, 122, 133–5, 197–8
elements, the 4–5
emotion 26–7
empirical 114–15
epilepsy 46–7, 185, 187, 190–2, 195, 197–8
epilogues (to medical writings) 77
ethics 143–4
experimenta 109–10, 191–2
eyes 55–6, 67–9, 92–3, 134–5
eyeskip 47

fabliaux 198–200
faeces 184–6
fear 110–11
Felski, Rita 163, 187
female medical literacy 11–12
fevers 161
finding aids 108, 110–24
Fissell, Mary 18–19
Fleming, Juliet 107, 126
formalism 24–5, 27–8, 86–7, 108–9
Foucault, Michel 36
fragments 25–6, 28, 31–7, 93, 107–8, 146–7, 181–2, 207–8, 212–13
Freedman, Paul 187

Galen 5–6, 114–15, 192
gender 11–12, 18–19
gentry medical engagement 11–13
Geoffrey of Vinsauf
   Poetria nova 24, 49–50, 53–5
Gilbert the Englishman
   Compendium medicinae 8–9, 44, 48, 52–3, 60–1, 65–6
Gilles of Corbeil
   Carmen de urinis 71, 78–81, 88, 92
Gillespie, Alexandra 108
Gillespie, Vincent 26–7, 102–3, 123
Goody, Jack 144

Gower, John
  Confessio Amantis 154–60
grammar 48–9
Gratian
  Decretum 180–1
Greek medicine 5–8, 71, 116–17
Green, Monica 11–12
Griffin, Carrie 18, 20, 112n.19, 135n.96
guild-trained surgeons 4
Guy de Chauliac 132

habit 26–7, 163, 173, 187
Hargreaves, Henry 18
Hawkins, Joy 65
headache 82–3, 92–4, 116–17, 163
head-to-toe order 115–19
Henri de Mondeville 64–5
Henryson, Robert 164–5
  'Sum Practysis of Medecyne' 34–7, 47–8, 69–70, 129, 132–3
  Testament of Cresseid 126–7
herbals 71, 75–7, 92–3, 98–102, 118, 197–8, 204–5
Hippocrates 5–6, 143–4, 162–3
hope 110–11, 172–3
Horace 80
  Ars poetica 32–4, 136
household book 9–10, 108–11, 149, 163, 178, 182, 200–1
Huizinga, John 25–6, 205
human remains 184–5, 190–200
humoral theory 4–6, 188–9, 191–2
Humphrey, Chris 145–6
Humphrey, Duke of Gloucester 11

imagination 32–7, 50–1
imaginative syllogism 26–7, 62–4
Ingham, Patricia 33
Isidore of Seville 2, 47–8, 143–4
itinerant practitioners 4, 116–17, 121–2

Jack and His Stepdame 202–3
Jacqueline of Hainault 11
jargon 20–1, 36–8, 156–7
Jarvis, Simon 95–6
John of Burgundy 111–12
John of Gaddesden 6–7, 194
John of Mirfield 131–2, 160–2, 172
Johnson, Eleanor 81–2
Jones, Claire 18

Julian of Norwich
  A Revelation of Love 60–1
Justice, Steven 172–3

Karnes, Michelle 33
Keiser, George 13, 77, 85–6
Kempe, Margery
  The Boke of 59–61
Kurtz, Patricia 17, 76–7
Kymer, Gilbert 11

labour 144–5, 147–60, 178
Lanfranc of Milan 118
Latour, Bruno 186
Lawton, David 100–2
Le Goff, Jacques 145–6
Leong, Elaine 18–19
leprosy 55–6, 167–8
Lévi-Strauss, Claude 153
linearity 142–3, 146–7, 150–1, 154, 170–2, 179
lists 37–40, 173
Lydgate, John 91–2
  'The Dietary' 74–7, 85–6, 141

Macer 71, 76–7
magic
  demonic magic 118–21, 155, 180–2, 188–9, 191–2, 194
  natural magic 40–1, 67, 155, 180–1, 189–94
Malory, Thomas
  Le Morte d'Arthur 170–2, 177–8
Mandeville, John
  The Book of 163–4
Mannyng, Robert 83, 99n.100
Marshall, Helen 108–9
marvellous 141–206
McDonald, Nicola 195–6
mechanical arts 34
Medea 154–60, 171
memory 71–2, 77–9, 82–3, 86, 89–90, 102–3, 123–4, 160–1
merchants 7–8, 13, 145–6, 187
metaphor 53–5, 62–3
Metham, John
  Amoryus and Cleopes 194–5
Metzler, Irina 142
Meyer-Lee, Robert 27–8
miracles 144–5, 163–4, 172–3

Mitchell, Laura 182, 197, 203–4
mnemonic aid 71–2, 77–9, 82–3, 86, 89–90, 102–3, 123–4, 160–1
mock recipes 34–7, 69–70
Mooney, Linne 18, 121–2, 145–6
mundane 141–206
Murphy, James Jerome 24
Murray Jones, Peter 10

narrative 19–21, 153–4
natural magic 40–1, 67, 155, 180–1, 189–94
necromancy 118–21, 155, 188–90, 194–5, 197
Nelson, Ingrid 108–9, 126–7
non-naturals 16, 64–5
numbering (of recipes) 119–21
Nuttall, Jenni 23–4, 54–5

occupatio 128–9
Odo de Meung 71, 76–7
Olsan, Lea 186–7
Olson, Glending 23–4, 54–5
orality 98–100
ordering 110–24
 alphabetical 115–16
 by number 119–21
 head-to-toe 115–19
ordinatio 22–3, 110–24
organization 110–24
Orlemanski, Julie 4, 12, 20–1, 34, 36–7, 40, 45–6, 157, 207
Ovid
 Metamorphoses 154–7
owners of remedy books 10–15
Oxford 6–7

paradise 163–4, 170–2
parody 20–1, 34–7, 157, 172
Paston family 11–12
Pearsall, Derek 85–6
Pennell, Sara 18–19
performance 98–9, 154–60
perspective 186, 190, 200–6
Petit, Catherine 192
Petrarch, Francesco 164–5
 Invective contra medicum 34–7
 Letters 130–1
physiognomy 4, 45–6, 207
placebo effect 3, 17, 41
plague 111–12, 144–5

play 25–6, 69–70, 99, 136–7, 200–6
playground 205
Pliny the Elder 5–6, 188–9
poetic
 definitions of 23–7
Poetria nova 24, 49–50, 53–5
Pouchelle, Marie-Christine 64–5
practice
 definitions of 22–3, 45–6, 153
 in relation to theory 8–9, 22–3, 44, 207–8
 material evidence of 18, 107, 121–2, 133
practitioners 4, 23–4
preservation 144
printing 212–13
prognosis 53, 55–6, 141–4
prologues (to medical writings) 2–3, 77–81, 84–6, 96–8
prose 31–70
 in relation to verse 75–8, 81–6, 88–9
 status of 71–2
 translation into and out of 71, 76–7, 88
prosopopoeia 96–8
proverbs 49, 59–60
prudence 143–4, 152–3
punctuation 42, 44, 83–4
punctus elevatus 44
puns 66–70
Pye, David 23

quack medical practitioner 34–7, 129–31
queerness
 queer time 142–3

race 193–7
regimen 4, 141, 143–4, 163
rejuvenation 154–60, 170–1
religion 11, 21–2, 59–61, 64, 102–3, 123, 151–3, 157–8, 170–9, 182, 191–2
repetition 31–2, 40–7
rhetoric 48–9, 80–2, 128–9
rhyme 71–3, 77, 80–1, 83–96
Richard Coeur de Lion 195–8
Richard of Salisbury 113
Rider, Catherine 186–7
Robertson, Kellie 158, 190
Rolle, Richard 64
romance 166–73, 208
roman medical writing 5–7, 71, 116–17
rubrication 41–2, 83, 98–9, 117–19, 174–7
running titles 115

GENERAL INDEX

Sadlek, Gregory 158
saints 164, 172–3, 193–4, 196–7
Samuels, Ellen 142
Sanok, Catherine 27–8
saracen 194–6
Sawyer, Daniel 83
scholasticism 44, 71, 130
scribal accuracy 41–2, 79, 83–4, 92–3
scribal confusion 46–7, 69, 79, 92–3
secrecy 168
senses, the 53
sequentiality 142–3, 146–7, 150–1, 154, 170–2, 179
similes 42–4, 47–66
Slack, Paul 212–13
sound patterning 39–47, 66–9
spectacle 153–4, 156–7, 165–6
spices 187–8
spider's web 51, 55–7, 64–6
Stallybrass, Peter 199–200
Stannard, Jerry 188–9
Star, Sarah 20–1, 45, 109–10
Steiner, Emily 109–10
Strohm, Paul 145–6
style 25–6
surgery
   surgeons 10, 23–4, 34, 114–15, 159–60
   surgical treatises 4
syntax 37–47, 72–3, 126, 149–50, 207–8

Taavitsainen, Irma 18
tables of contents (in remedy books) 111–12, 115–23
taboos 180–206
Tavormina, M. Teresa 58–9, 71, 80–1
temporality 19–20
theory
   medical 4–6, 8–9, 93–4, 130–2, 192–3, 207–8

theriac 147, 154–5
Thornton, Robert 13, 66–7, 136
time 19–20, 87–90, 136–7, 141–79
Timmerman, Anke 73
Tollemache Book of Secrets 201, 203–4
transplant 193–4
Trevisa, John
   translation of *De proprietatibus rerum* 45–6, 55, 63–6
Trigg, Stephanie 60
Turner, Marion 21n.81, 154n.40, 159n.57
tutty 187

university-educated physicians 4, 6–7
uroscopy 4, 45, 48, 52–3, 55–9, 71, 143–4
Urso of Salerno 194
usefulness 23

verbal homeopathy 67
vernacularization of science 7–8, 15–16
verse 37–9, 71–103
   verse herbal 71–8, 91–3, 98–102
   verse remedy book 73–4, 76–7, 82–3, 87–8, 91–6, 131
vervain 188–90, 203–4
veterinary medicine 118
voice 96–103
Voigts, Linda 17–18, 76–8

Wakelin, Daniel 41–2, 79, 108
Walker Bynum, Caroline 194
Wall, Wendy 18–19, 144, 178
Walsh Morrissey, Jake 75, 99n.98, 100n.103
water of Antioche 147
Weiss, Judith 169
White, Allon 199–200
Wise Book of Philosophy and Astronomy, the 111–12